Genetic Diversity of Coronaviruses: From SARS-CoV to SARS-CoV-2

(Part 2)

Edited by

Kamal Niaz
Department of Pharmacology and Toxicology, Faculty of Bio-Sciences, Cholistan University of Veterinary and Animal Sciences (CUVAS), Bahawalpur 63100, Pakistan

Muhammad Sajjad Khan
Department of Breeding and Genetics, Faculty of Animal Production and Technology, Cholistan University of Veterinary and Animal Sciences (CUVAS), Bahawalpur 63100, Pakistan

&

Muhammad Farrukh Nisar
Department of Physiology and Biochemistry, Faculty of Bio-Sciences, Cholistan University of Veterinary and Animal Sciences (CUVAS), Bahawalpur 63100, Pakistan

Genetic Diversity of Coronaviruses: From SARSCoV to SARS-CoV-2 – *(Part 2)*

Editors: Kamal Niaz, Muhammad Sajjad Khan & Muhammad Farrukh Nisar

ISBN (Online): 978-981-5322-19-4

ISBN (Print): 978-981-5322-20-0

ISBN (Paperback): 978-981-5322-21-7

First published in 2025.

need for a court order if at any point you breach any terms of this License Agreement. In no event will any delay or failure by Bentham Science Publishers in enforcing your compliance with this License Agreement constitute a waiver of any of its rights.

3. You acknowledge that you have read this License Agreement, and agree to be bound by its terms and conditions. To the extent that any other terms and conditions presented on any website of Bentham Science Publishers conflict with, or are inconsistent with, the terms and conditions set out in this License Agreement, you acknowledge that the terms and conditions set out in this License Agreement shall prevail.

Bentham Science Publishers Pte. Ltd.
No. 9 Raffles Place
Office No. 26-01
Singapore 048619
Singapore
Email: subscriptions@benthamscience.net

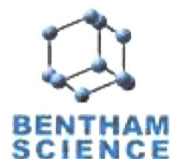

CONTENTS

Muhammad Safdar, Mehmet Ozaslan, Yasmeen Junejo, Umair Younas, Muhammad Zia Ahmad, Jannat Bibi and *Sobia Noreen*

Amjad Islam Aqib, Yasir Razzaq Khan, Tean Zaheer, Rabia Liaqat, Muhammad Luqman Sohail, Ahmad Ali, Hina Afzal Sajid, Firasat Hussain and *Saadia Muneer*

Amjad Islam Aqib, Tean Zaheer, Rabia Liaqat Khan, Yasir Razzaq Khan, Ahmad Ali, Hina Afzal Sajid, Vishal Kiran, C-Neen Fatima Zaheer, Firasat Hussain and *Muhammad Ashir Nabeel*

FOREWORD

The connection between human health, animals, and the environment has been widely recognized as important for the ecosystem we inherit and intend to improve for the generations to come. This, of course, is not a responsibility of a region or a country; rather is the responsibility of all of us. Efforts have to be collaborative and transboundary in approach. Of the many types of challenges, respiratory diseases have emerged as a real threat in the recent past. Scientists have been working to reduce their load and easily spread it from animals to human beings. Newly emerging respiratory diseases such as severe acute respiratory syndrome-coronavirus (SARS-CoV), Middle East respiratory syndrome (MERS), and severe acute respiratory syndrome-coronavirus-2 (SARS-CoV-2) pose a serious threat to the human population and are reported in the year 2003, 2012, and 2019, respectively.

This book is very relevant in this connection. This book consists of four key modules. The first module provides a clearly defined genetic mutation and progression of SARS-CoV in the human population. The second elaborates on the genetic mutational changes of MERS, and the third one summarizes the genetic mutation of SARS-CoV-2. The last one elaborated on the correlation of coronaviruses with various disorders, especially epigenetic, neurological disorders, and artificial intelligence. The learning outcomes of this book are developing knowledge, skills, and competencies in scientists, students, employers, and human resource specialists. This book focuses on developing a detailed set of guidelines regarding epidemiology, genetic alteration, a structural protein, quantitative analysis, and diagnostic approaches of SARS-CoV, MERS-CoV, and SARS-CoV-2, and will give step-by-step awareness to the researchers about these outbreaks. This book will be adopted to give reliable knowledge to all scientists globally. I hope that this book will be distributed widely in Pakistani higher institutions soon for thorough implementation at all levels of postgraduate studies.

Rakesh Srivastava
GLAX Health (Improve Health Through Innovation)
LLC, 8000 Innovation Park Drive, Baton Rouge
LA 70820, USA

PREFACE

Coronaviruses, such as severe acute respiratory syndrome-coronavirus (SARS-CoV), Middle East respiratory syndrome-coronavirus (MERS-CoV), and severe acute respiratory syndrome-coronavirus-2 (SARS-CoV-2) have posed significant public health threats in the last two decades. It has been revealed that bats act as natural reservoirs for these viruses, and periodic monitoring of coronaviruses in bats, dogs, civets, and other wild animals may thus provide important clues about emergent infectious viruses that transfer to humans. The Eastern bent-wing bat *Miniopterus fuliginosus* (*M. fuliginosus*) and genus *Rhinolophus* are distributed extensively throughout China and other countries. Therefore, there is a need to analyze the genetic diversity of coronaviruses transmitted to humans. The only coronavirus genus found was *alphacoronavirus*. The established *alphacoronavirus* genome sequences showed high similarity to other *alphacoronaviruses* found in other *Miniopterus* species and other animals. It suggests that their transmission in different *Miniopterus* species may provide opportunities for recombination with different *alphacoronaviruses*. The genetic information for these novel *alphacoronaviruses* will improve our understanding of the evolution and genetic diversity of coronaviruses, with potentially important implications for the transmission of human diseases. This virus is different from the previously isolated MERS-CoV and SARS-CoV and is the seventh that infects humans. SARS-CoV-2 spreads rapidly and infects a large number of the population globally. Besides, a new variant of coronavirus disease-19 (COVID-19) known as B.1.1.7 is spreading globally, especially in the United Kingdom (UK), with an unusually large number of mutations in the proteins. This variant spreads more easily and quickly than other variants. The new variant is defined by 14 mutations resulting in amino acid changes and three deletions, some of which are believed to influence the virus's transmissibility in humans. The World Health Organization (WHO) has reported that one of the mutations identified (N501Y) is altering an amino acid within the six key residues in the receptor-binding domain. It is indicated that the rate of transmission of the variant, known as B.1.1.7 or VUI 202012/01 (variant under investigation, the year 2020, month 12, variant 01), was 71% (95% confidence interval 67% to 75%), which is higher than for other variants. It may also have a higher viral load.

In this book proposal, we consolidated the genetic diversity/mutation that occurred in 2002-21. Since SARS-CoV-2 is the closest to SARS-CoV and MERS-CoV, the approaches discussed here will be similar and/or varying by a slight degree. In the last 18-19 years, this is the third outbreak of the same coronavirus with a slight mutation that shocked the whole world. This book should be prioritized as up-to-date literature on genetic mutations that have occurred in the form of SARS-CoV, MERS-CoV, and SARS-CoV-2. It will act as a suitable reference if any such virusappears in the future. This book proposal has been classified into four parts: Part I: Genetic Mutation of SARS-CoV, Part II: Genetic Mutation of MERS-CoV, Part III: Genetic Mutation of SARS-CoV-2, and Part IV: Correlation of Coronaviruses with Various Disorders.

With the emergence of new coronavirus variants, different host tropisms permit a thorough analysis of their genomic diversity/mutations that acquire adaptability to their host. Thus, in Part I, we start the book with chapters dealing with a mutation in SARS-CoV, the host genetic diversity of SARS-CoV, newly emerging variants of SARS-CoV, the genetic architecture of host proteins involved in SARS-CoV, and the landscape of host genetic factors correlating with SARS-CoV. In Part II, a critical analysis of the MERS-CoV involves the potential to mutate its genome by opposite genetics and to get better recombinant viruses with described mutations. Such processes will assist in studying the capabilities of particular genes and their effects on virus survival and pathogenesis. These strategies can even help in determining host factors correlating with MERS-CoV genome growth and proliferation. In Part III, we discuss mutation in SARS-CoV-2, the host genetic diversity of SARS-CoV-2, newly emerging variants of SARS-CoV-2, the genetic architecture of host proteins involved in SARS-CoV-2, and the landscape of host genetic factors correlating with SARS-CoV-2. Part IV includes the correlation of coronaviruses with various disorders, especially with epigenetic alteration, neurological disorders, and artificial intelligence.

This book will appear as a baseline for scientists and health professionals to better understand the genetic diversity of SARS-CoV, MERS-CoV, and SARS-CoV-2. However, this single book would not have succeeded without the enthusiasm and determination of publishers and investigators to take time from their hectic schedules and endow on time. We thank the scrutineers who contributed, directly and indirectly, to bring it to reality.

Kamal Niaz
Department of Pharmacology and Toxicology
Faculty of Bio-Sciences
Cholistan University of Veterinary and Animal Sciences (CUVAS)
Bahawalpur 63100, Pakistan

Muhammad Sajjad Khan
Department of Breeding and Genetics
Faculty of Animal Production and Technology
Cholistan University of Veterinary and Animal Sciences (CUVAS)
Bahawalpur 63100, Pakistan

&

Muhammad Farrukh Nisar
Department of Physiology and Biochemistry
Faculty of Bio-Sciences
Cholistan University of Veterinary and Animal Sciences (CUVAS)
Bahawalpur 63100, Pakistan

List of Contributors

Abdul Basit	Department of Microbiology, University of Jhang, Jhang 38000, Pakistan
Abdullah	Department of Pharmacy, University of Malakand, Chakdara Dir Lower, KP, Pakistan
Ahmad Ali	Department of Medicine, Faculty of Veterinary Science, Cholistan University of Veterinary and Animal Sciences (CUVAS), Bahawalpur 63100, Pakistan
Alam Zeb	Directorate of Livestock and Dairy Development Department, Khyber Pakhtunkhwa, Peshawar, Pakistan
Amjid Islam Aqib	Department of Medicine, Cholistan University of Veterinary and Animal Sciences (CUVAS), Bahawalpur 63100, Pakistan
Arooj Fatima	Department of Microbiology, Faculty of Veterinary Science, Cholistan University of Veterinary and Animal Sciences (CUVAS), Bahawalpur 63100, Pakistan
Ayesha Saeed	Department of Biochemistry, Govt. College University, Faisalabad, Pakistan
Aziz ur Rahman	Department of Pharmacy, University of Malakand, Chakdara Dir Lower, KP, Pakistan
Chen Shanyuan	School of Life Sciences, Yunnan University, Kunming 650091, China
C-Neen Fatima Zaheer	Faculty of Veterinary Science, University of Agriculture, Faisalabad, Pakistan
Fazlullah Khan	Department of Pharmacy, Faculty of Pharmacy, Capital University of Science and Technology (CUST), Islamabad, Pakistan
Firasat Hussain	Department of Microbiology, Cholistan University of Veterinary and Animal Sciences (CUVAS), Bahawalpur 63100, Pakistan
Furqan Shafqat	Department of Microbiology, Cholistan University of Veterinary and Animal Sciences (CUVAS), Bahawalpur 63100, Pakistan
Hina Afzal Sajid	Centre of Excellence in Molecular Biology, University of the Punjab, Lahore, Pakistan
Ihtisham Ulhaq	Department of Biosciences, COMSATS University, Islamabad, Pakistan
Ijaz Ahmad	Department of Human, Legal and Economic Sciences, Telematic University "Leonardo da Vinci", Chieti, Italy
Imtiaz Ali Khan	Department of Entomology, The University of Agriculture, Peshawar 25000, Pakistan
Jannat Bibi	Institute for Chinese Olympic Advanced Study, Beijing Sport University, Beijing 100084, China
Kamal Niaz	Department of Toxicology and Pharmacology, Faculty of Bio-Sciences, Cholistan University of Veterinary and Animal Sciences (CUVAS), Bahawalpur 63100, Pakistan
Kashif Prince	Department of Medicine, Faculty of Veterinary Science, Cholistan University of Veterinary and Animal Sciences (CUVAS), Bahawalpur 63100, Pakistan
Kashif Rahim	Department of Microbiology, Cholistan University of Veterinary and Animal Sciences (CUVAS), Bahawalpur 63100, Pakistan

Maryam Bashir	Department of Physiology and Biochemistry, Faculty of Bio-Sciences, Cholistan University of Veterinary and Animal Sciences (CUVAS), Bahawalpur 63100, Pakistan
Mehmet Ozaslan	Division of Molecular Biology and Genetics, Department of Biology, Gaziantep University, Gaziantep 27000, Turkey
Momin Khan	Directorate of Livestock and Dairy Development Department, Khyber Pakhtunkhwa, Peshawar, Pakistan
Muhammad Ashir Nabeel	Department of Theriogenology, University of Agriculture, Faisalabad, Pakistan
Muhammad Dilawar	Department of Zoology, Cholistan University of Veterinary and Animal Sciences (CUVAS), Bahawalpur 63100, Pakistan
Muhammad Farrukh Nisar	Department of Physiology and Biochemistry, Faculty of Bio-Sciences, Cholistan University of Veterinary and Animal Sciences (CUVAS), Bahawalpur 63100, Pakistan
Muhammad Farrukh Tahir	Department of Biochemistry, University of Jhang, Jhang 38000, Pakistan
Muhammad Humayun	Department of Biosciences, COMSATS University, Islamabad, Pakistan
Muhammad Ibrar	Department of Allied and Health Sciences, Iqra National University Swat Campus, Swat, Pakistan
Muhammad Kalim	Department of Microbiology and Immunology, Wake Forest University, Winston-Salem 27101, USA Houston Methodist Hospital Research Institute, Houston Methodist Hospital, Houston, Texas 77030, USA
Muhammad Luqman Sohail	Department of Medicine, Faculty of Veterinary Science, Cholistan University of Veterinary and Animal Sciences (CUVAS), Bahawalpur 63100, Pakistan
Muhammad Naveed	Department of Clinical Pharmacology, School of Pharmacy, Nanjing Medical University, Nanjing 211166, China
Muhammad Rafiq	Department of Physiology and Biochemistry, Faculty of Bio-Sciences, Cholistan University of Veterinary and Animal Sciences (CUVAS), Bahawalpur 63100, Pakistan
Muhammad Saeed	Department of Poultry Sciences, Faculty of Animal Production and Technology, Cholistan University of Veterinary and Animal Sciences (CUVAS), Bahawalpur 63100, Pakistan
Muhammad Safdar	Department of Breeding and Genetics, Cholistan University of Veterinary and Animal Sciences (CUVAS), Bahawalpur 63100, Pakistan
Muhammad Sajjad Khan	Department of Breeding and Genetics, Faculty of Animal Production and Technology, Cholistan University of Veterinary and Animal Sciences (CUVAS), Bahawalpur 63100, Pakistan
Muhammad Shuaib	School of Ecology and Environmental Science, Yunnan University, Kunming 650091, China
Muhammad Yasir Waqas	Department of Physiology and Biochemistry, Faculty of Bio-Sciences, Cholistan University of Veterinary and Animal Sciences (CUVAS), Bahawalpur 63100, Pakistan

Muhammad Zia Ahmad	Faculty of Social Sciences, University of Sargodha, Sargodha 40100, Punjab, Pakistan
Qurat ul Ain Babar	Department of Biochemistry, Govt. College University, Faisalabad, Pakistan
Rabia Liaqat	Department of Pathology, University of Agriculture, Faisalabad, Pakistan
Saadia Muneer	Institute of Microbiology, University of Agriculture, Faisalabad, Pakistan
Sana Tehseen	Department of Botany, Faculty of Science and Technology, Government College Women University, Faisalabad, Pakistan
Sartaj Ali	Department of Biosciences, COMSATS University, Islamabad, Pakistan
Shafeeq Ur Rehman	Department of Microbiology, Cholistan University of Veterinary and Animal Sciences (CUVAS), Bahawalpur 63100, Pakistan
Sobia Noreen	Department of Pharmaceutical Technology, University of Innsbruck, Innsbruck 6020, Austria
Tean Zaheer	Department of Parasitology, University of Agriculture, Faisalabad, Pakistan
Umair Younas	Department of Livestock Management, Cholistan University of Veterinary and Animal Sciences (CUVAS), Bahawalpur 63100, Pakistan
Vishal Kiran	Government College University Lahore, Lahore, Pakistan
Yasir Razzaq Khan	Department of Medicine, Faculty of Veterinary Science, Cholistan University of Veterinary and Animal Sciences (CUVAS), Bahawalpur 63100, Pakistan
Yasmeen Junejo	Department of Physiology and Biochemistry, Cholistan University of Veterinary and Animal Sciences (CUVAS), Bahawalpur 63100, Pakistan

CHAPTER 1

Genetic Architecture of Host Proteins Involved in MERS-CoV

Firasat Hussain[1,*], Muhammad Kalim[2,3], Kashif Rahim[1], Shafeeq Ur Rehman[1], Furqan Shafqat[1], Muhammad Shuaib[4], Umair Younas[5], Amjid Islam Aqib[6], Imtiaz Ali Khan[7] and Chen Shanyuan[8]

[1] *Department of Microbiology, Cholistan University of Veterinary and Animal Sciences (CUVAS), Bahawalpur 63100, Pakistan*

[2] *Department of Microbiology and Immunology, Wake Forest University, Winston-Salem, NC 27101, USA*

[3] *Houston Methodist Hospital Research Institute, Houston, Texas 77030, USA*

[4] *School of Ecology and Environmental Science, Yunnan University, Kunming 650091, China*

[5] *Department of Livestock Management, Cholistan University of Veterinary and Animal Sciences (CUVAS), Punjab, Bahawalpur 63100, Pakistan*

[6] *Department of Medicine, Cholistan University of Veterinary and Animal Sciences (CUVAS), Bahawalpur 63100, Pakistan*

[7] *Department of Entomology, The University of Agriculture, Peshawar 25000, Pakistan*

[8] *School of Life Sciences, Yunnan University, Kunming 650091, China*

Abstract: Middle East respiratory syndrome coronavirus (MERS-CoV), a novel coronavirus linked to severe respiratory tract illness, was initially identified in 2012. Since then, 1401 individuals have been infected with this virus in 26 countries, with 543 people (39%) dying. Severe respiratory infection, sometimes accompanying shock, acute renal damage, and coagulopathy are all symptoms of these disorders. This pandemic has sparked worldwide worry because of its human-to-human transmission *via* intimate contact. The Eastern Province, Riyadh, and Makkah were severely hit. In 2014, the pandemic progressed fastest in Makkah, Riyadh, and Eastern Province in 2013. Effective therapeutic and immunological solutions based on solid molecular research were critical, with the threat of an epidemic looming. The MERS-CoV intrinsic genetic heterogeneity across different clades may have set the way for cross-species transmission and alterations in inter-species and intra-species tropism. Host protease blockers include transmembrane serine protease 2 (TMPRSS2), cathepsin L, and furin. According to sequence comparison and modeling research, the viral spike features a putative receptor-binding domain (RBD) that enables this interaction.

* **Corresponding author Firasat Hussain:** Department of Microbiology, Cholistan University of Veterinary and Animal Sciences (CUVAS), Bahawalpur 63100, Pakistan;
E-mail: firasathussain@cuvas.edu.pk

The dipeptidyl-peptidase 4 (DPP4)-propeller engages with the receptor-binding subdomain but not the intrinsic hydrolase domain. The receptor binding subdomain of MERS CoV and severe acute respiratory syndrome coronavirus (SARS CoV) is drastically different. This chapter aims to explain the genetic architecture of host proteins involved in MERS-CoV and compare it with other coronaviruses.

Keywords: MERS-CoV, Protein S, Adaptive immune response, LY6E protein, DPP4, Dipeptidyl peptidase 4, CD26 protein.

INTRODUCTION

Given the present epidemic, the severe respiratory syndrome coronavirus-2 (SARS-CoV-2) has received a lot of study interest. Nonetheless, the Middle East respiratory syndrome-coronavirus (MERS-CoV), a formerly highly virulent coronavirus, remains a source of worry, particularly in Saudi Arabia and neighboring nations. Patients with mild to deadly MERS-CoV have a greater risk of spreading the virus because they shed more viral offspring than those with moderate symptoms [1, 2]. Reduced propagation and outbreak containment have been achieved by recognizing and isolating these individuals in healthcare institutions and instituting adequate infection control [3, 4]. Innovative MERS-CoV cases continue to be recorded, particularly in the Arabian Peninsula [4]. In the Arabian Peninsula, clade B viruses became common in dromedaries, producing zoonotic disease and, in some cases, clusters of human-to-human transmission. Camels in East Africa, Egypt, Ethiopia, Sudan, Djibouti, Kenya, North Africa, Morocco, West Africa, Nigeria, and Burkina Faso had viruses that belonged to different clade C sub-lineages [5, 6].

MERS-CoV is a zoonotic disease that causes asymptomatic to severe pneumonia in humans. The virus only produces a slight illness in dromedary camels but travels quickly amongst them. MERS-CoV, an innovative coronavirus, was discovered in people in the Middle East in 2012, followed by many European countries [7, 8]. A significant proportion of infected individuals (> 50%) experienced severe respiratory disease and clinical signs that were comparable to those reported during the 2003 SARS epidemic caused by the SARS-CoV [9]. Preliminary epidemiological studies show that this fatal virus may be spread from human to human, raising worldwide concerns about the opportunity of a MERS pandemic [10, 11]. The MERS-CoV virus requires a significant surface S glycoprotein to interact with and infiltrate the focus cell [12, 13].

According to recent studies, coronaviruses are exceptionally compatible with evading immune detection and decreasing immunological response [14]. This explains why they have such a lengthy incubation period, which may last 2 to 11 days. In a prior study, pegylated interferon (IFN) was more operative, contrary to

MERS-CoV, than SARS-CoV in cell culture in a macaque model [15]. MERS-CoV clearance from the respiratory system needs an IFN-mediated innate immune response. Overexpression of the LY6E (Lymphocyte Antigen 6 Family Member E) gene did not influence S1/S2 cleavage or the mutant MERS-CoV S pseudo-particle cell entrance level.

To summarize, LY6E is a CoV-restricting factor that prevents CoV invasion and defends the host from a severe viral illness. According to recent findings, coronaviruses appear unusually compatible with avoiding immune detection and lowering immunological reactivity. This helps to explain why they have such a long incubation period, ranging from 2 to 11 days [16]. Most processes, specifically the detection and signaling of IFN-I, depend on suppressing innate immune responses. Small and inexpensive measures are needed again for control, and comprehensive research is required to understand the pathogenesis and develop a vaccine against MERS-COV. Mice seem to be the most favorable small-animal species for this objective due to their abundance and the occurrence of a comprehensive level of knowledge, especially in heritability and serology. Unsurprisingly, rodents, gerbils, and badgers are immune to MERS-CoV because they lack the MERS-CoV binding site, sentient CD26 (hCD26), and synthetase activities occurred (DPP4) [17 - 19]. Receptor-binding domain (RBD)-protective trimer's immunity could be improved even more by stabilizing its trimeric configuration with disulfide bridges, trying to add other multimeric patterns, including GCN4, adapting spacer sequence data in between RBD and Fd, or incorporating such strategies, as has been completed for other virus particles [20]. Even though RBD-Fd influences the minimum concentration activation of cell-mediated immunity (data not shown), its robust control is primarily due to neutralizing antibodies. This supported the fact that almost all mice that withstood MERS-CoV infestation had reasonably extreme serum-thwarting levels of antibodies, implying that neutralizing antibodies, instead of cell-mediated immunity, could provide a significant function in attempting to avoid MERS-CoV infestation, which is based on RBD-trimeric form vaccine candidates.

The amplicon shares well with RBD–CD26 binding site interaction, and antibody adhesion prevents the viral RBD from conversing, including its cell surface receptor. As a result, one primary method of LCA60 suppression is the potent inhibition of virus–receptor interrelations. Algorithmic docking has proven experimental studies, and the creation of varieties enabled the identification of RBD toxins crucial for adhesion and neutralization. LCA60 has an innovative specific antigen that is unchanged by 3B11 and other phage-derived neutralizing antibodies. Proteins 7 and 8 are cofactors for polymerase activation, and protein 10 is a 20 O-methyltransferase. Three transmembrane proteins, 3, 4, and 6, function as membrane anchors for the replicative transcription complex. Protein

13 has a conserved region that contributes to the unwinding of RNA in the 50–30 direction [21]. Protein 9 is a coronavirus protein that protects the genome from damage during replication [22, 23]. The only protein translated is replicase transcriptase, which takes up 2/3 of the coding capacity. Conformational changes occur when the viral S protein interacts with its corresponding receptor, resulting in virion fusion with the cell membrane. Several coronaviruses' S protein is uncleaved in matured virions, necessitating a protease interaction during the infection entrance stage to dissociate the fusion S2 and binding S1 parts of the spike. Depending on MERS-CoV isolates from people and camels, Nsp3 is now undergoing selection [24]. In paired membranes, nsp3 and nsp4 collaborate to produce their effects. Non-structural protein 6 (nsp6) is assumed to enhance membrane proliferation by forming perinuclear vesicles, requiring full-length nsp3. MERS-CoV attaches to host cellular receptors when its S protein binds to them, resulting in infection. The S protein's N-terminal receptor-binding region has also influenced its ability to spread between species [25, 26].

MERS-CoV Host Interaction

Unlike some pathogenic coronaviruses, which primarily cause self-limited RT infections, MERS-CoV can induce severe disease with the involvement of lower RT and extra-pulmonary manifestations [27, 28]. In those with severe MERS, pneumonic indications such as cough, fever, and dyspnea are common, which can proceed to respiratory breakdown and acute respiratory distress syndrome (ARDS) [29, 30]. MERS primarily infects humans through the respiratory tract. MERS-CoV was shown to infect and reproduce successfully in the human respiratory epithelium [31]. In particular, *in vitro* research on human airway tissues consistently demonstrated that endothelial cells were highly vulnerable to MERS-CoV [32, 33], explaining that the infection of MERS-CoV in the respiratory tract can develop into a systemic or widespread infection. The respiratory epithelium is very tolerant to MERS-CoV when seen as a whole. Viral multiplication is resilient, and apoptosis is massively induced due to the effective infection. This research showed the pathophysiological background for MERS's key pulmonary manifestations, including pneumonia and severe lung damage. Immunodeficient people and patients with diseases are the most vulnerable to MERS-CoV infection, which can be fatal in many situations [34, 35].

Role of S Proteins

The MERS-CoV envelope contains the membrane, spike, and envelope proteins. By fusing and sticking to the receptor, the spike protein aids viral entrance. MERS-CoV host cell receptor CD 26, DPP4, has been recognized [36]. The spike protein is essential in MERS-CoV infection, promoting viral attachment to receptors and fusion. During infection, the MERS-S CoV protein is divided into a receptor-binding S1 and a membrane-fusion S2 subunit [37, 38]. A receptor-binding S1 subunit contacts with DPP4, allowing the virus to adhere to target cells [37, 39]. The S2 component of MERS-CoV is involved in membrane fusion, just like that of other coronaviruses like SARS-CoV. S2's heptad repeat 1 and 2 domains are significant and complementary in this process [40]. By experiencing substantial structural changes, S2 causes membrane fusion [41]. The S protein must be stimulated to enter the cells. One or more of the following proteases may be involved in this activation, based on cell type: Endosomal cathepsins, TMPRSS2, and proprotein convertases [42, 43].

Role of Adaptive and Immune Responses

Although SARS-cellular CoV's tropism in the human RT is related to MERS-CoV, immune cells showed unique vulnerability to SARS-CoV and MERS-CoV [44, 45]. Dendritic cells play a significant role in innate resistance and can release a slew of chemokines and cytokines. These cells can move from the periphery to lymphoid tissue, where they cause the activation of T cells [46]. MERS-CoV has developed approaches to modulate innate immunity and inhibit or stop Interferon synthesizing ways, which is rather interesting [47]. This feature could have a role in the high fatality ratios among MERS-CoV-affected individuals, particularly those with weakened immune systems [48]. According to an investigation on human macrophages, MERS-CoV may affect and proliferate in macrophages. MERS-CoV also dramatically increased the release of proinflammatory mediators in infected macrophages [49]. The virus assaults the immune defense and causes antigen-presenting cells (APC) to downregulate major histocompatibility complex I and II and CD80/86, inhibiting T cell response [50]. The amount of infected CD8+ T cells correlates with the seriousness of the illness. Severely infected patients have a lot of Tc cells, while Th cells and immunoglobulin responses are barely discernible at this point [51].

Network-Based Identification of Host Protein Complex

Coronavirus is +ve-sense, ssRNA virus that infects the respiratory tracts. Different strains have been identified, all of which elicit symptoms similar to the cold flu. Three new pathogenic strains have appeared since 2002: SARS-CoV, MERS-CoV, and SARS-CoV-2 [52 - 56]. Variable receptor binding can explain some of the differences in pathogenicity. SARS-CoV and SARS-CoV-2 use the angiotensin-converting enzyme2 (ACE2) receptor, whereas 229E adopts the aminopeptidase-N as a receptor [56 - 58]. These interactions change the cell's natural protein-protein interaction pattern and have been demonstrated to conduct various pro-viral functions, including immune evasion, by suppressing the type I interferon system [59 - 61]. With a genome length of around 30 kilobase pairs, one of the largest RNA virus genomes is a coronavirus. The three structural polypeptides utilized to build new viral particles and other auxiliary components found critical for pathogenesis are encoded in the genome. Two open reading frames make up two-thirds of the genome's 5′ encoding 16 nonstructural proteins that conduct a range of tasks, in addition to RNA genome replication and proofreading, as well as replication–transcription complex assembly. With roughly 2000 amino acids, Nsp 3 is the biggest of these proteins, whose papain-like-protease (PL2Pro) subunit has gotten the maximum attention. The PL2Pro domains have deubiquitinase and deacylation activity [62 - 64].

Furthermore, it was demonstrated that nsp3, in conjunction with other non-structural proteins, is sufficient for creating the membrane vesicles utilized by the replication cycle [65, 66]. However, the functions nsp3 outside of the PL2Pro are less clear [67]. The interactomes of isolated coronaviruses PL2pro domains were compared in another investigation [62]. The sections of nsp3 have been absent from SARS-CoV-2 research, most probably due to the difficulty and large size, which makes protein synthesis problematic. Based on a previous analysis of the SARS intraviral interactome, we split the nsp3 protein into three segments to avoid this problem [65, 68].

Lymphocyte Antigen 6 Complex Locus E Ly6e and Mers-CoV

LY6E is a 133-amino-acid glycosylphosphatidylinositol (GPI)-anchored cell surface protein called type-1 Thymic Shared Antigen. The ovary, uterus, liver, spleen, and brain are transcriptionally active tissues for LY6E [69], and Type I interferon can trigger its expression. LY6E has been linked to immune modulation, specifically influencing T cell activation, propagation, tumor metastasis, and differentiation [70, 71]. It was not until the early 2000s that LY6E was linked to viral infection, and there has been a surge in interest in the study of LY6E's role in viral interactions recently. The following points are discussed with LY6E's basic antiviral activity mechanisms. Firstly, it is a GPI-supported polypeptide abundant in the plasma membrane's lipid-raft micro-domain [72]. The indirect involvement of LY6E in cytoskeleton rearrangements could explain the boosting or suppressing effect of LY6E on virus infection [73, 74], which could have a cell and virus-specified impact. LY6E can control cell signaling and the immunological outcome necessary for infection defense. It is well understood that type I IFN signaling involves cytokines, chemokines, their corresponding receptors, and related adaptors, aiding the elimination of invading pathogenic microbes by signaling cascade series [75]. Recently, a particular link between LY6E and innate immunity was discovered. LY6E, in particular, has been found to inhibit CD14 [76] and enhance viral pathogenesis significantly. The latest surveillance of Kenyan camels, the primary viral reservoir for MERS-CoV, shows that the zoonotic virus persists [77]. LY6E in humans and camels controlled MERS-CoV infection. In an experiment to determine the availability of LY6E in respiratory cells impacted by human CoVs, single-cell RNA sequencing was used to evaluate the expression of LY6E in airway epithelium. LY6E was observed in all cell types, with goblet cells having the highest quantities. The next question was whether LY6E affects the spike protein's proteolytic activation. Host proteases break the spike protein once it attaches to the appropriate receptor, leading to membrane fusion [78]. The cell surface and endosomal protease inhibitors restricted infection but did not influence CoV infection restriction mediated by LY6E. Mutations at the cleavage site also inhibit proteolytic activation [79, 80]. Mutations lowered the spike protein's MERS-CoV activation in S1/S2 and S2'. Overexpression of the LY6E gene did not influence S1/S2 cleavage or the level of mutant MERS-CoV S pseudo-particle cell entrance. To summarize, LY6E is a CoV-restricting factor that prevents CoV invasion and defends the host from a severe viral illness.

Interferon Related Genes and MERS-CoV

While pathogenic human CoVs are believed to trigger severe pneumonia, the mechanisms underlying their increased morbidity and death remain a mystery. Virus replication is quick. High titers and concomitant increase in inflammatory responses play a significant role in severe pneumonia [81, 82]. The first-line defense that opposes various viral diseases is inborn immunity, namely the production of IFN-1. The induction of IFN-stimulated genes facilitates antiviral action by directly reducing virus multiplication and indirectly modifying the host immunological response to virus infection, both regulated by IFN-I [83, 84]. Type I IFNs have been identified to control the immune response to viruses as well as modulate the adaptive immune system's subsequent activation, which aids in the clearing of viral infection [85]. IFN- has recently been discovered to be necessary for the immune reaction to the respiratory viral invasion, with humans and mice lacking IFN-related innate immune responses being more prone to infection [86 - 88]. IFN-s like IFN-1, -2, -3, and -4 are key immune regulators against viral infection in the epithelial mucosa, according to information obtained, and IFN-s like IFN-1, -2, -3, and -4 activate the immune system in response to respiratory viruses. According to prior research, IFN is considered essential for the defense of viral invasions in the respiratory system and for performing a major part in localized antiviral immune responses [89]. According to recent findings, coronaviruses appear unusually compatible with avoiding immune detection and lowering immunological reactivity. This helps to explain why they have such a long incubation period, ranging from 2 to 11 days [16]. Most processes, specifically the detection and signaling of IFN-I, depend on suppressing innate immune responses. IFN-I suppresses the immune response to MERS-CoV and SARS-CoV invasions [90].

In a prior study, pegylated IFN was proven to be more efficient against different coronaviruses in cell culture in a macaque model [91, 92], and it was suggested that it owes to the unavailability of a MERS-CoV homolog of the SARS-CoV peptide, which leads to the expression of interferon associated anti-viral genes. IFN was combined with ribavirin in a macaque model, resulting in reduced clinical signs after infection, with microarray analysis indicating reduced inflammatory gene expression [92]. Consequently, MERS-CoV clearance from the respiratory system necessitates an innate immune response mediated by IFN. IFN-s, specifically IFN-4, caused an increase in ISG transcription and an efficient innate immune response in respiratory epithelial cells, implying superiority as a therapeutic possibility for suppressing MERS-CoV infection.

hACE and MERS-CoV

The receptor-binding domains on the carboxyl-terminus of the S1 subunit of the spike proteins are frequently used to evaluate specific receptor recognition of coronaviruses [93]. Three well-studied coronavirus targets, ACE2, DPP4, and aminopeptidase N, are S1-CTD binding exopeptidases [94 - 96]. The NL63-CoV uses ACE2 as an entrance receptor, also exploited by numerous arboviruses (beta-CoV lineage B) [97]. APN, similar to many alpha and delta coronaviruses, has a cross-genera receptor use profile (PDCoV) comparable to APN [98]. DPP4 use has only been detected in merbecoviruses such as HKU4, HKU25, and similar types [99, 100]. The type-I membrane-anchored dipeptidyl carboxypeptidase enzyme ACE, also known as peptidyldipeptidase A, helps control blood pressure by maintaining electrolyte balance through the renin-angiotensin mechanism [101]. Each human ACE functional domain has an active site containing a Zn+ bonding position (N and C) [102]. The N and C domains' substrate specificities, physiological forms, and inhibitors differ slightly [103]. On the one hand, the N and C regions both catalyze substrate breakdown with identical efficiency. Inhibiting the N domain of ACE, on the other hand, has been demonstrated not to affect blood pressure regulation [103, 104]. All inhibitors target the C domain because it was determined that targeting this site was sufficient for lowering blood pressure.

Transgenic Mouse Proteins and MERS-COV

Small and inexpensive measures are needed for control, and comprehensive research is required to understand pathogenesis and develop a vaccine against MERS-COV. Mice seem to be the most favorable small-animal species for this objective due to their abundance and the occurrence of a comprehensive level of knowledge, especially in heritability and serology. Unsurprisingly, rodents, gerbils, and badgers are immune to MERS-CoV because they lack the MERS-CoV binding site, sentient CD26 (hCD26), and synthetase activities (DPP4) [17 - 19]. Moreover, while research on model organisms (NHPs) such as cynomolgus and marsupials has shown their vulnerability to variable levels of MERS-CoV infectious disease, non-human primates are expensive frameworks of limited inventory [105, 106].

To study viral diseases, we mainly use animal models that play a central role in determining pathogenesis and assessing vaccines and therapies against the virus. However, the animal model should allow viral infections and the disease to develop. Its characteristics and pathology should be the same, just as Homo sapiens. MERS-CoV inflammation has been examined in different non-sentient mammal (NHP) designs, a macaque mammal, and the widely accepted lemur [92]. In rhesus macaques, MERS-CoV induces a brief respiratory tract illness. Infectious disease of rhesus macaques with the MERS coronavirus results in animal studies on MERS [107]. Virulence and spreading of MERS-CoV were observed in rhesus macaques with weak immunity [108]. MERS-CoV infection is possible in both species. Due to their orthologous, widely known small-scale lab models such as mice, ferrets, piglets, and gerbils are impervious to MERS-CoV infestation. DPP4 can be confined and used as a presenter binding site for MERS-CoV admittance [106]. The intrinsic blocker for DPP4-directed entrance of MERS-CoV is adenosine deaminase [109]. MERS-CoV is unlikely to be available in domestic pigs [110]. In Syrian hamsters, the MERS-CoV does not replicate [111].

MERS-CoV receptor, *via* its target, dipeptidyl peptidase 4 to the RBD, initiates the attachment to the host cell [112]. Many methods have been used to fight receptor incompatibility and make MERS-CoV transgenic mice. MERS-CoV's first mouse inflammation prototype was established in 2014 [113]. The airways of rodents were infected with enterovirus 5 chimeric encrypting sentient DPP4 (hDPP4). EBV functional annotation of hDPP4 provided mice vulnerable to MERS-CoV infestation for a brief period; however, the animals established lung problems. Transgenic mouse creation using a virus receptor to render mice vulnerable to illness is a common strategy.

Many other factions, along with ours, generated mice with hDPP4 transgenic interpretation that use distinct organizers—sensitivity to infections by genuine and pseudo-typed MERS-CoV in DPP4 knock-in mice. The disease intensity in transgenic mice after MERS-CoV illness was associated with the cellular allocation and hDPP4 interpretation trends. MERS-CoV mimics as well as induces transmissible disease and death rates. MERS-CoV infection resulted in only mild illness in mice given hDPP4 under the mortal apoprotein C (SPC) sponsor, which also limits representation to the upper airway and lung cellular membranes. In mice engineered for human dipeptidyl peptidase 4 and with respiratory disease in the MERS, coronavirus causes various organ injury and destruction. As a result, these modified mice must not recreate a severe lung disease phenotype comparable to MERS. The production of human DPP4 mice and adjusting the virus to the animals are two possible methods for generating mouse models of MERS-CoV infectious disease. Pascal *et al.* [114] described the framework that includes all of the rodent's DPP4 ORFs, which were humanized, as well as a new strategic plan for generating human monoclonal antibodies against the S protein.

MERS-CoV disease caused hypovolemia, vasculature handcuff, and upper airway sinus bulking, and a 20% loss of weight, entailing euthanasia. In transgenic mice of MERS, CD8+ T cells and macrophages govern the progression of the disease. One other MERS mouse model was developed using CRISPR-Cas9 to replace 2 amino acid residues in the DPP4 coding region of mice [115]. This model helped replicate MERS-CoV and did not cause any severe illness. The mouse model of DPP4 was also helpful in multiplying MERS-COV and did not cause any severe lung illness [116]. Following the HCoV-EMC/2012 role inside the respiratory system of 2 humanized transgenic mice, 2 different cursor (MA) segregates of MERS-CoV were isolated [54]. Transmittable syndrome, which was established in a template of the mouse, as well as the related death rates, resembled severe forms of MERS-CoV. In human DPP4 knock-in mice, the mouse-adapted MERS coronavirus produces deadly chest infections [117].

A genetically engineered mouse prototype demonstrates MERS of coronavirus receptor, CoV's hDPP4 (hDPP4-Tg), because MERS-CoV does not cause infection in wild-type mice [111]. The primer hDPP4 gene is converted into exotic mice, and the resulting Tg mice exhibit hDPP4 inflection across the body. A transgenic model of mice is entirely susceptible to the infection of MERS-CoV, leading to serious chest disease and some causes of severe viral replication observed in the airways, kidneys, and CNS. Genetically engineered mice infected with MERS-CoV also have consistent weight reduction and start dying. In hDPP4-Tg mice, RBD-Fd protein evoked protracted lifelong immunity against MERS-CoV infection. We used an aluminum adjuvant to immunize hDPP4-Tg mice, which are genetically-modified C57BL/6 rodents susceptible to MERS-CoV infection, with this protein to assess the efficacy of RBD-Fd heterodimers in eliciting immunological responses against MERS-CoV [118]. We then contested the vaccinated rodents with a lethal dose of MERS-CoV and assessed their longevity, weight, and clinical manifestations. According to the findings, 83% of RBD-Fd-immunized mice withstood fatal MERS-CoV infectious disease. Before the actual virus contest, such mice had deactivating levels of antibodies, which resided in MERS-CoV. Even though the questioned mice lost weight for 8–14 weeks after being afflicted with MERS-CoV, they quickly regained their average weight.

Conversely, regulated mice with a baseline level of autoantibodies in their serum samples lost weight continuously upon virus contest, and all mice (100%) died on day 11. Clinical findings in the mouse lungs showed lung tissue tissues in RBD-Fd-immunized mice. There is little pathological difference between this challenged mouse and other mice with normal healthy lungs, except for the alveolar wall thickness. In contrast, MERS-CoV-infected PBS-regulated mice developed intercellular pneumonia, including inflammatory cell invasion, upper airway sinus bulking, pivotal extravasation, and hemorrhage. RBD-Fd was administered to the hDPP4-Tg mice when they were 4 months old. They got a booster dose four weeks later. The mice were exposed to MERS-CoV twelve weeks following their first vaccination. Before being sacrificed to evaluate clinical signs, they were observed for a further three weeks. As a result, the above results indicate that RBD-Fd can stimulate lengthy resistance mechanisms against the MERS-CoV virus in aging mice. People would be unable to obtain enough isomeric RBD nutrients and use them as regulators in this study owing to the minor affirmation of receptor-binding domain monomer inside the human cell plasmid vector.

The RBD-Fd-immunized hDPP4-Tg mice's 83% survival rate and limited pathological processes prove its elevated preventive effect against deadly MERS-CoV contests. RBD-protective trimer's immunity can be improved even more by stabilizing its trimeric configuration with disulfide bridges, trying to add other multimeric patterns, including GCN4, adapting spacer sequence data in between RBD and Fd, or incorporating such strategies as has been completed for other virus particles [20]. Even though RBD-Fd influences the minimum concentration activation of cell-mediated immunity, its robust control is primarily due to neutralizing antibodies. It supports that the majority of the mice that withstood MERS-CoV infestation had high levels of antibodies, implying that neutralizing antibodies, instead of cell-mediated immunity, can provide a significant function in attempting to avoid MERS-CoV infestation, which is based on RBD-trimeric form vaccine candidates.

Human Receptor DPP4 and MERS-COV Spike RBD

For cell membrane entrance and viral propagation, MERS-CoV uses DPP4 [119]. DPP4 binds to itself to form a homodimer. Each subunit comprises alpha and beta hydrolase and beta propulsor domains. The comprehensive DPP4 protein is a type-2 transmembrane peptide with a membrane-spanning region of amino acids 7–28. The alpha and beta hydrolase domain nearest the membrane comprises amino acids 506–766 and 39–51 and includes the influential quartet His740, Ser630, and Asp708 [120]. Each propeller has a 4-stranded alternatively spliced layer motif and blade-4 with an extra non-parallel sheet motif between strands 3 and 4 [120, 121]. As per structural studies, the spike protein RBD moderates illnesses by connecting purely to propellers 4 and 5 of the DPP4 receptor's amino-terminal propulsor domain [121]. The recognition of 16 amino acid residues in the DPP4 with spike protein was facilitated by the settlement of the comprehensive protein crystalline orientation of the DPP4 binding to the MERS-CoV spike protein complex [38, 39]. Humans, camels, and bats use the DPP4 receptor to bind with the spike protein [122]. The genetic drift of these DPP4 amino acid sequences in immediate communication with MERS-CoV between many animal strains was a crucial variable for preventing MERS-CoV's entry into certain species [123]. The DPP4 cellular binding site is found in a variety of living tissues. It is present in many cellular functions, with metabolic glucose homeostasis [124]. The enzyme activity was already linked to the legislation of the recombinant activity of various hormones, chemokines, and T-cells [125 - 127]. Significant public health circumstances, including hyperglycemia and coronary artery disease, have been strenuously correlated with the involvement of DPP4 genomic drifts or SNPs [128, 129]. Nevertheless, there is an effective way to find the insufficient information on epigenetic homo sapiens DPP4 variance, particularly the signatory spike protein, which may influence the DPP4-S protein intricate interactions by provoking systemic senate confirmation changes.

MERS-CoV spike (S) protein is vital in virus infection and etiology. It unites the cellular receptor DPP through the RBD in the S1 component, resulting in virus-cell fusion membranes *via* the S2 subunit [93, 94, 130]. Moreover, by utilizing RBD-specific neutralizing monoclonal antibodies, numerous essential antibodies flee genetic changes in the MERS-CoV RBD, like those at contaminants 511 and 513 [131, 132]. MERS-CoV RBD's proclivity to morph over time can aid in the highly contagious avoidance of cross-neutralizing monoclonal antibodies found in camels and humans initially afflicted with MERS-CoV. Knowing which RBD-based MERS vaccines being developed are efficacious against MERS-CoV strains currently prevalent in humans is critical. The S1 subunit has determinants of cell phenotypic plasticity and communication with the recipient cell, whereas the S2 subunit encompasses facilitators of transfection [41, 133]. Raj and colleagues discovered that DPP4, also recognized as CD26, is a cell surface target for MERS-CoV through a combined-purification process with the MERS-CoV S1 subunit [12]. DDP4, like ACE2, is present in the incitation of different types of cells, such as those discovered in living beings' air passages, and has ectopeptidase interaction. However, this enzymatic role does not appear to be needed for viral entry [134]. A potential MERS-CoV RBD has been recognized through contouring assessments of S glycoproteins from many human coronaviruses [13]. Nevertheless, due to the relatively low extent of structural similarity among S glycoprotein patterns and techniques of communication with unique cell receptors, structural characteristics among all respective receptor pairs seem to vary substantially.

Human Receptor CD26 and MERS-COV

The relatively newer MERS-CoV can potentially cause respiratory illness in humans and is the 2nd type of a successful infective CoV; the first is SARS-CoV [7, 54, 135]. CD 26 had been formerly recognized as the cell surface target for MERS-CoV4 [12]. The interaction of the MERS-CoV flare protease with CD 26 modulates the virus, resulting in organized cells and virus-cell merging, causing illness. We present the first crystalline formation of the MERS-CoV S protein's unrestricted RBD and its interaction with CD26 to demarcate the molecular mechanism of this direct association. Moreover, with a degree of unsaturation of 16.7 nM, connecting the RBD and CD26 is assessed utilizing an accurate spectral response. The viral RBD comprises a whole subnet comparable with that of the SARS-CoV spike peptide and a distinct filament exterior receptor binding archetype that acknowledges propellers 4 and 5 of the cluster of differentiation 26 b-propeller. The nuclear specifics at the intersection of these two signatory units expose an unexpected protein-protein interaction facilitated primarily by water-soluble byproducts. Sequence analysis reveals potential structural sustainability for such a territory that is genetically identical to the MERS-CoV RBD, which is vital between many beta-coronaviruses but has high variability in the exterior binding affinity pattern region for virus-specific pathophysiology, including receptor determination. SARS-CoV and MERS-CoV are beta-coronaviruses found to entangle the cell receptors ACE2 and CD26.

SARS-CoV infects highly folded pulmonary cells, category 1 and category 2 pneumocytes, and non-ciliated pulmonary cells, although MERS-CoV afflicts type-2 pneumocytes and pulmonary cells without cilia. These distinctions may compensate for the disparities in living beings' transmission rates, which were greater for SARS-CoV and relatively small for MERS-CoV. The 2 pathogens also vary in the length of their outbreaks, which is brief for SARS-CoV and lengthy for MERS-CoV, which also emerged in 2012 and is still circulating in the Mideast. In terms of the zoonoses cistern, MERS-CoV and SARS-CoV are imagined to have evolved in bats, with filarial mammals representing the definitive host for human MERS-CoV disease and civets and squirrel dogs for SARS-CoV infection [136 - 138]. Notably, although MERS-CoV permeates the lower respiratory tract in living beings, actively making transmission ineffective, the virus spreads to the respiratory tract. It is available in large amounts in the respiratory secretions of camels, causing infection in humans and other camels.

MERS-trimeric CoV S protein modulates receptor signaling and membrane merging but is the prime goal for protection [42, 139]. X-ray computational modeling is used to characterize the shape of the cell surface receptor (CD26), which would be preserved throughout many life forms, and the complicated CD 26 with the bonding affinity receptor binding domain of the S subunit [12, 38, 39]. Recently, two sides isolated antibody responses to MERS-CoV using nonimmune human autoantibodies monitor modules [132, 140]. LCA60 unites sub-nanomolar particles to an adhesin in the S peptide RBD and efficaciously nullifies MERS-CoV infectious disease in numerous isolated strains. The amplicon shares well with RBD–CD26 binding site interaction, and antibody adhesion precludes the viral RBD from conversing, including its cell surface receptor. As a result, one primary method of LCA60 suppression is the potent inhibitor of virus–receptor interrelations. Algorithmic docking has proven experimental studies, and the creation of varieties enabled the identification of RBD toxins crucial for adhesion and neutralization. LCA60 has an innovative specific antigen that is unchanged by 3B11 and other virus-derived neutralizing antibodies. It is demonstrated in cultured cells for LCA60 and another immunoglobulin characterized by the need for a solitary thwarting antibody, which raises the chances of picking flee replicants *in vivo*. This issue can be resolved by using two immunoglobulins against non-overlapped locations. Many of the MERS-CoV combating immunoglobulin have indeed been discovered to merge, which may not provide a rationalization for integrating such immunoglobulin. While the full range of MERS-CoV antigen presentation is already being studied, it should be mentioned that its LCA60 signatory fragments are preserved throughout all MERS-CoV isolated strains. The 3B11 is unsuccessful in acknowledging the London1_novel CoV/2012 (a coronavirus strain identified in 2012 in a patient in London who was among the first to contract the virus now known as MERS-CoV) due to mutation.

Recently, coronaviral genetic codes found in dromedary nasopharyngeal swabs have been the same as the genomic sequences of human MERS-CoV isolated strains [138, 141, 142]. However, one genetic code was extracted from such a mammal effectively in a person trying to care for a sick dromedary [143]. Furthermore, MERS-CoV has been secluded explicitly from a dromedary in Qatar [144]. The origin of dromedary MERS-CoV infectious disease is unidentified. However, it is not inconceivable that those serving are just intermediating hosts. Additional MERS-CoV hosts, such as bats, have been suggested [145]. MERS-CoV might be preserved in nature by bats, who might often afflict dromedaries and transmit the virus [146, 147]. CD26, also recognized as dipeptidyl peptidase 4, has been recently recognized as that of the living thing MERS-CoV cell entrance ligand as well as a binding site for Tylonycteris bat coronavirus HKU4 [148 - 150]. The CD26/DPP4 antibody is retained between many mammals, and MERS-potentially CoV broad organisms' phenotypic plasticity could be partly due to this sustainability [23, 148], revealing that the affirmation of acceptable CD26 homologs may entirely dictate MERS-CoV host tissue tropism. Also, bats cannot be governed with MERS-CoV boreholes at this time.

Genetic Evolution of MERS-CoV

Viral respiratory infections have been the primary cause of sickness and mortality in people and animals worldwide since the early 1930s [151 - 153]. Human respiratory sickness is caused by almost 200 antigenically diverse types of influenza viruses, rhinoviruses, adenoviruses, coronaviruses, *metapneumoviruses*, and *orthopneumoviruses* [152]. One of the most prevalent viruses that cause deadly respiratory infections belongs to the Coronaviridae family [154]. They are RNA viruses with crown-shaped envelopes that can infect humans and other animals [155, 156]—grouped into four sub-groups: alpha, beta, gamma, and delta viruses, with the Betacoronavirus genus being the most virulent [157, 158]. The seven types of Betacoronoviruses genus are HCoV-OC43, HCoV-229E, HCoV-HKU1, HCoV-NL63, SARS-CoV, MERS-CoV, and the recently discovered SARS-CoV-2 (otherwise known as COVID-19) [157, 159]. SARS-CoV, MERS-CoV, and SARS-CoV-2 are probable Betacoronoviridae family members well-recognized for their pandemic outbreaks of deadly respiratory illnesses in humans. In contrast, the other forms are linked to moderate respiratory sickness [160].

RNA viruses, notably the Coronaviridae family of the order Nidovirales with genome lengths of less than 30 Kb, have a rapid genetic development compared to all other animals [161]. Because of their rapid genetic development, these lethal virus types can cross species borders and cause severe sickness and fatality in humans. Viral genomes generally encode proteins that perform three functions: replication and transcription, structural proteins, and infectivity-enabling proteins. ORF 1a and b are located in the viral genome. They are translated into the non-structural RNA-dependent-RNA-polymerase, also known as R protein, which assists in viral genome transcription and replication [162, 163]. These proteins are responsible for 2/3rd of the viral RNA and help in replication and produce a nested set of sg mRNAs (sub-genomic mRNA) that code for various structural and auxiliary proteins [22, 164]. Nsps encoded by ORF 1b (proteins 12–16) are less expressed than structural proteins encoded by ORF 1a (proteins 1–11) [165]. Non-structural proteins involved in viral proliferation include the following: Protein 12 is involved in genome transcription and replication [166]. Protein 14 was identified as a 30–50 exonuclease with proofreading activity [167]. Protein 15 endo-ribonuclease activity is unknown [21]; proteins 7 and 8 are cofactors for polymerase activation, and protein 10 is a 20 O-methyltransferase. Three transmembrane proteins, proteins 3, 4, and 6, function as membrane anchors for the replicative transcription complex; protein 13 has a conserved region that contributes to the unwinding of RNA in the 50–30 direction [21], and protein 9 is a coronavirus protein that protects the genome from damage during replication [22, 23].

MERS-CoV sequencing requires reverse transcription and PCR amplification to convert the 30,000 nucleotide RNA genome to DNA. MERS-CoV RNA from a patient in Bisha (EMC/2012) and a Jordanian patient who was diagnosed retrospectively in April 2012 are the first to be disclosed (Jordan-N3) [168]. All epidemiologically unrelated viruses with more than 70% RNA were used to create a time-resolved phylogeny (Fig. **1**). The spread of MERS-geographical CoV and its phylogenetic connection in Saudi Arabia were investigated over time. MERS-CoV isolates from the Al-Hasa area exhibit a tight phylogenetic grouping, indicating that human-to-human transmission is possible [169]. Based on this larger sample of MERS-CoV sequences, calculations indicate a broad credible range for MERS-debut CoVs in July 2011. According to a short sequencing study, the MERS-CoV virus may have a bat ancestor [7, 10, 14, 26].

Genomic Architecture

Serologic evidence of human MERS-CoV infection is less widespread in Africa than in the Saudi Arabia [170 - 172]. MERS-CoV is divided into three groups depending on its evolutionary relationships: A, B, and C [5, 6]. Clade A of the MERS-CoV virus, initially discovered in Saudi Arabia (human/EMC/2012) (EMC), is no longer distinguishable in humans or dromedaries. In the Arabian Peninsula, Clade B viruses became common in dromedaries, producing zoonotic disease and, in some cases, clusters of human-to-human transmission. Camels in East Africa, Egypt, Ethiopia, Sudan, Djibouti, Kenya, North Africa, Morocco, West Africa, Nigeria, and Burkina Faso all had viruses that belonged to different clade C sub-lineages [5, 6]. Coronaviruses have a non-segmented +ve-sense RNA that is 30 kb long. The RNA features a 5′ cap and a 3′ poly-A tail, making it suitable for use as mRNA for replicase polyprotein synthesis. Compared to structural and accessory proteins, the replicase gene encodes nsp, which takes up 2/3rd of the genome. Numerous stem-loop structures are found in a leader sequence and a UTR at the 5′ ends of the RNA, which are needed for RNA replication and transcription.

Furthermore, transcription control sequence was discovered at the origination of structural or auxiliary genes and is required for their expression. In addition, the 3′-UTR contains RNA needed for RNA replication and translation. There is a 3′-

UTR-poly (A) tail on the 3′ of the RNA with auxiliary genes scattered among the structural genes. Although auxiliary proteins are not required for viral replication in cell lines, some are essential in virulence [173].

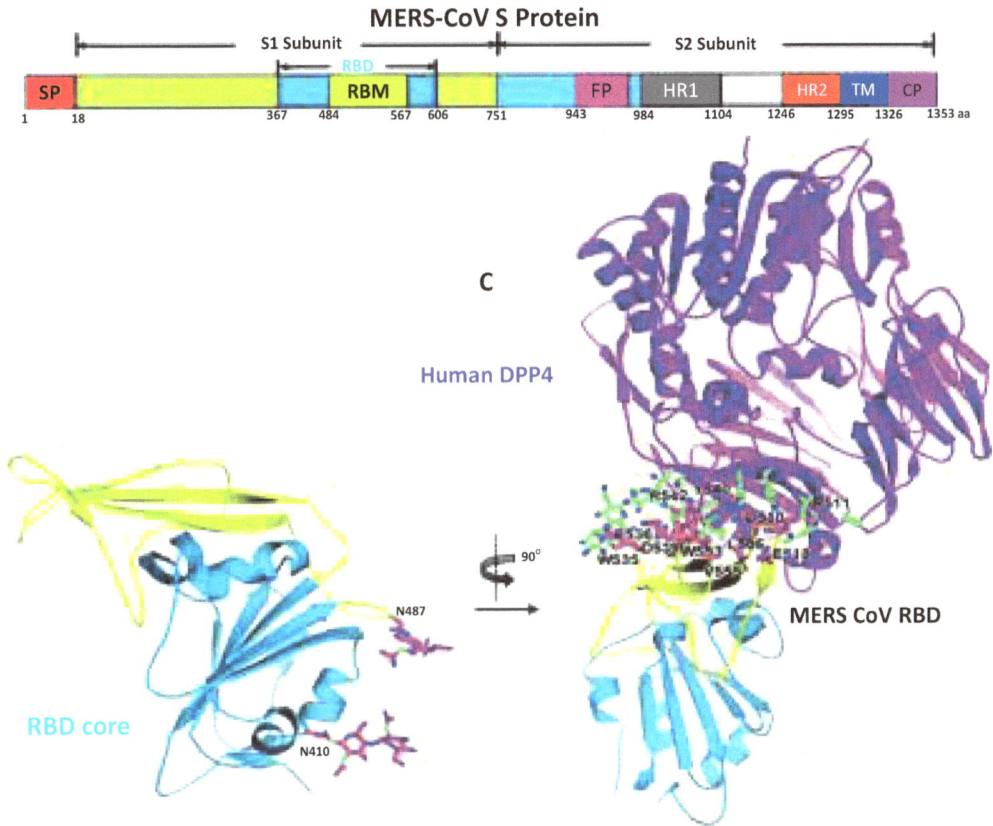

Fig. (1). MERS-CoV S protein functional domains and the structural foundation of receptor binding for MERS CoV [38, 193].

MERS-CoV Critical Residue and Viral Entry

According to phylogenetic analysis, the MERS coronavirus is intrinsically linked to the clade 2c beta-coronavirus seen in camels and bats [174]. However, the exact viral reservoir is unclear. Even though the two viruses employ specific receptors, MERS-CoV causes symptoms comparable to severe acute respiratory syndrome-producing coronaviruses. MERS-CoV uses dipeptidyl peptidase 4, while SARS-CoV uses ACE2. Strains from hamsters [17], ferrets [175], and mice [176] are frequent small laboratory strains in which MERS-CoV infection is resistant. The restricted range of hosts for MERS-limited CoV has impeded the buildout of a sufficient laboratory model for investigating the virus's virulence and assessing the effectiveness of therapies. Raj *et al.* (2014) discovered that the human DPP4 could make the ferret DPP4 domain susceptible to MERS-CoV disease. Zhao *et al.* [177] are the first to report a strategy for introducing an animal MERS-CoV model. An adeno-V expressing DPP4 was used to convert mice's respiratory cells and create mice liable for MERS-CoV disease. DPP4 is presently shown to play a crucial part in the reported species tropism of MERS-CoV infection by van Doremalen *et al.* [178], and residues in DPP4 were determined to be responsible for this restriction. According to these discoveries, the failure of MERS-CoV to bind to DPP4 of non-permissive cell culture is a critical predictor of infection susceptibility. According to an earlier study, the extracellular domain of hDPP4 comprises a changeable N-terminal propeller surface and a preserved C-terminal domain [120, 179]. However, nothing is known regarding the involvement of critical hDPP4 residues in MERS-CoV interplay and entrance. The binding efficiency of the MERS-CoV receptor binding domain to hDDP4 was estimated by employing the SPR method to evaluate the linking efficacy among these proteins. Various hDPP4 variants were produced utilizing the complex between RBD and hDPP4 [180]. MERS-CoV can significantly reduce viral entry and binding efficiency.

MERS-CoV Spike Proteins Structure Architecture

MERS CoV's S protein comprises S1 and S2 subunits [181]. The S1 component, identical to other coronaviruses and consisting of an RBD with a central subdomain and a receptor-binding motif (RBM), is required to enter host cells. MERS-CoV has a different RBM than SARS-CoV, which states that it exploits the DPP4 receptor rather than the ACE-2 receptor DPP4, which is extensively represented in organs comprising the lungs and kidneys and is important in MERS-CoV infection organism's tropism; for instance, MERS-CoV infection is favorable in camel, human, bat, and swine cells, but not in mouse, hamster, or ferret cells [178, 182]. Glycosylation of mouse DPP4 has also been linked to MERS-CoV infection suppression, with variations in 5 amino acids constituting DPP4-RBD binding being associated with hosting species limitation [178, 182, 183]. The human DPP4 receptor, particularly anti-DPP4 mAbs, is a promising aim for MERS-CoV-specific therapies [181, 183]. Adenosine deaminase (ADA) participates with MERS-CoV for DPP4 adherence, making it a natural MERS-CoV competitor that might develop therapeutic antagonists [182]. The RBD of the MERS-CoV's-S1 region attaches to the permeable host cell DPP4, which is a principal focus for potential MERS-CoV therapies [183]. MERS-CoV then employs the S2 component for virus-host membrane fusion, much like other coronaviruses. Host proteases cut the S protein at the S1/S2 border due to fusion [184]. The fusion peptide, two HR1 and HR2 heptad repeat domains, and a transmembrane domain are all found in the S2 subunit [184]. The S1 protein of the MERS-CoV is made up of four independently folded domains, $S1^A$ through $S1^{D\,2,3}$. The $S1^A$ domain attaches to glycotopes containing α2,3-sialic acids, while the $S1^B$ identifies DPP4, a host exopeptidase, and the viral receptor [185, 186]. In the shortage of DPP4, cells are immune to MERS-CoV. Removing sialic acids from vulnerable cell lines decreases MERS-CoV disease dramatically. The following results suggest that α2,3-sialic acids and DPP4, the MERS-functional CoV's entrance receptor, operate as an attachment receptor [185, 186].

Structure and Function of MERS-CoV S Proteins

MERS-CoV S protein comprises S1 and S2 subunits [181]. The S protein is important in MERS-CoV disease because it regulates viral adherence to host and membrane combination cells. During illness, the MERS-CoV S protein is split into receptor-attachments components S1 and S2 [37, 40]. MERS-CoV S1 and S2 subunits, with their operational domains like RBD, have a range of activities in MERS-CoV disease and pathological processes. MERS-CoV vaccines and therapeutic antibodies can target S1, RBD, and S protein, whereas anti-MER--CoV fusion inhibitors can target S2 [181, 187]. The genome of MERS CoV is the biggest among all RNA viruses and contains an essential collection of genes in the constant order 5`replicase -S-E-M-N-3`. The only protein translated is replicase transcriptase, which takes up 2/3 of the coding capacity. Conformational changes occur when the viral S protein interacts with its corresponding receptor, resulting in virion fusion with the cell membrane. Several coronavirus's S proteins are uncleaved in matured virions, necessitating a protease interaction during the infection's entrance stage to dissociate the fusion S2 and binding S1 parts of the spike. The position of proteolytic activation varies. Coronaviruses bind to host extracellular components and penetrate target cells *via* their S protein. The N terminal component of the S protein is essential for viral adherence to the host cells. In contrast, the C terminal portion is essential for the fusion of the virus to the host's cells following attachment [58]. Indeed, in inoculated animals, the MERS-CoV S protein may elicit robust antibody and/or cellular immune responses, with S-specific neutralizing antibodies significantly limiting MERS-CoV infection [188, 189].

MERS-CoV S1 Protein Subunit Structure and Function

S1-RBD-mediated MERS-CoV Receptor Binding

Unlike SARS-CoV, which uses the ACE2 receptor to engage target cells, MERS-CoV uses the DPP4 receptor to attach to targeted cells [190]. RBD in the MERS-CoV S1 subunit engages DPP4 and mediates viral adherence to target cells [37, 191, 192]. MERS CoV RBD can join DPP4 from various hosts, including bats, camels, and humans. The engaging capacity varies depending on which DPP4 is present in the host [123, 150]. This determines MERS-CoV host species limitation and vulnerability.

MERS CoV RBD and DPP4/RBD Complex Structures

MERS CoV RBD has a central subdomain, and it is identical to SARS-CoV RBD. The core subdomains of SARS CoV and MERS CoV RBDS are structurally alike, but their RBMs are significantly dissimilar, suggesting that the receptors are different [38, 193]. The center subdomain comprises an antiparallel β sheet of five stranded and many linking helices balanced by three disulfide bonds [38, 39, 193].

The core and RBM, correspondingly, contain two glycans of N-linked (N410 and N487), as shown in Fig. (**1B**) [193]. The RBM is specifically responsible for interacting with DPP4's extracellular domain of the β propeller (Fig. **1C**) [38, 39].

MERS CoV S Protein S2 Subunit Structure and Function

Mechanism of MERS CoV S2 Mediated Membrane Fusion

MERS CoV S2 subunit with other coronaviruses like SARS CoV is necessary for membrane fusion. In these mechanisms, both sections of S2 (HR1 and HR2) perform crucial and corresponding activities [40, 194]. S2 facilitates membrane fusion through many conformational alterations [40, 194]. The S protein appears on the viral surface as a natural trimeric form prior to membrane fusion. A 6-helix bundle (6HB) fusion core is formed when S2 splits from S1 during the process of membrane fusion, disclosing a hydrophobic fusion peptide injected into the membrane of the host for fusing and carrying the viral and host membranes closer together (Fig. **2**). The rational design of MERS CoV fusion blockers and anti-MERS CoV therapies mainly aimed at S2 can be guided by an understanding of the structure of this fusion core.

Structure and Function of Other Regions of MERS-CoV Protein

Membrane (M) Protein

The MERS-CoV M protein is critical for viral assemblage, development of the viral cover, and production of the virus's core by collaborating with the N protein [196, 197]. As a result, developing fusion peptides and IFN inhibitors might be a valuable therapy approach.

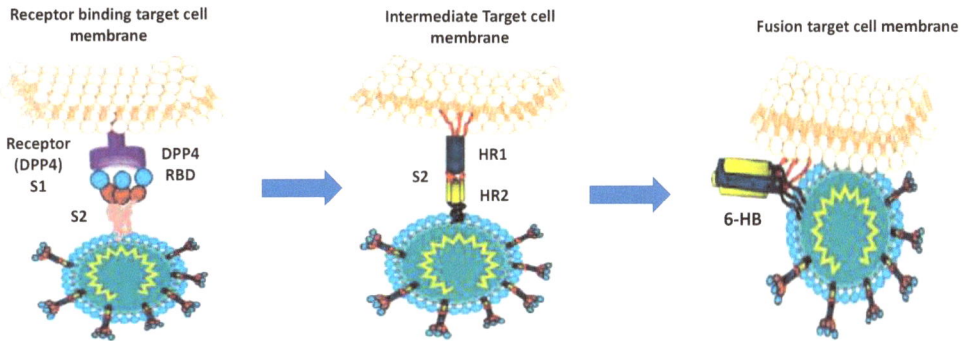

Fig. (2). Representation of S targeting mAbs and peptides of MERS CoV and MERS CoV S protein-mediated membrane fusion [194, 195].

Envelope (E) Protein

The MERS-CoV E protein is an internal barrier protein that is a minor structural protein. It comprises 82 amino acids and is projected to have at least one transmembrane helix [198]. CoVs' E protein is involved in intracellular transportation, host identification, virus packaging, and virus release [198]. The CoV E protein's function during infection is unclear. In the lipid bilayer, pure E proteins of MERS CoV construct a pentameric ion pathway. Channel functionality may be lost if the E protein is missing. Depending on the expected channel role as a virulence component, the E protein of MERS CoV might be a potential antiviral therapy target [198].

Nucleocapsid (N) Protein

MERS-CoV's N protein is a phosphorylated basic protein with 413 amino acid residues, making it the second most prominent structural protein. The N protein forms a nucleocapsid by linking to the RNA genome, which is necessary for viral multiplication and assembly [176]. The N-terminus (residues 39–165) of the N protein might be an RNA-binding domain, whereas the C-terminus could be a self-binding oligomer-forming area [199]. The nucleocapsid structure needs not just identification of the viral RNA's unique sequences but also detection of attachment to proteins present in the structure of the virus. The RNA is shielded from nucleases in the host cell when the N protein binds to the viral genomic RNA and forms a complex [200].

Accessory Proteins (Ap)

MERS-CoV contains a massive range of genomes, each encoding a different AP. These Aps are ORF3, ORF4a, ORF4b, and ORF5. Even amongst highly similar

CoVs, the quantity and sequence of their genes vary, resulting in host shift and the formation of HCoV [201]. *In vivo* and *in vitro*, the MERS-CoV AP ORF is essential for viral copying. It indicates that these ORFs may be utilized as vaccine goals and that MERS-CoV APs could be used for monitoring and therapy. Furthermore, simultaneous interruption of the AP ORF offers a quick reaction platform for emerging SARS or MERS-CoV AP ORF mutations [202]. The MERS-CoV ORF 4a protein is thought to interfere with IFNs' antiviral activities [203].

Nonstructural Proteins

ORF1a and ORF1b are located at the 50 termini of the genome coded for polyprotein 1a and 1b of CoV that may be divided into 16 nsps. The multiplication and transcription of viruses need these proteins [204]. Nsp3, which suppresses the IFN reaction by deubiquitination and de-esterification, is involved in most adaptive processes [64]. Depending on MERS-CoV isolates from people and camels, Nsp3 is now undergoing selection [24]. In paired membranes, nsp3 and nsp4 collaborate to produce their effects. Nsp6 is assumed to enhance membrane proliferation by forming perinuclear vesicles, which requires the presence of full-length nsp3.

MERS-CoV Molecular Dynamics

MERS-CoV has a genomic profile of almost 30,000 nucleotides, with 7 projected ORFs (ORF1a, ORF1b, ORF3, ORF4a, ORF4b, ORF5, and ORF8b) [38, 205]. The replicase complex is encoded by two ORFs (ORF1a, ORF1b), while the other five supplementary ORFs encode five Aps that are critical in infection and pathogenesis [202]. S, E, M, and N proteins are coded by the four structural genes S, E, M, and N, respectively [38, 206]. S protein is found on the exterior of the cell. Two subunits, S1 and S2, make up MERS-S CoV's protein, which is transmembrane. The RBD of the S1 subunit interconnects to the host's DPP4 receptor [207, 208]. MERS-CoV enters cells by attaching to the host's cellular DPP4 receptor with its S protein [12]. HR1 and HR2 of the S2 subunit constitute the primary membrane fusion unit [36]. MERS-CoV organization, intracellular transport, and budding are all aided by the E protein, while the M protein is necessary for viral arrangement and morphology [196]. All structural proteins interact to create a full viral particle [209]. MERS-CoV attaches to host cellular receptors when its S protein binds to them, resulting in infection. The S protein's N-terminal receptor-binding region also influences its ability to spread between species [25, 26]. As proven by ultracentrifugation investigations, Glu169 is required for dimerization and catalysis to show that MERS-CoV Mpro undergoes a conversion process that changes it from a monomer to a dimer [169, 210]. The latest research shows that this coronavirus's nsp1 has an end nucleolytic RNA breakage activity. Translation suppression and endonucleolytic breakage initiation of host mRNAs contribute to producing infectious virus units in specialized human cell lines. Nsp1's translation restriction and endonucleolytic RNA breakage triggering function have been confirmed in wild-type MERS-CoV and two mutant MERS-CoV strains deficient in one or both functions. According to the studies, nsp1 is the first coronavirus gene 1 protein adequate in virus duplication and RNA breakage influencing activity [169, 211].

Virus-Host Cell Interactions and Implications on Pathogenesis

Most coronaviruses invade sensitive hosts through respiratory or oral-fecal routes, with multiplication beginning in epithelial cells. Whereas most MERS-CoV was transmitted from person to person, the principal instances in clusters were probably obtained through non-human origins of the virus [212]. MERS-CoV was first found in bats. MERS-CoV infects bat cells using the evolutionarily retained DPP4 protein of Pipistrellus bats and DPP4 or CD26, found in the lower respiratory tracts of humans, as an effective receptor. Given the rarity of direct human encounters with bat secretion, intermediary hosts like camels and goats have been used [12]. Given the synchronized parturition trend of dormitory camels, which results in births throughout the winter months, a rise in epizootic action after some delay during the first half of each year was predicted [213]. MERS-CoV replication was permissive in goat and camel cell lines [214]. MERS-CoV has been transmitted from person to person in multiple clusters of infections in France, the UAE, Italy, the UK, Qatar, Jordan, and Tunisia, most notably among family members and healthcare personnel [215].

MERS-CoV Cellular Tropism in the Respiratory System and the Innate Immune Response to Infection

The human respiratory system is the major infection location for MERS. MERS-CoV can infect and replicate the human respiratory epithelium [44, 45]. *Ex vivo* findings on MERS-CoV cellular tropism in human respiratory tract tissues were also investigated [32, 33]. According to the research, MERS-CoV infection was found in non-ciliated bronchial and bronchiolar epithelium cells, alveolar epithelial cells, and pulmonary artery endothelial cells [32]. Furthermore, uninfected cells suffered substantial apoptosis with widespread caspase 3 activation after infection with MERS-CoV in *ex vivo* lung tissues, suggesting that a paracrine pathway may lead to suicide induction [32]. One further examination was performed on human *ex vivo* lung tissue [33] to determine the occurrence of MERS-CoV infection and multiplication in addition to infection-induced apoptosis.

Extrapulmonary Organ Involvement after MERS-CoV Infection

Research suggests that the virus may have transferred from person to person through bodily fluids such as feces, urine, and blood samples [216]. MERS-CoV was evidenced to be permissive in endothelial cells of blood vessels in human *ex vivo* lung tissues [32, 49], which might offer the pathophysiological foundation for viral propagation. MERS-CoV has also been revealed to invade human monocyte-derived dendritic cells and promote viral multiplication [217]. MERS-CoV is also easily transferred to human primary T cells [218]. In the human body, dendritic cells and T cells are migratory cells. As a result, dendritic cells and T cells infected with MERS-CoV may enable the virus to spread systemically across the respiratory tract. MERS-CoV infection *in vivo* is likely to affect extrapulmonary organs and tissues. However, no human autopsy studies have been published to date. Even though none of these animals can completely mimic human MERS illness, we need data from MERS-CoV-infected experimental animals to assess the possibility of extrapulmonary participation.

MERS-CoV RBD and SARS-CoV RBD Comparative Studies

MERS-CoV RBD is made up of a core subdomain and a receptor-binding subdomain. A five-stranded antiparallel β sheet (β1, β2, β3, β4, and β9) with two small helices in the interconnecting loops makes up the core subdomain (Fig. **3C** and **E**). Three disulfide bonds maintain the fold in the core subdomain (Fig. **3E**). A four-stranded antiparallel β sheet serves as the receptor-binding subdomain. It is located between the core domain's strands β4 and β9 (Fig. **3C** and **E**). A long loop connects the β6 and β7 strands and spans the β sheet perpendicularly (Fig. **3C** and **E**). This loop is attached to strand β5 **(Fig. 3E)** by a disulfide link between C503 and C526, offering structural assistance for the β sheet to form a link with DPP4. The core and receptor-binding subdomains are likewise present in the SARS-CoV RBD (Fig. **3D** and **2F**) [219]. The RBDs of MERS and SARS-CoV are structurally comparable despite the minimal amino acid sequence homology. Moreover, there are significant changes between MERS-CoV and SARS-CoV in the receptor-binding subdomain. While the former contains 84 amino acids (Fig. **3A**) that form a four-stranded antiparallel β sheet (Fig. **3C** and **E**), the latter has 68 amino acids that form two short antiparallel β strands and one disulfide link between C467 and C474 (Fig. **3D** and **F**) [38].

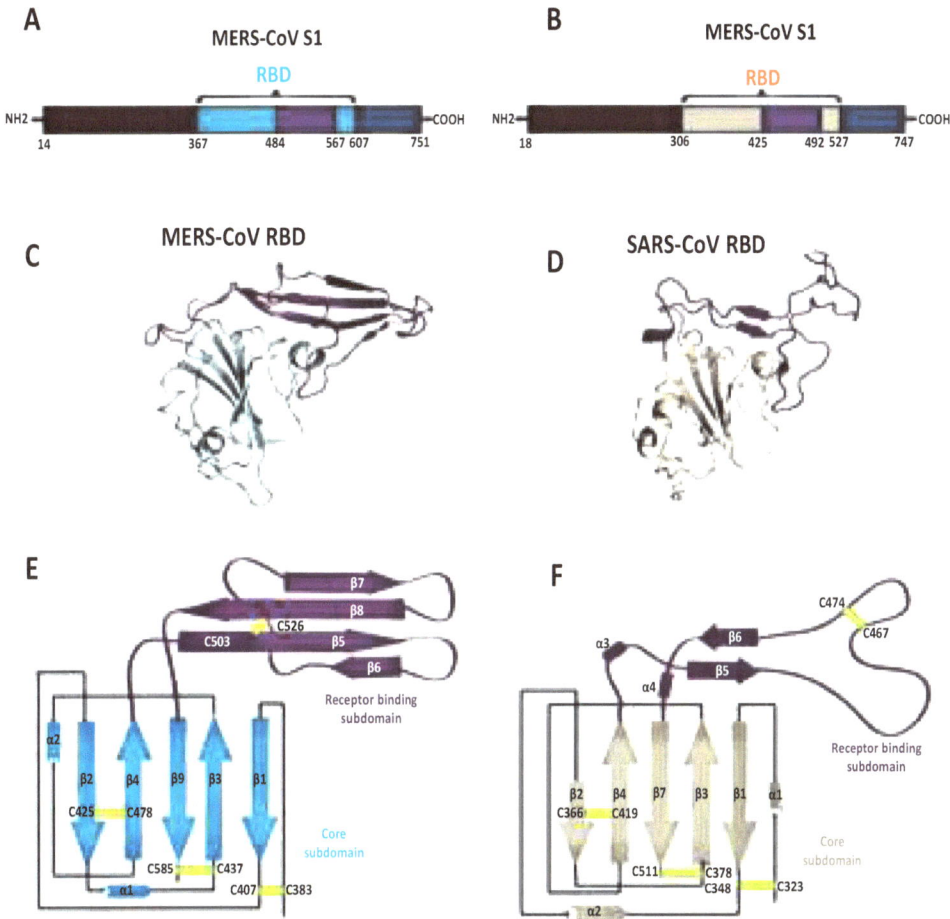

Fig. (3). MERS-CoV RBD structural comparison with SARS-CoV RBD. MERS-CoV S1 (**A**) and SARS-CoV S1 (**B**) domain structures (B). (**C**) MERS-CoV RBD structure.

CONCLUSION AND FUTURE PERSPECTIVE

MERS-CoV outbreaks pose a severe danger to global public health, highlighting the requirement for additional study on the virus's epidemiology and pathogenesis and the establishment of efficient MERS-CoV treatment and prevention drugs. Novel MERS-CoV instances continue to be documented despite breakthroughs in diagnostics and public health interventions. This shows that several treatments targeting various impacted groups may be required to halt these epidemics. The structural knowledge linked with MERS-CoV proteins may be exploited to design several possible therapies to diminish the epidemic. The pathogenesis of MERS-CoV must be better understood to discover viral and host variables that contribute to the establishment of MERS in humans, which might lead to novel therapy and intervention options. MERS-CoV, SARS-CoV, and other emerging diseases are still on WHO Blueprint 2020 priority list. MERS-CoV is highly endemic in camels from various African and Middle Eastern countries, mainly Saudi Arabia. New viral strains that may infect new hosts and evade their immune systems are just a matter of time because of the rapid recombination events that have taken place among the members of this beta coronavirus family. Identifying MERS-CoV from respiratory secretions requires RT-PCR; nonetheless, there is currently no effective antiviral medication. Since investigations have linked glucocorticoid medication to an increased risk of death, the administration is mainly supportive.

REFERENCES

[1]   Moon S, Son JS. Infectivity of an asymptomatic patient with Middle East respiratory syndrome coronavirus infection. Clin Infect Dis 2017; 64(10): 1457-8.
[http://dx.doi.org/10.1093/cid/cix170] [PMID: 28444154]

[2]   Kim SW, Park JW, Jung H-D, et al. Risk factors for transmission of Middle East respiratory syndrome coronavirus infection during the 2015 outbreak in South Korea. Clin Infect Dis 2017; 64(5): 551-7.
[PMID: 27940937]

[3]   Normile D. South Korea finally MERS-free. Science 2015.
[http://dx.doi.org/10.1126/science.aae0157]

[4]   Widagdo W, Sooksawasdi Na Ayudhya S, Hundie GB, Haagmans BL. Host determinants of MERS-CoV transmission and pathogenesis. Viruses 2019; 11(3): 280.
[http://dx.doi.org/10.3390/v11030280] [PMID: 30893947]

[5]   El-Kafrawy SA, Corman VM, Tolah AM, et al. Enzootic patterns of Middle East respiratory syndrome coronavirus in imported African and local Arabian dromedary camels: a prospective genomic study. Lancet Planet Health 2019; 3(12): e521-8.
[http://dx.doi.org/10.1016/S2542-5196(19)30243-8] [PMID: 31843456]

[6]   Chu DKW, Hui KPY, Perera RAPM, et al. MERS coronaviruses from camels in Africa exhibit region-dependent genetic diversity. Proc Natl Acad Sci USA 2018; 115(12): 3144-9.
[http://dx.doi.org/10.1073/pnas.1718769115] [PMID: 29507189]

[7]   Bermingham A, Chand MA, Brown CS, et al. Severe respiratory illness caused by a novel coronavirus, in a patient transferred to the United Kingdom from the Middle East, September 2012. Euro Surveill 2012; 17(40): 20290.
[http://dx.doi.org/10.2807/ese.17.40.20290-en] [PMID: 23078800]

[8]   de Groot RJ, Baker SC, Baric RS, et al. Middle East respiratory syndrome coronavirus (MERS-CoV): announcement of the Coronavirus Study Group. J Virol 2013; 87(14): 7790-2.
[http://dx.doi.org/10.1128/JVI.01244-13] [PMID: 23678167]

[9]   Danielsson N, on behalf of the ECDC Internal Response Team , Catchpole M. Novel coronavirus associated with severe respiratory disease: Case definition and public health measures. Euro Surveill 2012; 17(39): 20282.
[http://dx.doi.org/10.2807/ese.17.39.20282-en] [PMID: 23041021]

[10]   Chan JFW, Li KSM, To KKW, Cheng VCC, Chen H, Yuen KY. Is the discovery of the novel human betacoronavirus 2c EMC/2012 (HCoV-EMC) the beginning of another SARS-like pandemic? J Infect 2012; 65(6): 477-89.
[http://dx.doi.org/10.1016/j.jinf.2012.10.002] [PMID: 23072791]

[11]   Memish ZA, Zumla AI, Assiri A. Middle East respiratory syndrome coronavirus infections in health care workers. N Engl J Med 2013; 369(9): 884-6.
[http://dx.doi.org/10.1056/NEJMc1308698] [PMID: 23923992]

[12] Raj VS, Mou H, Smits SL, *et al.* Dipeptidyl peptidase 4 is a functional receptor for the emerging human coronavirus-EMC. Nature 2013; 495(7440): 251-4.
[http://dx.doi.org/10.1038/nature12005] [PMID: 23486063]

[13] Jiang S, Lu L, Du L, Debnath AK. A predicted receptor-binding and critical neutralizing domain in S protein of the novel human coronavirus HCoV-EMC. J Infect 2013; 66(5): 464-6.
[http://dx.doi.org/10.1016/j.jinf.2012.12.003] [PMID: 23266463]

[14] Karikalan B, Darnal HK. Immune Status of COVID-19 Patients with Reference to SARS and MERS. J Pure Appl Microbiol 2020; 14 (Suppl. 1): 817-21.
[http://dx.doi.org/10.22207/JPAM.14.SPL1.18]

[15] Li HS, Kuok DIT, Cheung MC, *et al.* Effect of interferon alpha and cyclosporine treatment separately and in combination on Middle East Respiratory Syndrome Coronavirus (MERS-CoV) replication in a human *in-vitro* and *ex-vivo* culture model. Antiviral Res 2018; 155: 89-96.
[http://dx.doi.org/10.1016/j.antiviral.2018.05.007] [PMID: 29772254]

[16] Lessler J, Reich NG, Brookmeyer R, Perl TM, Nelson KE, Cummings DAT. Incubation periods of acute respiratory viral infections: a systematic review. Lancet Infect Dis 2009; 9(5): 291-300.
[http://dx.doi.org/10.1016/S1473-3099(09)70069-6] [PMID: 19393959]

[17] Coleman CM, Matthews KL, Goicochea L, Frieman MB. Wild-type and innate immune-deficient mice are not susceptible to the Middle East respiratory syndrome coronavirus. J Gen Virol 2014; 95(2): 408-12.
[http://dx.doi.org/10.1099/vir.0.060640-0] [PMID: 24197535]

[18] Widagdo W, Okba NMA, Li W, *et al.* Species-specific colocalization of Middle East respiratory syndrome coronavirus attachment and entry receptors. J Virol 2019; 93(16): e00107-19.
[http://dx.doi.org/10.1128/JVI.00107-19] [PMID: 31167913]

[19] Scobey T, Yount BL, Sims AC, *et al.* Reverse genetics with a full-length infectious cDNA of the Middle East respiratory syndrome coronavirus. Proc Natl Acad Sci USA 2013; 110(40): 16157-62.
[http://dx.doi.org/10.1073/pnas.1311542110] [PMID: 24043791]

[20] Tai W, Zhao G, Sun S, *et al.* A recombinant receptor-binding domain of MERS-CoV in trimeric form protects human dipeptidyl peptidase 4 (hDPP4) transgenic mice from MERS-CoV infection. Virology 2016; 499: 375-82.
[http://dx.doi.org/10.1016/j.virol.2016.10.005] [PMID: 27750111]

[21] Ivanov KA, Thiel V, Dobbe JC, van der Meer Y, Snijder EJ, Ziebuhr J. Multiple enzymatic activities associated with severe acute respiratory syndrome coronavirus helicase. J Virol 2004; 78(11): 5619-32.
[http://dx.doi.org/10.1128/JVI.78.11.5619-5632.2004] [PMID: 15140959]

[22] Snijder EJ, Bredenbeek PJ, Dobbe JC, *et al.* Unique and conserved features of genome and proteome of SARS-coronavirus, an early split-off from the coronavirus group 2 lineage. J Mol Biol 2003; 331(5): 991-1004.
[http://dx.doi.org/10.1016/S0022-2836(03)00865-9] [PMID: 12927536]

[23] Buzon MJ, Seiss K, Weiss R, *et al.* Inhibition of HIV-1 integration in *ex vivo*-infected CD4 T cells from elite controllers. J Virol 2011; 85(18): 9646-50.
[http://dx.doi.org/10.1128/JVI.05327-11] [PMID: 21734042]

[24] Forni D, Cagliani R, Mozzi A, *et al.* Extensive positive selection drives the evolution of nonstructural proteins in lineage C betacoronaviruses. J Virol 2016; 90(7): 3627-39.
[http://dx.doi.org/10.1128/JVI.02988-15] [PMID: 26792741]

[25] Lu X, Whitaker B, Sakthivel SKK, *et al.* Real-time reverse transcription-PCR assay panel for Middle East respiratory syndrome coronavirus. J Clin Microbiol 2014; 52(1): 67-75.
[http://dx.doi.org/10.1128/JCM.02533-13] [PMID: 24153118]

[26] Shahkarami M, Yen C, Glaser C, Xia D, Watt J, Wadford DA. Laboratory testing for Middle East

respiratory syndrome coronavirus, California, USA, 2013–2014. Emerg Infect Dis 2015; 21(9): 1664-6.
[http://dx.doi.org/10.3201/eid2109.150476] [PMID: 26291839]

[27]   Chan JFW, Lau SKP, Woo PCY. The emerging novel Middle East respiratory syndrome coronavirus: The "knowns" and "unknowns". J Formos Med Assoc 2013; 112(7): 372-81.
[http://dx.doi.org/10.1016/j.jfma.2013.05.010] [PMID: 23883791]

[28]   Chan JFW, Choi GKY, Tsang AKL, *et al.* Development and evaluation of novel real-time reverse transcription-PCR assays with locked nucleic acid probes targeting leader sequences of human-pathogenic coronaviruses. J Clin Microbiol 2015; 53(8): 2722-6.
[http://dx.doi.org/10.1128/JCM.01224-15] [PMID: 26019210]

[29]   Assiri A, Al-Tawfiq JA, Al-Rabeeah AA, *et al.* Epidemiological, demographic, and clinical characteristics of 47 cases of Middle East respiratory syndrome coronavirus disease from Saudi Arabia: a descriptive study. Lancet Infect Dis 2013; 13(9): 752-61.
[http://dx.doi.org/10.1016/S1473-3099(13)70204-4] [PMID: 23891402]

[30]   Al-Tawfiq JA, Hinedi K, Ghandour J, *et al.* Middle East respiratory syndrome coronavirus: a case-control study of hospitalized patients. Clin Infect Dis 2014; 59(2): 160-5.
[http://dx.doi.org/10.1093/cid/ciu226] [PMID: 24723278]

[31]   Chu DKW, Peiris JSM, Chen H, Guan Y, Poon LLM. Genomic characterizations of bat coronaviruses (1A, 1B and HKU8) and evidence for co-infections in Miniopterus bats. J Gen Virol 2008; 89(5): 1282-7.
[http://dx.doi.org/10.1099/vir.0.83605-0] [PMID: 18420807]

[32]   Chan RWY, Chan MCW, Agnihothram S, *et al.* Tropism of and innate immune responses to the novel human betacoronavirus lineage C virus in human *ex vivo* respiratory organ cultures. J Virol 2013; 87(12): 6604-14.
[http://dx.doi.org/10.1128/JVI.00009-13] [PMID: 23552422]

[33]   Hocke AC, Becher A, Knepper J, *et al.* Emerging human middle East respiratory syndrome coronavirus causes widespread infection and alveolar damage in human lungs. Am J Respir Crit Care Med 2013; 188(7): 882-6.
[http://dx.doi.org/10.1164/rccm.201305-0954LE] [PMID: 24083868]

[34]   Alsahafi AJ, Cheng AC. The epidemiology of Middle East respiratory syndrome coronavirus in the Kingdom of Saudi Arabia, 2012–2015. Int J Infect Dis 2016; 45: 1-4.
[http://dx.doi.org/10.1016/j.ijid.2016.02.004] [PMID: 26875601]

[35]   Cotten M, Watson SJ, Kellam P, *et al.* Transmission and evolution of the Middle East respiratory syndrome coronavirus in Saudi Arabia: a descriptive genomic study. Lancet 2013; 382(9909): 1993-2002.
[http://dx.doi.org/10.1016/S0140-6736(13)61887-5] [PMID: 24055451]

[36]   Xia S, Liu Q, Wang Q, *et al.* Middle East respiratory syndrome coronavirus (MERS-CoV) entry inhibitors targeting spike protein. Virus Res 2014; 194: 200-10.
[http://dx.doi.org/10.1016/j.virusres.2014.10.007] [PMID: 25451066]

[37]   Li F. Receptor recognition mechanisms of coronaviruses: a decade of structural studies. J Virol 2015; 89(4): 1954-64.
[http://dx.doi.org/10.1128/JVI.02615-14] [PMID: 25428871]

[38]   Wang N, Shi X, Jiang L, *et al.* Structure of MERS-CoV spike receptor-binding domain complexed with human receptor DPP4. Cell Res 2013; 23(8): 986-93.
[http://dx.doi.org/10.1038/cr.2013.92] [PMID: 23835475]

[39]   Lu G, Hu Y, Wang Q, *et al.* Molecular basis of binding between novel human coronavirus MERS-CoV and its receptor CD26. Nature 2013; 500(7461): 227-31.
[http://dx.doi.org/10.1038/nature12328] [PMID: 23831647]

[40]   Gao J, Lu G, Qi J, *et al.* Structure of the fusion core and inhibition of fusion by a heptad repeat peptide derived from the S protein of Middle East respiratory syndrome coronavirus. J Virol 2013; 87(24): 13134-40.
[http://dx.doi.org/10.1128/JVI.02433-13] [PMID: 24067982]

[41]   Du L, He Y, Zhou Y, Liu S, Zheng BJ, Jiang S. The spike protein of SARS-CoV — a target for vaccine and therapeutic development. Nat Rev Microbiol 2009; 7(3): 226-36.
[http://dx.doi.org/10.1038/nrmicro2090] [PMID: 19198616]

[42]   Gierer S, Bertram S, Kaup F, *et al.* The spike protein of the emerging betacoronavirus EMC uses a novel coronavirus receptor for entry, can be activated by TMPRSS2, and is targeted by neutralizing antibodies. J Virol 2013; 87(10): 5502-11.
[http://dx.doi.org/10.1128/JVI.00128-13] [PMID: 23468491]

[43]   Qian Z, Dominguez SR, Holmes KV. Role of the spike glycoprotein of human Middle East respiratory syndrome coronavirus (MERS-CoV) in virus entry and syncytia formation. PLoS One 2013; 8(10): e76469.
[http://dx.doi.org/10.1371/journal.pone.0076469] [PMID: 24098509]

[44]   Kindler E, Jónsdóttir HR, Muth D, *et al.* Efficient replication of the novel human betacoronavirus EMC on primary human epithelium highlights its zoonotic potential. MBio 2013; 4(1): e00611-12.
[http://dx.doi.org/10.1128/mBio.00611-12] [PMID: 23422412]

[45]   Zielecki F, Weber M, Eickmann M, *et al.* Human cell tropism and innate immune system interactions of human respiratory coronavirus EMC compared to those of severe acute respiratory syndrome coronavirus. J Virol 2013; 87(9): 5300-4.
[http://dx.doi.org/10.1128/JVI.03496-12] [PMID: 23449793]

[46]   Crespo HJ, Lau JTY, Videira PA. Dendritic cells: a spot on sialic Acid. Front Immunol 2013; 4: 491.
[http://dx.doi.org/10.3389/fimmu.2013.00491] [PMID: 24409183]

[47]   Balachandran S, Roberts PC, Brown LE, *et al.* Essential role for the dsRNA-dependent protein kinase PKR in innate immunity to viral infection. Immunity 2000; 13(1): 129-41.
[http://dx.doi.org/10.1016/S1074-7613(00)00014-5] [PMID: 10933401]

[48]   Breban R, Riou J, Fontanet A. Interhuman transmissibility of Middle East respiratory syndrome coronavirus: estimation of pandemic risk. Lancet 2013; 382(9893): 694-9.
[http://dx.doi.org/10.1016/S0140-6736(13)61492-0] [PMID: 23831141]

[49]   Zhou J, Chu H, Li C, *et al.* Active replication of Middle East respiratory syndrome coronavirus and aberrant induction of inflammatory cytokines and chemokines in human macrophages: implications for pathogenesis. J Infect Dis 2014; 209(9): 1331-42.
[http://dx.doi.org/10.1093/infdis/jit504] [PMID: 24065148]

[50]   Han J, Sun J, Zhang G, Chen H. DCs-based therapies: potential strategies in severe SARS-CoV-2 infection. Int J Med Sci 2021; 18(2): 406-18.
[http://dx.doi.org/10.7150/ijms.47706] [PMID: 33390810]

[51]   Shin HS, Kim Y, Kim G, *et al.* Immune responses to Middle East respiratory syndrome coronavirus during the acute and convalescent phases of human infection. Clin Infect Dis 2019; 68(6): 984-92.
[http://dx.doi.org/10.1093/cid/ciy595] [PMID: 30060038]

[52]   Ksiazek TG, Erdman D, Goldsmith CS, *et al.* A novel coronavirus associated with severe acute respiratory syndrome. N Engl J Med 2003; 348(20): 1953-66.
[http://dx.doi.org/10.1056/NEJMoa030781] [PMID: 12690092]

[53]   Drosten C, Günther S, Preiser W, *et al.* Identification of a novel coronavirus in patients with severe acute respiratory syndrome. N Engl J Med 2003; 348(20): 1967-76.
[http://dx.doi.org/10.1056/NEJMoa030747] [PMID: 12690091]

[54]   Zaki AM, van Boheemen S, Bestebroer TM, Osterhaus ADME, Fouchier RAM. Isolation of a novel coronavirus from a man with pneumonia in Saudi Arabia. N Engl J Med 2012; 367(19): 1814-20.

[http://dx.doi.org/10.1056/NEJMoa1211721] [PMID: 23075143]

[55] Wu F, Zhao S, Yu B, *et al.* A new coronavirus associated with human respiratory disease in China. Nature 2020; 579(7798): 265-9.
[http://dx.doi.org/10.1038/s41586-020-2008-3] [PMID: 32015508]

[56] Zhou P, Yang X-L, Wang X-G, *et al.* A pneumonia outbreak associated with a new coronavirus of probable bat origin. Nature. 2020; 579(7798): 270-273.
[http://dx.doi.org/10.1038/s41586-020-2012-7]

[57] Letko M, Marzi A, Munster V. Functional assessment of cell entry and receptor usage for SARS-Co-2 and other lineage B betacoronaviruses. Nat Microbiol 2020; 5(4): 562-9.
[http://dx.doi.org/10.1038/s41564-020-0688-y] [PMID: 32094589]

[58] Fehr AR, Perlman S. Coronaviruses: an overview of their replication and pathogenesis. Methods Mol Biol 2015; 1282: 1-23.
[http://dx.doi.org/10.1007/978-1-4939-2438-7_1] [PMID: 25720466]

[59] Chan YK, Gack MU. A phosphomimetic-based mechanism of dengue virus to antagonize innate immunity. Nat Immunol 2016; 17(5): 523-30.
[http://dx.doi.org/10.1038/ni.3393] [PMID: 26998762]

[60] Hou Z, Zhang J, Han Q, *et al.* Hepatitis B virus inhibits intrinsic RIG-I and RIG-G immune signaling *via* inducing miR146a. Sci Rep 2016; 6(1): 26150.
[http://dx.doi.org/10.1038/srep26150] [PMID: 27210312]

[61] Shi CS, Qi HY, Boularan C, *et al.* SARS-coronavirus open reading frame-9b suppresses innate immunity by targeting mitochondria and the MAVS/TRAF3/TRAF6 signalosome. J Immunol 2014; 193(6): 3080-9.
[http://dx.doi.org/10.4049/jimmunol.1303196] [PMID: 25135833]

[62] Shin D, Mukherjee R, Grewe D, *et al.* Papain-like protease regulates SARS-CoV-2 viral spread and innate immunity. Nature 2020; 587(7835): 657-62.
[http://dx.doi.org/10.1038/s41586-020-2601-5] [PMID: 32726803]

[63] Clementz MA, Chen Z, Banach BS, *et al.* Deubiquitinating and interferon antagonism activities of coronavirus papain-like proteases. J Virol 2010; 84(9): 4619-29.
[http://dx.doi.org/10.1128/JVI.02406-09] [PMID: 20181693]

[64] Báez-Santos YM, St John SE, Mesecar AD. The SARS-coronavirus papain-like protease: structure, function and inhibition by designed antiviral compounds. Antiviral Res 2015; 115: 21-38.
[http://dx.doi.org/10.1016/j.antiviral.2014.12.015] [PMID: 25554382]

[65] Angelini MM, Akhlaghpour M, Neuman BW, Buchmeier MJ. Severe acute respiratory syndrome coronavirus nonstructural proteins 3, 4, and 6 induce double-membrane vesicles. MBio 2013; 4(4): e00524-13.
[http://dx.doi.org/10.1128/mBio.00524-13] [PMID: 23943763]

[66] Oostra M, Hagemeijer MC, van Gent M, *et al.* Topology and membrane anchoring of the coronavirus replication complex: not all hydrophobic domains of nsp3 and nsp6 are membrane spanning. J Virol 2008; 82(24): 12392-405.
[http://dx.doi.org/10.1128/JVI.01219-08] [PMID: 18842706]

[67] Lei J, Kusov Y, Hilgenfeld R. Nsp3 of coronaviruses: Structures and functions of a large multi-domain protein. Antiviral Res 2018; 149: 58-74.
[http://dx.doi.org/10.1016/j.antiviral.2017.11.001] [PMID: 29128390]

[68] Pan JA, Peng X, Gao Y, *et al.* Genome-wide analysis of protein-protein interactions and involvement of viral proteins in SARS-CoV replication. PLoS One 2008; 3(10): e3299.
[http://dx.doi.org/10.1371/journal.pone.0003299] [PMID: 18827877]

[69] Mao M, Yu M, Tong JH, *et al.* RIG-E, a human homolog of the murine Ly-6 family, is induced by retinoic acid during the differentiation of acute promyelocytic leukemia cell. Proc Natl Acad Sci USA

1996; 93(12): 5910-4.
[http://dx.doi.org/10.1073/pnas.93.12.5910] [PMID: 8650192]

[70] Noda S, Kosugi A, Saitoh S, Narumiya S, Hamaoka T. Protection from anti-TCR/CD3-induced apoptosis in immature thymocytes by a signal through thymic shared antigen-1/stem cell antigen-2. J Exp Med 1996; 183(5): 2355-60.
[http://dx.doi.org/10.1084/jem.183.5.2355] [PMID: 8642345]

[71] Hanke T, Mitnacht R, Boyd R, Hünig T. Induction of interleukin 2 receptor beta chain expression by self-recognition in the thymus. J Exp Med 1994; 180(5): 1629-36.
[http://dx.doi.org/10.1084/jem.180.5.1629] [PMID: 7964450]

[72] Head BP, Patel HH, Insel PA. Interaction of membrane/lipid rafts with the cytoskeleton: Impact on signaling and function. Biochim Biophys Acta Biomembr 2014; 1838(2): 532-45.
[http://dx.doi.org/10.1016/j.bbamem.2013.07.018] [PMID: 23899502]

[73] Mar KB, Rinkenberger NR, Boys IN, *et al.* LY6E mediates an evolutionarily conserved enhancement of virus infection by targeting a late entry step. Nat Commun 2018; 9(1): 3603.
[http://dx.doi.org/10.1038/s41467-018-06000-y] [PMID: 30190477]

[74] Hackett BA, Cherry S. Flavivirus internalization is regulated by a size-dependent endocytic pathway. Proc Natl Acad Sci USA 2018; 115(16): 4246-51.
[http://dx.doi.org/10.1073/pnas.1720032115] [PMID: 29610346]

[75] Samuel CE. Antiviral actions of interferons. Clin Microbiol Rev 2001; 14(4): 778-809.
[http://dx.doi.org/10.1128/CMR.14.4.778-809.2001] [PMID: 11585785]

[76] Xu X, Qiu C, Zhu L, *et al.* IFN-stimulated gene LY6E in monocytes regulates the CD14/TLR4 pathway but inadequately restrains the hyperactivation of monocytes during chronic HIV-1 infection. J Immunol 2014; 193(8): 4125-36.
[http://dx.doi.org/10.4049/jimmunol.1401249] [PMID: 25225669]

[77] Yu J, Liang C, Liu SL. Interferon-inducible LY6E protein promotes HIV-1 infection. J Biol Chem 2017; 292(11): 4674-85.
[http://dx.doi.org/10.1074/jbc.M116.755819] [PMID: 28130445]

[78] Heald-Sargent T, Gallagher T. Ready, set, fuse! The coronavirus spike protein and acquisition of fusion competence. Viruses 2012; 4(4): 557-80.
[http://dx.doi.org/10.3390/v4040557] [PMID: 22590686]

[79] Park JE, Li K, Barlan A, *et al.* Proteolytic processing of Middle East respiratory syndrome coronavirus spikes expands virus tropism. Proc Natl Acad Sci USA 2016; 113(43): 12262-7.
[http://dx.doi.org/10.1073/pnas.1608147113] [PMID: 27791014]

[80] Kleine-Weber H, Elzayat MT, Hoffmann M, Pöhlmann S. Functional analysis of potential cleavage sites in the MERS-coronavirus spike protein. Sci Rep 2018; 8(1): 16597.
[http://dx.doi.org/10.1038/s41598-018-34859-w] [PMID: 30413791]

[81] Baseler LJ, Falzarano D, Scott DP, *et al.* An acute immune response to Middle East respiratory syndrome coronavirus replication contributes to viral pathogenicity. Am J Pathol 2016; 186(3): 630-8.
[http://dx.doi.org/10.1016/j.ajpath.2015.10.025] [PMID: 26724387]

[82] Channappanavar R, Fehr AR, Vijay R, *et al.* Dysregulated type I interferon and inflammatory monocyte-macrophage responses cause lethal pneumonia in SARS-CoV-infected mice. Cell Host Microbe 2016; 19(2): 181-93.
[http://dx.doi.org/10.1016/j.chom.2016.01.007] [PMID: 26867177]

[83] Schneider WM, Chevillotte MD, Rice CM. Interferon-stimulated genes: a complex web of host defenses. Annu Rev Immunol 2014; 32(1): 513-45.
[http://dx.doi.org/10.1146/annurev-immunol-032713-120231] [PMID: 24555472]

[84] Totura AL, Baric RS. SARS coronavirus pathogenesis: host innate immune responses and viral antagonism of interferon. Curr Opin Virol 2012; 2(3): 264-75.

[http://dx.doi.org/10.1016/j.coviro.2012.04.004] [PMID: 22572391]

[85]   Cakebread JA, Xu Y, Grainge C, *et al.* A fluorene-terminated hole-transporting material for highly efficient and stable perovskite solar cells Nature Energy 2018; 3(8): 682-9.
[http://dx.doi.org/10.1038/s41560-018-0200-6]

[86]   Jeon NJ, Na H, Jung EH, *et al.* A fluorene-terminated hole-transporting material for highly efficient and stable perovskite solar cells. Nat Energy 2018; 3(8): 682-9.
[http://dx.doi.org/10.1038/s41560-018-0200-6]

[87]   Galani IE, Triantafyllia V, Eleminiadou E-E, *et al.* Interferon-λ mediates non-redundant front-line antiviral protection against influenza virus infection without compromising host fitness. Immunity, 2017; 46(5): 875-90.
[http://dx.doi.org/10.1016/j.immuni.2017.04.025]

[88]   Kim S, Chen J, Cheng T, *et al.* PubChem 2019 update: improved access to chemical data. Nucleic Acids Res 2019; 47(D1): D1102-9.
[http://dx.doi.org/10.1093/nar/gky1033] [PMID: 30371825]

[89]   Kim H, Lee J-H, Na S-H. Proceedings of the Second Conference on Machine Translation 2017; 562-8.

[90]   Kindler E, Thiel V, Weber F. Interaction of SARS and MERS coronaviruses with the antiviral interferon response. Adv Virus Res 2016; 96: 219-43.
[http://dx.doi.org/10.1016/bs.aivir.2016.08.006] [PMID: 27712625]

[91]   Dewilde WJM, Oirbans T, Verheugt FWA, *et al.* Use of clopidogrel with or without aspirin in patients taking oral anticoagulant therapy and undergoing percutaneous coronary intervention: an open-label, randomised, controlled trial. Lancet 2013; 381(9872): 1107-15.
[http://dx.doi.org/10.1016/S0140-6736(12)62177-1] [PMID: 23415013]

[92]   Falzarano D, de Wit E, Rasmussen AL, *et al.* Treatment with interferon-α2b and ribavirin improves outcome in MERS-CoV–infected rhesus macaques. Nat Med 2013; 19(10): 1313-7.
[http://dx.doi.org/10.1038/nm.3362] [PMID: 24013700]

[93]   Xu RH, He JF, Evans MR, *et al.* Epidemiologic clues to SARS origin in China. Emerg Infect Dis 2004; 10(6): 1030-7.
[http://dx.doi.org/10.3201/eid1006.030852] [PMID: 15207054]

[94]   Raj, V.; Mou, H.; Smits, S.; Dekkers, D.; Muller, M.; Dijkman, R.; Muth, D.; Demmers, J.; Zaki, A., 440 Fouchier RA, Thiel V, Drosten C, Rottier PJ, Osterhaus AD, Bosch BJ, Haagmans BL. Dipeptidyl, 2013, 544, 251-254.

[95]   Pitek AS, Wen AM, Shukla S, Steinmetz NF. The protein corona of plant virus nanoparticles influences their dispersion properties, cellular interactions, and *in vivo* fates. Small 2016; 12(13): 1758-69.
[http://dx.doi.org/10.1002/smll.201502458] [PMID: 26853911]

[96]   Yeager CL, Ashmun RA, Williams RK, *et al.* Human aminopeptidase N is a receptor for human coronavirus 229E. Nature 1992; 357(6377): 420-2.
[http://dx.doi.org/10.1038/357420a0] [PMID: 1350662]

[97]   Hofmann H, Pyrc K, van der Hoek L, Geier M, Berkhout B, Pöhlmann S. Human coronavirus NL63 employs the severe acute respiratory syndrome coronavirus receptor for cellular entry. Proc Natl Acad Sci USA 2005; 102(22): 7988-93.
[http://dx.doi.org/10.1073/pnas.0409465102] [PMID: 15897467]

[98]   Li W, Hulswit RJG, Kenney SP, *et al.* Broad receptor engagement of an emerging global coronavirus may potentiate its diverse cross-species transmissibility. Proc Natl Acad Sci USA 2018; 115(22): E5135-43.
[http://dx.doi.org/10.1073/pnas.1802879115] [PMID: 29760102]

[99]   Yang Y, Baranov E, Jiang P, *et al.* Natl Acad Sci USA. V111 P, 2014, 12516.

[100] Luo CM, Wang N, Yang XL, *et al.* Discovery of novel bat coronaviruses in South China that use the same receptor as Middle East respiratory syndrome coronavirus. J Virol 2018; 92(13): e00116-18.
[http://dx.doi.org/10.1128/JVI.00116-18] [PMID: 29669833]

[101] Natesh R, Schwager SLU, Sturrock ED, Acharya KR. Crystal structure of the human angiotensin-converting enzyme–lisinopril complex. Nature 2003; 421(6922): 551-4.
[http://dx.doi.org/10.1038/nature01370] [PMID: 12540854]

[102] Soubrier F, Alhenc-Gelas F, Hubert C, *et al.* Two putative active centers in human angiotensin I-converting enzyme revealed by molecular cloning. Proc Natl Acad Sci USA 1988; 85(24): 9386-90.
[http://dx.doi.org/10.1073/pnas.85.24.9386] [PMID: 2849100]

[103] Junot C, Gonzales M-F, Ezan E, *et al.* RXP 407, a selective inhibitor of the N-domain of angiotensin I-converting enzyme, blocks *in vivo* the degradation of hemoregulatory peptide acetyl-Ser-Asp--ys-Pro with no effect on angiotensin I hydrolysis. J Pharmacol Exp Ther 2001; 297(2): 606-11.
[PMID: 11303049]

[104] Esther CR, Marino EM, Howard TE, *et al.* The critical role of tissue angiotensin-converting enzyme as revealed by gene targeting in mice. J Clin Invest 1997; 99(10): 2375-85.
[http://dx.doi.org/10.1172/JCI119419] [PMID: 9153279]

[105] de Wit E, Rasmussen AL, Falzarano D, *et al.* Middle East respiratory syndrome coronavirus (MERS-CoV) causes transient lower respiratory tract infection in rhesus macaques. Proc Natl Acad Sci USA 2013; 110(41): 16598-603.
[http://dx.doi.org/10.1073/pnas.1310744110] [PMID: 24062443]

[106] Falzarano D, de Wit E, Feldmann F, *et al.* Infection with MERS-CoV causes lethal pneumonia in the common marmoset. PLoS Pathog 2014; 10(8): e1004250.
[http://dx.doi.org/10.1371/journal.ppat.1004250] [PMID: 25144235]

[107] Li F, Du L. Multidisciplinary Digital Publishing Institute 2019; 11: 663.

[108] Singh A, Singh RS, Sarma P, *et al.* A comprehensive review of animal models for coronaviruses: SARS-CoV-2, SARS-CoV, and MERS-CoV. Virol Sin 2020; 35(3): 290-304.
[http://dx.doi.org/10.1007/s12250-020-00252-z] [PMID: 32607866]

[109] Avanzato VA, Matson MJ, Seifert SN, *et al.* Case study: prolonged infectious SARS-CoV-2 shedding from an asymptomatic immunocompromised individual with cancer. Cell 2020; 1901-12.
[http://dx.doi.org/10.1016/j.cell.2020.10.049]

[110] de Wit E, Feldmann F, Horne E, *et al.* Domestic pig unlikely reservoir for MERS-CoV. Emerg Infect Dis 2017; 23(6): 985-8.
[http://dx.doi.org/10.3201/eid2306.170096] [PMID: 28318484]

[111] Zhao G, Jiang Y, Qiu H, *et al.* Multi-organ damage in human dipeptidyl peptidase 4 transgenic mice infected with Middle East respiratory syndrome-coronavirus. PLoS One 2015; 10(12): e0145561.
[http://dx.doi.org/10.1371/journal.pone.0145561] [PMID: 26701103]

[112] Letko M, Miazgowicz K, McMinn R, *et al.* Adaptive evolution of MERS-CoV to species variation in DPP4. Cell Rep 2018; 24(7): 1730-7.
[http://dx.doi.org/10.1016/j.celrep.2018.07.045] [PMID: 30110630]

[113] Liu Y, Zhao J, Li Z, *et al.* Aggregation and morphology control enables multiple cases of high-efficiency polymer solar cells. Nat Commun 2014; 5(1): 5293.
[http://dx.doi.org/10.1038/ncomms6293] [PMID: 25382026]

[114] Pascal KE, Coleman CM, Mujica AO, *et al.* Pre- and postexposure efficacy of fully human antibodies against Spike protein in a novel humanized mouse model of MERS-CoV infection. Proc Natl Acad Sci USA 2015; 112(28): 8738-43.
[http://dx.doi.org/10.1073/pnas.1510830112] [PMID: 26124093]

[115] Cockrell AS, Yount BL, Scobey T, *et al.* A mouse model for MERS coronavirus-induced acute

respiratory distress syndrome. Nat Microbiol 2016; 2(2): 16226.
[http://dx.doi.org/10.1038/nmicrobiol.2016.226] [PMID: 27892925]

[116]   Huttlin EL, Bruckner RJ, Paulo JA, *et al.* Architecture of the human interactome defines protein communities and disease networks. Nature 2017; 545(7655): 505-9.
[http://dx.doi.org/10.1038/nature22366] [PMID: 28514442]

[117]   Li K, Wohlford-Lenane CL, Channappanavar R, *et al.* Mouse-adapted MERS coronavirus causes lethal lung disease in human DPP4 knockin mice. Proc Natl Acad Sci USA 2017; 114(15): E3119-28.
[http://dx.doi.org/10.1073/pnas.1619109114] [PMID: 28348219]

[118]   Zhao Z, Nelson AR, Betsholtz C, Zlokovic BV. Establishment and dysfunction of the blood-brain barrier. Cell 2015; 163(5): 1064-78.
[http://dx.doi.org/10.1016/j.cell.2015.10.067] [PMID: 26590417]

[119]   Raj V, Mou H, Smits S, *et al.* La dipeptidil peptidasa 4 es un receptor funcional para el emergente coronavirus-EMC humano. Naturaleza 2013; 495: 251-4.
[http://dx.doi.org/10.1038/nature12005]

[120]   Rasmussen HB, Branner S, Wiberg FC, Wagtmann N. Crystal structure of human dipeptidyl peptidase IV/CD26 in complex with a substrate analog. Nat Struct Biol 2003; 10(1): 19-25.
[http://dx.doi.org/10.1038/nsb882] [PMID: 12483204]

[121]   Alaofi AL. Exploring structural dynamics of the MERS-CoV receptor DPP4 and mutant DPP4 receptors. J Biomol Struct Dyn 2022; 40(2): 752-63.
[http://dx.doi.org/10.1080/07391102.2020.1818626] [PMID: 32909925]

[122]   Widagdo W, Raj VS, Schipper D, *et al.* Differential expression of the Middle East respiratory syndrome coronavirus receptor in the upper respiratory tracts of humans and dromedary camels. J Virol 2016; 90(9): 4838-42.
[http://dx.doi.org/10.1128/JVI.02994-15] [PMID: 26889022]

[123]   Barlan A, Zhao J, Sarkar MK, *et al.* Receptor variation and susceptibility to Middle East respiratory syndrome coronavirus infection. J Virol 2014; 88(9): 4953-61.
[http://dx.doi.org/10.1128/JVI.00161-14] [PMID: 24554656]

[124]   Deacon CF. Physiology and pharmacology of DPP-4 in glucose homeostasis and the treatment of type 2 diabetes. Front Endocrinol (Lausanne) 2019; 10: 80.
[http://dx.doi.org/10.3389/fendo.2019.00080] [PMID: 30828317]

[125]   Mentlein R. Dipeptidyl-peptidase IV (CD26)-role in the inactivation of regulatory peptides. Regul Pept 1999; 85(1): 9-24.
[http://dx.doi.org/10.1016/S0167-0115(99)00089-0] [PMID: 10588446]

[126]   Mortier A, Gouwy M, Van Damme J, Proost P, Struyf S. CD26/dipeptidylpeptidase IV—chemokine interactions: double-edged regulation of inflammation and tumor biology. J Leukoc Biol 2016; 99(6): 955-69.
[http://dx.doi.org/10.1189/jlb.3MR0915-401R] [PMID: 26744452]

[127]   Ohnuma K, Dang NH, Morimoto C. Revisiting an old acquaintance: CD26 and its molecular mechanisms in T cell function. Trends Immunol 2008; 29(6): 295-301.
[http://dx.doi.org/10.1016/j.it.2008.02.010] [PMID: 18456553]

[128]   Ahmed RH, Huri HZ, Al-Hamodi Z, Salem SD, Al-absi B, Muniandy S. Association of DPP4 gene polymorphisms with type 2 diabetes mellitus in Malaysian subjects. PLoS One 2016; 11(4): e0154369.
[http://dx.doi.org/10.1371/journal.pone.0154369] [PMID: 27111895]

[129]   Aghili N, Devaney JM, Alderman LO, Zukowska Z, Epstein SE, Burnett MS. Polymorphisms in dipeptidyl peptidase IV gene are associated with the risk of myocardial infarction in patients with atherosclerosis. Neuropeptides 2012; 46(6): 367-71.
[http://dx.doi.org/10.1016/j.npep.2012.10.001] [PMID: 23122333]

[130]   Huai W, Zhao R, Song H, *et al.* Aryl hydrocarbon receptor negatively regulates NLRP3

inflammasome activity by inhibiting NLRP3 transcription. Nat Commun 2014; 5(1): 4738.
[http://dx.doi.org/10.1038/ncomms5738] [PMID: 25141024]

[131] Jiang L, Wang N, Zuo T, *et al.* 2014.

[132] Tang XC, Agnihothram SS, Jiao Y, *et al.* Identification of human neutralizing antibodies against MERS-CoV and their role in virus adaptive evolution. Proc Natl Acad Sci USA 2014; 111(19): E2018-26.
[http://dx.doi.org/10.1073/pnas.1402074111] [PMID: 24778221]

[133] Weiss SR, Navas-Martin S. Coronavirus pathogenesis and the emerging pathogen severe acute respiratory syndrome coronavirus. Microbiol Mol Biol Rev 2005; 69(4): 635-64.
[http://dx.doi.org/10.1128/MMBR.69.4.635-664.2005] [PMID: 16339739]

[134] Gallagher T, Perlman S. Broad reception for coronavirus. Nature 2013; 495(7440): 176-7.
[http://dx.doi.org/10.1038/495176a] [PMID: 23486053]

[135] Yuen K, Chan W, Fan D, Chong K, Sung J, Lam D. Ocular screening in severe acute respiratory syndrome. Am J Ophthalmol 2004; 137(4): 773-4.
[http://dx.doi.org/10.1016/S0002-9394(03)01148-6] [PMID: 15059730]

[136] Ge XY, Li JL, Yang XL, *et al.* Isolation and characterization of a bat SARS-like coronavirus that uses the ACE2 receptor. Nature 2013; 503(7477): 535-8.
[http://dx.doi.org/10.1038/nature12711] [PMID: 24172901]

[137] Memish ZA, Mishra N, Olival KJ, *et al.* Middle East respiratory syndrome coronavirus in bats, Saudi Arabia. Emerg Infect Dis 2013; 19(11): 1819-23.
[http://dx.doi.org/10.3201/eid1911.131172] [PMID: 24206838]

[138] Haagmans BL, Al Dhahiry SHS, Reusken CBEM, *et al.* Middle East respiratory syndrome coronavirus in dromedary camels: an outbreak investigation. Lancet Infect Dis 2014; 14(2): 140-5.
[http://dx.doi.org/10.1016/S1473-3099(13)70690-X] [PMID: 24355866]

[139] Hofmann H, Hattermann K, Marzi A, *et al.* S protein of severe acute respiratory syndrome-associated coronavirus mediates entry into hepatoma cell lines and is targeted by neutralizing antibodies in infected patients. J Virol 2004; 78(12): 6134-42.
[http://dx.doi.org/10.1128/JVI.78.12.6134-6142.2004] [PMID: 15163706]

[140] Ying T, Du L, Ju TW, *et al.* Exceptionally potent neutralization of Middle East respiratory syndrome coronavirus by human monoclonal antibodies. J Virol 2014; 88(14): 7796-805.
[http://dx.doi.org/10.1128/JVI.00912-14] [PMID: 24789777]

[141] Briese T, Mishra N, Jain K, *et al.* Middle East respiratory syndrome coronavirus quasispecies that include homologues of human isolates revealed through whole-genome analysis and virus cultured from dromedary camels in Saudi Arabia. MBio 2014; 5(3): e01146-14.
[http://dx.doi.org/10.1128/mBio.01146-14] [PMID: 24781747]

[142] Alagaili AN, Briese T, Mishra N, *et al.* Middle East respiratory syndrome coronavirus infection in dromedary camels in Saudi Arabia. MBio 2014; 5(2): e00884-14.
[http://dx.doi.org/10.1128/mBio.00884-14] [PMID: 24570370]

[143] Azhar EI, El-Kafrawy SA, Farraj SA, *et al.* Evidence for camel-to-human transmission of MERS coronavirus. N Engl J Med 2014; 370(26): 2499-505.
[http://dx.doi.org/10.1056/NEJMoa1401505] [PMID: 24896817]

[144] Raj VS, Farag EABA, Reusken CBEM, *et al.* Isolation of MERS coronavirus from a dromedary camel, Qatar, 2014. Emerg Infect Dis 2014; 20(8): 1339-42.
[http://dx.doi.org/10.3201/eid2008.140663] [PMID: 25075761]

[145] Corman VM, Ithete NL, Richards LR, *et al.* Rooting the phylogenetic tree of middle East respiratory syndrome coronavirus by characterization of a conspecific virus from an African bat. J Virol 2014; 88(19): 11297-303.
[http://dx.doi.org/10.1128/JVI.01498-14] [PMID: 25031349]

[146] Pulliam JRC, Epstein JH, Dushoff J, *et al.* Agricultural intensification, priming for persistence and the emergence of Nipah virus: a lethal bat-borne zoonosis. J R Soc Interface 2012; 9(66): 89-101.
[http://dx.doi.org/10.1098/rsif.2011.0223] [PMID: 21632614]

[147] Plowright RK, Foley P, Field HE, *et al.*

[148] Ohnuma K, Haagmans BL, Hatano R, *et al.* Inhibition of Middle East respiratory syndrome coronavirus infection by anti-CD26 monoclonal antibody. J Virol 2013; 87(24): 13892-9.
[http://dx.doi.org/10.1128/JVI.02448-13] [PMID: 24067970]

[149] Wang Q, Qi J, Yuan Y, *et al.* Bat origins of MERS-CoV supported by bat coronavirus HKU4 usage of human receptor CD26. Cell Host Microbe 2014; 16(3): 328-37.
[http://dx.doi.org/10.1016/j.chom.2014.08.009] [PMID: 25211075]

[150] Yang Y, Du L, Liu C, *et al.* Receptor usage and cell entry of bat coronavirus HKU4 provide insight into bat-to-human transmission of MERS coronavirus. Proc Natl Acad Sci USA 2014; 111(34): 12516-21.
[http://dx.doi.org/10.1073/pnas.1405889111] [PMID: 25114257]

[151] Cesario TC. Viruses associated with pneumonia in adults. Clin Infect Dis 2012; 55(1): 107-13.
[http://dx.doi.org/10.1093/cid/cis297] [PMID: 22423119]

[152] Jartti T, Jartti L, Ruuskanen O, Söderlund-Venermo M. New respiratory viral infections. Curr Opin Pulm Med 2012; 18(3): 271-8.
[http://dx.doi.org/10.1097/MCP.0b013e328351f8d4] [PMID: 22366993]

[153] Vareille M, Kieninger E, Edwards MR, Regamey N. The airway epithelium: soldier in the fight against respiratory viruses. Clin Microbiol Rev 2011; 24(1): 210-29.
[http://dx.doi.org/10.1128/CMR.00014-10] [PMID: 21233513]

[154] Desforges M, Le Coupanec A, Stodola JK, Meessen-Pinard M, Talbot PJ. Human coronaviruses: Viral and cellular factors involved in neuroinvasiveness and neuropathogenesis. Virus Res 2014; 194: 145-58.
[http://dx.doi.org/10.1016/j.virusres.2014.09.011] [PMID: 25281913]

[155] Cavanagh P. The artist as neuroscientist. Nature 2005; 434(7031): 301-7.
[http://dx.doi.org/10.1038/434301a] [PMID: 15772645]

[156] Talbot HK, Griffin MR, Chen Q, Zhu Y, Williams JV, Edwards KM. Effectiveness of seasonal vaccine in preventing confirmed influenza-associated hospitalizations in community dwelling older adults. J Infect Dis 2011; 203(4): 500-8.
[http://dx.doi.org/10.1093/infdis/jiq076] [PMID: 21220776]

[157] Chan P, Chan M, Publications AME. 2013.

[158] de Groot RJ, Baker SC, Baric RS, *et al.* Middle East respiratory syndrome coronavirus (MERS-CoV): announcement of the Coronavirus Study Group. J Virol 2013; 87(14): 7790-2.
[http://dx.doi.org/10.1128/JVI.01244-13] [PMID: 23678167]

[159] Vijaykrishna D, Smith GJD, Zhang JX, Peiris JSM, Chen H, Guan Y. Evolutionary insights into the ecology of coronaviruses. J Virol 2007; 81(8): 4012-20.
[http://dx.doi.org/10.1128/JVI.02605-06] [PMID: 17267506]

[160] Desforges M, Le Coupanec A, Dubeau P, Bourgouin A, Lajoie L, Dubé M. Coronavirus humanos y otros virus respiratorios:¿ patógenos oportunistas subestimados del sistema nervioso central? Virus 2019; 12: 14.
[http://dx.doi.org/10.3390/v12010014]

[161] Sevajol M, Subissi L, Decroly E, Canard B, Imbert I. Insights into RNA synthesis, capping, and proofreading mechanisms of SARS-coronavirus. Virus Res 2014; 194: 90-9.
[http://dx.doi.org/10.1016/j.virusres.2014.10.008] [PMID: 25451065]

[162] Mizutani T, Repass JF, Makino S. Nascent synthesis of leader sequence-containing subgenomic

mRNAs in coronavirus genome-length replicative intermediate RNA. Virology 2000; 275(2): 238-43.
[http://dx.doi.org/10.1006/viro.2000.0489] [PMID: 10998322]

[163] Weidmann M, Zanotto PMDA, Weber F, Spiegel M, Brodt HR, Hufert FT. High-efficiency detection of severe acute respiratory syndrome virus genetic material. J Clin Microbiol 2004; 42(6): 2771-3.
[http://dx.doi.org/10.1128/JCM.42.6.2771-2773.2004] [PMID: 15184466]

[164] Rota P, Oberste M, Monroe S, *et al.* 2003.

[165] Pasternak AO, Spaan WJM, Snijder EJ. Nidovirus transcription: how to make sense…? J Gen Virol 2006; 87(6): 1403-21.
[http://dx.doi.org/10.1099/vir.0.81611-0] [PMID: 16690906]

[166] Gorbalenya AE, Enjuanes L, Ziebuhr J, Snijder EJ. Nidovirales: Evolving the largest RNA virus genome. Virus Res 2006; 117(1): 17-37.
[http://dx.doi.org/10.1016/j.virusres.2006.01.017] [PMID: 16503362]

[167] Minskaia E, Hertzig T, Gorbalenya AE, *et al.* Discovery of an RNA virus $3'{\rightarrow}5'$ exoribonuclease that is critically involved in coronavirus RNA synthesis. Proc Natl Acad Sci USA 2006; 103(13): 5108-13.
[http://dx.doi.org/10.1073/pnas.0508200103] [PMID: 16549795]

[168] Ithete NL, Stoffberg S, Corman VM, *et al.* Close relative of human Middle East respiratory syndrome coronavirus in bat, South Africa. Emerg Infect Dis 2013; 19(10): 1697-9.
[http://dx.doi.org/10.3201/eid1910.130946] [PMID: 24050621]

[169] van Boheemen S, de Graaf M, Lauber C, *et al.* Genomic characterization of a newly discovered coronavirus associated with acute respiratory distress syndrome in humans. MBio 2012; 3(6): e00473-12.
[http://dx.doi.org/10.1128/mBio.00473-12] [PMID: 23170002]

[170] Alshukairi AN, Zheng J, Zhao J, *et al.* High prevalence of MERS-CoV infection in camel workers in Saudi Arabia. MBio 2018; 9(5): e01985-18.
[http://dx.doi.org/10.1128/mBio.01985-18] [PMID: 30377284]

[171] Abbad A, Perera RAPM, Anga L, *et al.* Middle East respiratory syndrome coronavirus (MERS-CoV) neutralising antibodies in a high-risk human population, Morocco, November 2017 to January 2018. Euro Surveill 2019; 24(48): 1900244.
[http://dx.doi.org/10.2807/1560-7917.ES.2019.24.48.1900244] [PMID: 31796154]

[172] Liljander A, Meyer B, Jores J, *et al.* MERS-CoV antibodies in humans, Africa, 2013–2014. Emerg Infect Dis 2016; 22(6): 1086-9.
[http://dx.doi.org/10.3201/eid2206.160064] [PMID: 27071076]

[173] Zhao L, Jha BK, Wu A, *et al.* Antagonism of the interferon-induced OAS-RNase L pathway by murine coronavirus ns2 protein is required for virus replication and liver pathology. Cell Host Microbe 2012; 11(6): 607-16.
[http://dx.doi.org/10.1016/j.chom.2012.04.011] [PMID: 22704621]

[174] Ithete NL, Stoffberg S, Corman VM, *et al.* Close relative of human Middle East respiratory syndrome coronavirus in bat, South Africa. Emerg Infect Dis 2013; 19(10): 1697-9.
[http://dx.doi.org/10.3201/eid1910.130946] [PMID: 24050621]

[175] de Wit E, Prescott J, Baseler L, *et al.* The Middle East respiratory syndrome coronavirus (MERS-CoV) does not replicate in Syrian hamsters. PLoS One 2013; 8(7): e69127.
[http://dx.doi.org/10.1371/journal.pone.0069127] [PMID: 23844250]

[176] Lin SC, Ho CT, Chuo WH, Li S, Wang TT, Lin CC. Effective inhibition of MERS-CoV infection by resveratrol. BMC Infect Dis 2017; 17(1): 144.
[http://dx.doi.org/10.1186/s12879-017-2253-8] [PMID: 28193191]

[177] Zhao J, Li K, Wohlford-Lenane C, *et al.* Rapid generation of a mouse model for Middle East respiratory syndrome. Proc Natl Acad Sci USA 2014; 111(13): 4970-5.
[http://dx.doi.org/10.1073/pnas.1323279111] [PMID: 24599590]

[178] van Doremalen N, Miazgowicz KL, Milne-Price S, *et al.* Host species restriction of Middle East respiratory syndrome coronavirus through its receptor, dipeptidyl peptidase 4. J Virol 2014; 88(16): 9220-32.
[http://dx.doi.org/10.1128/JVI.00676-14] [PMID: 24899185]

[179] Engel M, Hoffmann T, Wagner L, *et al.* The crystal structure of dipeptidyl peptidase IV (CD26) reveals its functional regulation and enzymatic mechanism. Proc Natl Acad Sci USA 2003; 100(9): 5063-8.
[http://dx.doi.org/10.1073/pnas.0230620100] [PMID: 12690074]

[180] Wang J, Duncan D, Shi Z, Zhang B. WEB-based gene set analysis toolkit (WebGestalt): update 2013. Nucleic Acids Res 2013; 41(W1): W77-83.
[http://dx.doi.org/10.1093/nar/gkt439] [PMID: 23703215]

[181] Du L, Yang Y, Zhou Y, Lu L, Li F, Jiang S. MERS-CoV spike protein: a key target for antivirals. Expert Opin Ther Targets 2017; 21(2): 131-43.
[http://dx.doi.org/10.1080/14728222.2017.1271415] [PMID: 27936982]

[182] Raj VS, Smits SL, Provacia LB, *et al.* Adenosine deaminase acts as a natural antagonist for dipeptidyl peptidase 4-mediated entry of the Middle East respiratory syndrome coronavirus. J Virol 2014; 88(3): 1834-8.
[http://dx.doi.org/10.1128/JVI.02935-13] [PMID: 24257613]

[183] Peck KM, Cockrell AS, Yount BL, Scobey T, Baric RS, Heise MT. Glycosylation of mouse DPP4 plays a role in inhibiting Middle East respiratory syndrome coronavirus infection. J Virol 2015; 89(8): 4696-9.
[http://dx.doi.org/10.1128/JVI.03445-14] [PMID: 25653445]

[184] Durai P, Batool M, Shah M, Choi S. Middle East respiratory syndrome coronavirus: transmission, virology and therapeutic targeting to aid in outbreak control. Exp Mol Med 2015; 47(8): e181-1.
[http://dx.doi.org/10.1038/emm.2015.76] [PMID: 26315600]

[185] Mou H, Raj VS, van Kuppeveld FJM, Rottier PJM, Haagmans BL, Bosch BJ. The receptor binding domain of the new Middle East respiratory syndrome coronavirus maps to a 231-residue region in the spike protein that efficiently elicits neutralizing antibodies. J Virol 2013; 87(16): 9379-83.
[http://dx.doi.org/10.1128/JVI.01277-13] [PMID: 23785207]

[186] Li W, Hulswit RJG, Widjaja I, *et al.* Identification of sialic acid-binding function for the Middle East respiratory syndrome coronavirus spike glycoprotein. Proc Natl Acad Sci USA 2017; 114(40): E8508-17.
[http://dx.doi.org/10.1073/pnas.1712592114] [PMID: 28923942]

[187] Du L, Tai W, Zhou Y, Jiang S. Vaccines for the prevention against the threat of MERS-CoV. Expert Rev Vaccines 2016; 15(9): 1123-34.
[http://dx.doi.org/10.1586/14760584.2016.1167603] [PMID: 26985862]

[188] Haagmans BL, van den Brand JMA, Raj VS, *et al.* An orthopoxvirus-based vaccine reduces virus excretion after MERS-CoV infection in dromedary camels. Science 2016; 351(6268): 77-81.
[http://dx.doi.org/10.1126/science.aad1283] [PMID: 26678878]

[189] Zhang N, Channappanavar R, Ma C, *et al.* Identification of an ideal adjuvant for receptor-binding domain-based subunit vaccines against Middle East respiratory syndrome coronavirus. Cell Mol Immunol 2016; 13(2): 180-90.
[http://dx.doi.org/10.1038/cmi.2015.03] [PMID: 25640653]

[190] Li Y, Zhang Z, Yang L, *et al.* The MERS-CoV receptor DPP4 as a candidate binding target of the SARS-CoV-2 spike. iScience 2020; 23(6): 101160.
[http://dx.doi.org/10.1016/j.isci.2020.101160] [PMID: 32405622]

[191] Zhang N, Jiang S, Du L. Current advancements and potential strategies in the development of MERS-CoV vaccines. Expert Rev Vaccines 2014; 13(6): 761-74.

[http://dx.doi.org/10.1586/14760584.2014.912134] [PMID: 24766432]

[192] Du L, Zhao G, Kou Z, *et al.* Identification of a receptor-binding domain in the S protein of the novel human coronavirus Middle East respiratory syndrome coronavirus as an essential target for vaccine development. J Virol 2013; 87(17): 9939-42.
[http://dx.doi.org/10.1128/JVI.01048-13] [PMID: 23824801]

[193] Chen Y, Rajashankar KR, Yang Y, *et al.* Crystal structure of the receptor-binding domain from newly emerged Middle East respiratory syndrome coronavirus. J Virol 2013; 87(19): 10777-83.
[http://dx.doi.org/10.1128/JVI.01756-13] [PMID: 23903833]

[194] Lu L, Liu Q, Zhu Y, *et al.* Structure-based discovery of Middle East respiratory syndrome coronavirus fusion inhibitor. Nat Commun 2014; 5(1): 3067.
[http://dx.doi.org/10.1038/ncomms4067] [PMID: 24473083]

[195] Ying T, Prabakaran P, Du L, *et al.* Junctional and allele-specific residues are critical for MERS-CoV neutralization by an exceptionally potent germline-like antibody. Nat Commun 2015; 6(1): 8223.
[http://dx.doi.org/10.1038/ncomms9223] [PMID: 26370782]

[196] Liu J, Sun Y, Qi J, *et al.* The membrane protein of severe acute respiratory syndrome coronavirus acts as a dominant immunogen revealed by a clustering region of novel functionally and structurally defined cytotoxic T-lymphocyte epitopes. J Infect Dis 2010; 202(8): 1171-80.
[http://dx.doi.org/10.1086/656315] [PMID: 20831383]

[197] de Haan CAM, Rottier PJM. Molecular interactions in the assembly of coronaviruses. Adv Virus Res 2005; 64: 165-230.
[http://dx.doi.org/10.1016/S0065-3527(05)64006-7] [PMID: 16139595]

[198] Surya W, Li Y, Verdià-Bàguena C, Aguilella VM, Torres J. MERS coronavirus envelope protein has a single transmembrane domain that forms pentameric ion channels. Virus Res 2015; 201: 61-6.
[http://dx.doi.org/10.1016/j.virusres.2015.02.023] [PMID: 25733052]

[199] Szelazek B, Kabala W, Kus K, *et al.* Structural characterization of human coronavirus NL63 N protein. J Virol 2017; 91(11): e02503-16.
[http://dx.doi.org/10.1128/JVI.02503-16] [PMID: 28331093]

[200] Grunewald ME, Fehr AR, Athmer J, Perlman S. The coronavirus nucleocapsid protein is ADP-ribosylated. Virology 2018; 517: 62-8.
[http://dx.doi.org/10.1016/j.virol.2017.11.020] [PMID: 29199039]

[201] Forni D, Cagliani R, Clerici M, Sironi M. Molecular evolution of human coronavirus genomes. Trends Microbiol 2017; 25(1): 35-48.
[PMID: 27743750]

[202] Menachery VD, Mitchell HD, Cockrell AS, *et al.* MERS-CoV accessory ORFs play key role for infection and pathogenesis. MBio 2017; 8(4): e00665-17.
[PMID: 28830941]

[203] Yang Y, Zhang L, Geng H, *et al.* The structural and accessory proteins M, ORF 4a, ORF 4b, and ORF 5 of Middle East respiratory syndrome coronavirus (MERS-CoV) are potent interferon antagonists. Protein Cell 2013; 4(12): 951-61.
[PMID: 24318862]

[204] Zumla A, Chan JF, Azhar EI, Hui DS, Yuen K-Y. Coronaviruses - drug discovery and therapeutic options. Nat Rev Drug Discov 2016; 15(5): 327-47.
[PMID: 26868298]

[205] Skariyachan S, Challapilli SB, Packirisamy S, Kumargowda ST, Sridhar VS. Recent aspects on the pathogenesis mechanism, animal models and novel therapeutic interventions for Middle East respiratory syndrome coronavirus infections. Front Microbiol 2019; 10: 569.
[PMID: 30984127]

[206] Eckerle I, Müller MA, Kallies S, Gotthardt DN, Drosten C. *In-vitro* renal epithelial cell infection

reveals a viral kidney tropism as a potential mechanism for acute renal failure during Middle East Respiratory Syndrome (MERS) Coronavirus infection. Virol J 2013; 10(1): 359.
[PMID: 24364985]

[207]   Momattin H, Al-Ali AY, Mohammed K, Al-Tawfiq JA. Benchmarking of antibiotic usage: An adjustment to reflect antibiotic stewardship program outcome in a hospital in Saudi Arabia. J Infect Public Health 2018; 11(3): 310-3.
[PMID: 28864362]

[208]   Zumla A, Hui DS, Perlman S. Middle East respiratory syndrome. Lancet 2015; 386(9997): 995-1007.
[PMID: 26049252]

[209]   Sripa B, Kaewkes S, Intapan PM, Maleewong W, Brindley PJ. Food-borne trematodiases in Southeast Asia epidemiology, pathology, clinical manifestation and control. Adv Parasitol 2010; 72: 305-50.
[PMID: 20624536]

[210]   Needle D, Lountos GT, Waugh DS. Structures of the Middle East respiratory syndrome coronavirus 3C-like protease reveal insights into substrate specificity. Acta Crystallogr D Biol Crystallogr 2015; 71(Pt 5): 1102-11.
[PMID: 25945576]

[211]   Melchiorre MG, Chiatti C, Lamura G, *et al.* Social support, socio-economic status, health and abuse among older people in seven European countries. PLoS One 2013; 8(1): e54856.
[PMID: 23382989]

[212]   Group, W.M.-C.R., State of knowledge and data gaps of Middle East respiratory syndrome coronavirus (MERS-CoV) in humans. PLoS Curr 2013; 5.
[http://dx.doi.org/10.1371/currents.outbreaks.0bf719e352e7478f8ad85fa30127ddb8]

[213]   Memish ZA, Cotten M, Meyer B, *et al.* Human infection with MERS coronavirus after exposure to infected camels, Saudi Arabia, 2013. Emerg Infect Dis 2014; 20(6): 1012-5.
[PMID: 24857749]

[214]   Eckerle I, Corman VM, Müller MA, Lenk M, Ulrich RG, Drosten C. Replicative capacity of MERS coronavirus in livestock cell lines. Emerg Infect Dis 2014; 20(2): 276-9.
[PMID: 24457147]

[215]   Cotten M, Lam TT, Watson SJ, *et al.* Full-genome deep sequencing and phylogenetic analysis of novel human betacoronavirus. Emerg Infect Dis 2013; 19(5): 736-42B.
[PMID: 23693015]

[216]   Corman V. Viral shedding and antibody response in 37 patients with MERS-coronavirus infection. Clin Infect Dis 2015; 10.
[http://dx.doi.org/10.1093/cid/civ951]

[217]   Chu H, Zhou J, Wong BH-Y, *et al.* Productive replication of Middle East respiratory syndrome coronavirus in monocyte-derived dendritic cells modulates innate immune response. Virology 2014; 454-455: 197-205.
[PMID: 24725946]

[218]   Chu H, Zhou J, Wong BH-Y, *et al.* Middle East respiratory syndrome coronavirus efficiently infects human primary T lymphocytes and activates the extrinsic and intrinsic apoptosis pathways. J Infect Dis 2016; 213(6): 904-14.
[PMID: 26203058]

[219]   Li F, Li W, Farzan M, Harrison SC. Structure of SARS coronavirus spike receptor-binding domain complexed with receptor. Science 2005; 309(5742): 1864-8.
[PMID: 16166518]

CHAPTER 2

Landscape of Host Genetic Factors Correlating with MERS-CoV

Abdullah[1], Aziz ur Rahman[1], Muhammad Ibrar[2] and **Fazlullah Khan[3,*]**

[1] *Department of Pharmacy, University of Malakand, Chakdara Dir Lower, KP, Pakistan*

[2] *Department of Allied and Health Sciences, Iqra National University Swat Campus, Swat, Pakistan*

[3] *Department of Pharmacy, Faculty of Pharmacy, Capital University of Science and Technology (CUST), Islamabad, Pakistan*

Abstract: The current outbreak of SARS-CoV-2 has raised various clinical and scientific questions, including the effect of host genetic factors on pathogenesis and disease susceptibility. MERS-CoV is a highly pathogenic virus in humans, causing high mortality (30-40%) and morbidity. CoVs are found to be widespread in man, poultry, and mammals. MERS-CoV enters the host cells by attachment with DPP4 receptors; it hijacks the host cell cycle, which helps in its survival and proliferation. Understanding the innate immune response against MERS-CoV is essential in the treatment development and precautionary measures. Nonstructural protein 1 (nsp1) has attracted greater attention as a potential virulence factor and a possible target for vaccine development. Downregulation of Th2, inadequate Th1 immune response, and overexpression of inflammatory cytokines IL-1α IL-1β, and IL-8 occur in the lower respiratory tract of patients infected with MERS-CoV. Research has shown that high viral load, high expression of inflammatory cytokines, and the downregulation of Th1 and Th2 response result in severe infection, contribute to lung inflammation, develop acute respiratory distress syndrome (ARDS) and pneumonia, and cause high fatality.

Keywords: Cell cycle, Genetic, Interleukin, MERS-CoV, Nonstructural protein.

INTRODUCTION

Several unique features characterize infectious diseases, such as a single agent causes them, they can cause an epidemic due to person-to-person transmission, and they can strongly impact human evolution [1, 2]. Moreover, infectious diseases may be eradicated, but new ones may emerge, thus forming a dynamic stage for human-infection interplay [3]. Innovative research on infectious diseases

* **Corresponding author Fazlullah Khan:** Department of Pharmacy, Faculty of Pharmacy, Capital University of Science and Technology (CUST), Islamabad, Pakistan; Tel: +92-3469433155; E-mail: fazlullahdr@gmail.com

Kamal Niaz, Muhammad Sajjad Khan & Muhammad Farrukh Nisar (Eds.)

has shown strong inter-individual differences attributed to host genetic makeup. Heritability studies have provided the primary evidence to corroborate this [4, 5], consequently increasing interest in understanding the genetic background of infectious diseases in the last decade of the 20th century [4, 5]. Consequently, more than 4000 gene studies focusing on respiratory infections were published between 2001 and 2010 [6]. As respiratory infectious diseases have the potential to cause epidemics and pandemics, extensive interest in the host factors has developed. In this connection, the Spanish influenza of 1918 has been recorded as the largest recorded pandemic, causing approximately 25-100 million deaths [7, 8].

Similarly, the severe acute respiratory syndrome-coronavirus (SARS-CoV) outbreak in 2003 showed how quickly a novel respiratory pathogen could spread on a global scale [9]. In September 2012, a beta coronavirus was found in the Middle East that causes severe respiratory infection in humans [10]. The International Committee on Taxonomy of Viruses named the virus Middle East Respiratory Syndrome-coronavirus (MERS-CoV) in 2013 [11]. Camel is the vector for MERS-CoV [12]. CoVs have a positive-sense, large, single-stranded RNA genome with a length of 27-32 kb, the largest among other viruses [13, 14]. Gene 1, which occupies two-thirds of the genome, consists of 2 large overlapping open reading frames (ORFs), ORF1a and ORF1b, having a ribosomal frameshifting signal at the junction of the 2 ORFs [15]. As the virus enters the host cell, its genome translation generates 2 large precursor polyproteins 1a (pp1a) and 1ab (pp1ab), which are processed by ORF1a-encoded viral proteinases 3C-like proteinase (3CL[pro]) and papain-like proteinase (PL[pro]) into 16 nonstructural proteins (nsp1-16). These are numbered according to their order from the N-terminus to the C-terminus of the ORF [15]. The nsps play a key role during viral RNA transcription and replication [16 - 18]. In addition, protease, helicase, RNA-dependent RNA polymerase, and some nsps are RNA processing enzymes [15, 19]. MERS-CoV infection is characterized by elevated systemic inflammatory chemokines/cytokines and immunopathology [20 - 22]. The high level of inflammatory chemokines and cytokines correlates with poor disease outcomes, increased infiltration of inflammatory cells into the lungs, and immunopathology [23, 24]. In addition, cytokine storms may occur due to stimulating chemokines, cytokines, and innate immune cells [25, 26]. Moreover, the high interleukin 8 (IL-8) level plays a vital role in acute SARS infection, severe immunopathology, and viral bronchiolitis pathogenesis [27, 28]. The high level of inflammatory IL-1α and IL-1β cytokines is linked with acute inflammatory response and tissue damage, consequently causing severe pathogenesis, mortality, and inflammatory loop induction [29, 30]. MERS-CoV evades the interferon (IFN) signaling cascade and nuclear factor-κB (NF-B) signaling pathway and antagonizes the antiviral immune response [31, 32]. Pathogenesis of MERS-CoV infection is complex, involving the dissemination of the virus to other organs and severe damage to the lungs [33, 34]. As susceptibility to infectious agents lies at least partly hidden or masked in immune response or inborn errors, an insight into host genetic factors may prove invaluable [35]. This makes infectious disease a high research priority, keeping in view the mobility of modern humans and the changing nature of the pathogen.

Species Susceptibility

MERS-CoV can infect humans, bats, and camels. While guinea pigs, mice, hamsters, and ferrets are unaffected. SARS-CoV-2 better replicates in cats and ferrets than in pigs, dogs, ducks, and chickens [36]. Bats have been extensively investigated as they serve as natural reservoirs of many coronaviruses. Studies have focused on co-evolutionary aspects between CoVs and the bat genome and other studies related to host genetic factors [37]. These include well-known genes such as ACE2 receptor genes for SARS-CoV-1 [38] and the DPP4 receptor genes for MERS-CoV [39].

Host Receptors Involved in MERS-CoV Entry

MERS-CoV enters its host near or at the plasma membrane or endosomes. The spike protein of MERS-CoV binds with dipeptidyl peptidase 4 (DDP4). Because of this interaction, the protein cleavage sites of S protein are exposed. In the presence of cell surface proteases (hTMPRSS2), cleavage of S protein occurs, and thus, the fusion of the virus occurs at or near the plasma membrane. In the absence of cell surface proteases, endocytosis of MERS-CoV occurs, facilitated by endosomal proteases (cathepsin L) [40]. It has been found that MERS-CoV prefers plasma membrane entry instead of endosomal entry [41, 42].

Translation and the Unfolded Protein Response in MERS-CoV-Infected Cells

To facilitate virus assembly and replication of the viral genome, virus infection alters cellular gene expression. CoVs utilize the translational machinery of the host cell for viral protein synthesis. The host mRNA translation is stopped, the host antiviral response is inhibited, and the translational machinery is used for the non-canonical mode of protein synthesis of the virus [43]. During replication of CoV, the increased modification and production of viral proteins and virion budding-related endoplasmic reticulum (ER) membrane depletion cause overloading of the folding capacity of the ER, which results in ER stress [44]. This causes the activation of the unfolded protein response (UPR), causing the cell to reverse to homeostasis and reducing the risk posed by protein misfolding for the correct functioning of the cell [45]. In humans, three ER-resident transmembrane sensors control the UPR that are activating transcription factor-6

(ATF6), the protein kinase R (PKR)-like ER-kinase (PERK), and the inositol requiring enzyme-1 (IRE1). These sensors recognize the unfolded/misfolded proteins inside the ER and a signal is transmitted to the nucleus for specific gene transcribing whose products increase ER folding capacity and reduce protein synthesis [45]. It has been found by ribosome profiling and parallel RNASeq studies that the host activates UPR to combat virus infection while the virus, in turn, manipulates the UPR to promote pathogenesis and replication [46 - 48]. The interplay between ER and MERS-CoV during replication results in ER stress responses when the cell attempts to regain homeostasis [49 - 52].

MERS-CoV-Induced Modification of Host Cell Membranes

CoV infection alters the structure and lipid composition of the membrane, trafficking, and topology of host cells to facilitate replication and proliferation of the virus [53]. CoVs induce multiple changes in lipid membrane architecture in host cells. CoVs cause remodeling in ER cisternae with the detachment of closed vesicular objects known as double-membrane vesicles (DMVs) [54]. In addition to the formation of DMV lipid envelops called CoVs replication organelles, the host membrane adopts a 3D topology known as a convoluted membrane [54, 55]. These are produced by multiple DMV fusion or other structural transitions [55]. Different terminologies are for the production of 3D non-lamellar assemblies of folded membranes [56]. These are known as tubule-reticular structures (TRS) in SARS-CoV [57] and MERS-CoV [58].

Host Proteins Interacting with the MERS-CoV Genome and its Replication or Expression

The fusion of the host cell membrane and the virus is the crucial step in the viral entry that is mediated by S protein in CoVs [59]. The binding of MERS-CoV to target cells *via* surface receptors (DPP4) occurs through large class 1 fusion proteins (S proteins) [60]. Therefore, tissue tropism and host range are defined by receptor distribution and the CoV-S receptor interaction [61]. The S protein is composed of S1 and S2 subunits; the S1 at the N terminus is responsible for receptor binding, and the S2 at the C-terminus for viral fusion [59]. Host cell proteases, cathepsin, and the transmembrane protease serine 2 (TMPRSS2) cause cleavage of subunits from the complete S [62]. After binding with DPP4 by S1, the fusion and uptake mechanism into vesicles by S2 bring the cellular and viral membranes much closer than when only fusion occurs [63]. As a result, a conformational change occurs in the clathrin-coated vesicle that is endocytosed, consequently releasing the fusion peptide to interact with the vesicle membrane, provided cleavage of S into subdomains has occurred [64]. The S2 collapse that bridges the cellular membranes and virus pulls the two membranes together with two conserved heptad repeats (HR1 and HR2), resulting in the formation of a 6-helix canonical bundle [65]. Until now, the fusion peptide (FP) precise location and sequence have not been fully elucidated for all CoVs due to the difficulty of recognizing the FP motif within large spike proteins [66]. Yet, bioinformatics analysis has demonstrated that a part of FP is located near the N-terminus of S2 [67]. Some S protein cleavage maps show that the motif is not located at the N-terminus of HR1 [63] but is immediately located at the second S2 cleavage site, mapped in SAR-CoV S and later in MERS-CoV S [68, 69]. A sequence that shows that this motif acts as FP has been shown for SARS-CoV as observed in an *in vitro* binding assay in multilamellar vesicles where it re-orders membrane in a calcium-dependent manner [70]. The S2 endodomain is divided into two regions: a carboxy-terminal region that is rich in charge residues and the N-terminus region rich in cysteine residues [71, 72]. The palmitoylation of S needs cysteine residues [73]. In addition, it has been found that the cysteine rich residue is important for syncytium formation during viral infection [74, 75]. Membrane deformation and binding is the property of FP sequence, propelled into the membrane by conformational changes in S, while palmitoylation of S make the protein stable as it interacts with lipid rafts in target membrane to provide sufficient time for fusion. Recently the structures of several SARS-CoV-S and MERS-CoV-S proteins have been determined by atomic resolution following imaging *via* cryo-electron microscopy [76 - 78].

Host Innate Immune Responses Against MERS-CoV

MERS-CoV mainly infects the human respiratory tract. It has been found that MERS-CoV can infect and replicate in the airway epithelium of humans [79, 80]. MERS-CoV infects the non-ciliated bronchial epithelial cells, alveolar epithelial cells, bronchiolar epithelial cells, and endothelial cells of pulmonary vessels [81]. The first line of innate immune response is the neutrophils. In the lower respiratory tract of the patient, neutrophil chemoattractant chemokine IL-8 is highly expressed [82]. IL-8 is a key player in the activation, accumulation, and attraction of neutrophils in the infection site that subsequently forms neutrophil extracellular traps. These traps directly cause inflammation and further increase IL-8 secretion, resulting in the recruitment of more neutrophils at the injection site [83]. Macrophages and dendritic cells are also involved in innate immune functioning. The virus or its derivatives activates plasmacytoid dendritic cells and secrete a large amount of interferon type-1 (IFN-I) that produces an antiviral response in the host cell [84]. Macrophages secrete proinflammatory cytokines and IFN-I that trigger a protective response against the virus and pathologic complications of the disease [85].

Upon infection with MERS-CoV, human epithelial cells are activated to produce pro-inflammatory chemokines and cytokines (IL-6 and CXCL-10) to get rid of the offending pathogen [86, 87]. Interferon type 1 response is inhibited by MERS-CoV [88]. The invading MERS-CoV virion is cleared by CD8+ T cells, while antibodies are developed that protect against subsequent infection [89, 90]. The spectrum of the immune response against MERS-CoV and SARA-CoV are very similar. As in SARS-CoV infection, lymphodepletion also occurs in severe MERS during the acute phase [91]. Moreover, with an increase in the severity of SARS-CoV and MERS-CoV infection, the serum level of inflammatory cytokines and chemokines, as well as humoral immune response, is increased [92]. In severe/ moderate MERS-CoV infection, B-cell and T-cell responses are increased [22].

MERS-CoV-Induced Deregulation of the Cell Cycle

The control and prevention of CoVs emergence and re-emergence have been a major challenge nowadays. Therefore, in addition to the development of vaccines, antiviral drugs, and diagnostics, it is mandatory to get a deeper insight into the mechanism of interaction between CoVs and host cells. Recently, cell cycle arrest has been the hot spot in CoV research. To enhance replication efficiency and provide favourable conditions for growth, viruses have evolved several mechanisms to manipulate the cell cycle [93].

Other Immune Genes and MERS-CoV

The major histocompatibility complex (MHC) has been explored in studies of multiple species related to CoVs, including cats, cheetahs, and chickens [94 - 96]. Similarly, in humans, the HLA gene has been studied concerning SARS-CoV-1. HLA alleles are thought to relate to susceptibility and outcome of COVID-19 in humans [97]. In case-control hosts, genetic studies on affinities of peptide binding between hundreds of HLA class I and class II proteins and proteomes of CoVs have been described. Similarly, in work on ACE2 and other genes in humans, the peptide-binding affinity of HLA alleles has been investigated [98]. The viral peptide-MHC class I binding affinity about HLA genotypes for SARS-CoV-2 peptides in an *in silico* study was found to be related to the vulnerability of COVID-19 [99]. Besides HLA genes, other important genes that play a role in immune processes have been studied in host genetic investigations. In mouse models, the majority of research work is focused on the pathways involved in viral infection susceptibility. While in humans, the studies are mainly concentrated on key immune genes [100].

Evidence of MER-CoV and Host Genetic Factors

Endogenous RNA Network

Circular RNAs (circRNAs) are non-coding RNAs that exhibit unique splicing reactions, forming covalently closed-loop structures [101, 102]. These are in abundance in human cells, playing key regulatory functions, including micro RNA (miRNA) sponges, interacting with RNA binding proteins (RBPs), and modulating parental gene transcription by interacting with RNA polymerase II [102 - 104]. It has been suggested by the competitive endogenous RNA (ceRNA) hypothesis that RNA transcripts, including mRNAs, circRNAs, and long non-coding RNAs (lncRNAs), contain miRNA response elements (MREs) that compete for miRNA binding among themselves to regulate each other's expression [105, 106]. In a recent investigation, the circRNA-miRNA-mRNA network determined seven important differential expression circRNAs decreased MERS-CoV load significantly and also reduced the mRNA expression that modulates different biological pathways, including ubiquitination and mitogen-activated protein kinase (MAPK) pathways [107].

Genes Encoding Th1 and Th2 Cytokines

The expression of genes encoding Th1 and Th2 cytokines is downregulated in the lower respiratory tract of patients infected by MERS-CoV. About 26 genes encoding Th1 and Th2 cytokines were downregulated. In early immunity, IFNγ induces apoptosis of infected cells and stimulates natural killer cells and CD8$^+$ [86, 108]. It has been demonstrated that IFNγ and the level of Th1-associated cytokine mRNA expression were downregulated in the lower respiratory tract of MERS-CoV-infected patients, while 6 Th1-related chemokines and cytokines were overexpressed in the lungs, and 15 Th2-related cytokines were downregulated [82]. The humoral immune response and antibody production are mediated by Th2 cytokines. The Th2 response was downregulated by MERS-CoV infection [82]. In acute SARS-CoV infection, a strong inflammatory response was observed despite the downregulation of genes involved in mRNA expression [27]. Downregulation of Th1/Th2 chemokines/cytokines is responsible for the inefficient clearing of infection, pathological change, and the susceptibility of the host to immune-mediated diseases. Upregulation of Th1 chemokines/cytokines has been linked with virus-induced immunopathology and inflammation of the lungs [109].

MERS-CoV Nsp1 and Host Gene

CoVs have 16 nonstructural proteins (nsps), nsp 1-16, which are required for replication of the virus at various stages of the life cycle [110]. The nsp1 of

MERS-CoV contains 193 amino acids, while that of SARS-CoV contains 180 amino acids [111]. The sequence observed for nsp1 of MERS-CoV was LRKxGxGG. In addition, both the CoVs possess RNA cleavage activity in nsp1 [112, 113]. No effect on interaction with the 5′ UTR of viral RNA was observed by substitution of R146A in MERS-CoV nsp1. However, the mutation of R13A in MERS-CoV nsp1 abrogated the interaction with the 5′ UTR of viral RNA, suggesting that the binding domain in nsp1 with the 5′ UTR of viral RNA is different between MERS-CoV and SARS-CoV [111]. Several studies have shown the role of CoV nsp1 in the regulation of gene expression and viral replication. SARS-CoV nsp1 is the most studied of the CoVs nsp and is the focus of research [114]. After infection, the nsp1 of MERS-CoV diffuses into the nucleus and cytoplasm [113]. The nsp1 of MERS-CoV and SARS-CoV inhibit protein synthesis of the host *via* suppression of translational machinery and digestion of mRNA by endonuclease [113, 115]. It has been suggested that the MERS-CoV has evolved to utilize R13 of nsp1 for interaction with 5′ UTR of viral RNA to circumvent the nsp1-mediated shutoff [116]. The 5′ UTR of MERS-CoV contains four stem-loops (SL), SL1, SL2, SL4-1, and SL4-2, that are conserved among beta CoVs. The nsp1 of MERS-CoV interacts with cyclophilin, resulting in the degradation of host mRNA, which is thought to be a major virulence factor. Moreover, some residues of nsp1 are important for evading translational shutdown [116]. The escape of MERS-CoV mRNA from inhibition by MERS-CoV nsp1 is promoted by their cytoplasmic origin [113].

Different Animals and MER-CoV

DPP4 (an exopeptidase) is the receptor for MERS-CoV. However, some laboratory animals such as mice, ferrets, and Syrian hamsters are not susceptible to MERS-CoV as the DPP4 orthologs do not bind spike protein of the virus and, thus, do not facilitate viral entry [117, 118]. Asymptomatic infection was caused by inoculation of MERS-CoV into rabbits. The virus was detectable in the lung tissues of rabbits but no histopathological and clinical symptoms were observed [119]. MERS-CoV isolated from a human can cause infection in camels and vice versa. Mild signs of disease were observed in camels even though infected camels shed a large amount of virus from the upper respiratory tract [120]. Mild to moderate respiratory infection occurs in Rhesus macaques [121, 122], while moderate to severe infection occurs in common marmosets [123]. The MERS-CoV infection in marmosets was a disseminated one as viral DNA was detected in almost all tested tissues, such as the kidney, liver, blood, spleen, intestine, *etc.* Among these organs, the infectious virus was only isolated from the respiratory tract [123].

Human Studies and MERS-CoV

A large number of research articles involving humans have been published. About 75 research studies involved humans; 36 of these involved analysis of specific genes or loci, while 39 involved computational, case reports, or biological studies on human host genetic factors. Thirty involved non-human and human host genetic factors. These studies aimed to focus on the areas that are relevant to COVID-19 and humans [124, 125].

CONCLUSION

The respiratory epithelium of humans is susceptible to MERS-CoV infection and may support viral replication. However, the human immune system has evolved several mechanisms to produce antiviral and proinflammatory cytokines by infected epithelial cells. MERS-CoV causes apoptosis after infection of human T cells. Altogether, the high expression of inflammatory chemokines/cytokines in the lower respiratory tract of patients infected with MERS-CoV confirms immunopathology of the lung. Therefore, the downregulation of Th1 and Th2 and high expression of inflammatory cytokines may result in more severe infection.

REFERENCES

[1]   Fauci AS, Morens DM. The perpetual challenge of infectious diseases. N Engl J Med 2012; 366(5): 454-61.
        [http://dx.doi.org/10.1056/NEJMra1108296] [PMID: 22296079]

[2]   Fumagalli M, Pozzoli U, Cagliani R, *et al.* Genome-wide identification of susceptibility alleles for viral infections through a population genetics approach. PLoS Genet 2010; 6(2): e1000849.
        [http://dx.doi.org/10.1371/journal.pgen.1000849] [PMID: 20174570]

[3]   Morens DM, Folkers GK, Fauci AS. Emerging infections: a perpetual challenge. Lancet Infect Dis 2008; 8(11): 710-9.
        [http://dx.doi.org/10.1016/S1473-3099(08)70256-1] [PMID: 18992407]

[4]   Cooke GS, Hill AVS. Genetics of susceptibitlity to human infectious disease. Nat Rev Genet 2001; 2(12): 967-77.
        [http://dx.doi.org/10.1038/35103577] [PMID: 11733749]

[5]   Burgner D, Jamieson SE, Blackwell JM. Genetic susceptibility to infectious diseases: big is beautiful, but will bigger be even better? Lancet Infect Dis 2006; 6(10): 653-63.
        [http://dx.doi.org/10.1016/S1473-3099(06)70601-6] [PMID: 17008174]

[6]   Rowell JL, Dowling NF, Yu W, Yesupriya A, Zhang L, Gwinn M. Trends in population-based studies of human genetics in infectious diseases. PLoS One 2012; 7(2): e25431.
        [http://dx.doi.org/10.1371/journal.pone.0025431] [PMID: 22347358]

[7]   Patterson KD, Pyle GFJBHM. The geography and mortality of the 1918 influenza pandemic. Bull Hist Med 1991; 65(1): 4-21.
        [PMID: 2021692]

[8]   Johnson NPAS, Mueller J. Updating the accounts: global mortality of the 1918-1920 "Spanish" influenza pandemic. Bull Hist Med 2002; 76(1): 105-15.
        [http://dx.doi.org/10.1353/bhm.2002.0022] [PMID: 11875246]

[9]   Li W, Moore MJ, Vasilieva N, *et al.* Angiotensin-converting enzyme 2 is a functional receptor for the SARS coronavirus. Nature 2003; 426(6965): 450-4.
[http://dx.doi.org/10.1038/nature02145] [PMID: 14647384]

[10]   Zaki AM, van Boheemen S, Bestebroer TM, Osterhaus ADME, Fouchier RAM. Isolation of a novel coronavirus from a man with pneumonia in Saudi Arabia. N Engl J Med 2012; 367(19): 1814-20.
[http://dx.doi.org/10.1056/NEJMoa1211721] [PMID: 23075143]

[11]   de Groot RJ, Baker SC, Baric RS, *et al.* Middle East respiratory syndrome coronavirus (MERS-CoV): announcement of the Coronavirus Study Group. J Virol 2013; 87(14): 7790-2.
[http://dx.doi.org/10.1128/JVI.01244-13] [PMID: 23678167]

[12]   Reusken CBEM, Haagmans BL, Müller MA, *et al.* Middle East respiratory syndrome coronavirus neutralising serum antibodies in dromedary camels: a comparative serological study. Lancet Infect Dis 2013; 13(10): 859-66.
[http://dx.doi.org/10.1016/S1473-3099(13)70164-6] [PMID: 23933067]

[13]   Lee HJ, Shieh CK, Gorbalenya AE, *et al.* The complete sequence (22 kilobases) of murine coronavirus gene 1 encoding the putative proteases and RNA polymerase. Virology 1991; 180(2): 567-82.
[http://dx.doi.org/10.1016/0042-6822(91)90071-I] [PMID: 1846489]

[14]   Lomniczi B, Kennedy I. Genome of infectious bronchitis virus. J Virol 1977; 24(1): 99-107.
[http://dx.doi.org/10.1128/jvi.24.1.99-107.1977] [PMID: 198590]

[15]   J Ziebuhr. The coronavirus replicase. Curr Top Microbiol Immunol. 2005; 287: 57-94.
[http://dx.doi.org/10.1007/3-540-26765-4_3]

[16]   Fan K, Wei P, Feng Q, *et al.* Biosynthesis, purification, and substrate specificity of severe acute respiratory syndrome coronavirus 3C-like proteinase. J Biol Chem 2004; 279(3): 1637-42.
[http://dx.doi.org/10.1074/jbc.M310875200] [PMID: 14561748]

[17]   Imbert I, Guillemot JC, Bourhis JM, *et al.* A second, non-canonical RNA-dependent RNA polymerase in SARS Coronavirus. EMBO J 2006; 25(20): 4933-42.
[http://dx.doi.org/10.1038/sj.emboj.7601368] [PMID: 17024178]

[18]   Saikatendu KS, Joseph JS, Subramanian V, *et al.* Structural basis of severe acute respiratory syndrome coronavirus ADP-ribose-1″-phosphate dephosphorylation by a conserved domain of nsP3. Structure 2005; 13(11): 1665-75.
[http://dx.doi.org/10.1016/j.str.2005.07.022] [PMID: 16271890]

[19]   Thiel V, Ivanov KA, Putics Á, *et al.* Mechanisms and enzymes involved in SARS coronavirus genome expression. J Gen Virol 2003; 84(9): 2305-15.
[http://dx.doi.org/10.1099/vir.0.19424-0] [PMID: 12917450]

[20]   Kindler E, Thiel V, Weber F. Interaction of SARS and MERS coronaviruses with the antiviral interferon response. Adv Virus Res 2016; 96: 219-43.
[http://dx.doi.org/10.1016/bs.aivir.2016.08.006] [PMID: 27712625]

[21]   Channappanavar R, Perlman S. Pathogenic human coronavirus infections: causes and consequences of cytokine storm and immunopathology Semin Immunopathol, 2017; 39: 529–539.
[http://dx.doi.org/10.1007/s00281-017-0629-x]

[22]   Shin HS, Kim Y, Kim G, *et al.* Immune responses to Middle East respiratory syndrome coronavirus during the acute and convalescent phases of human infection. Clin Infect Dis 2019; 68(6): 984-92.
[http://dx.doi.org/10.1093/cid/ciy595] [PMID: 30060038]

[23]   Lau SKP, Lau CCY, Chan KH, *et al.* Delayed induction of proinflammatory cytokines and suppression of innate antiviral response by the novel Middle East respiratory syndrome coronavirus: implications for pathogenesis and treatment. J Gen Virol 2013; 94(12): 2679-90.
[http://dx.doi.org/10.1099/vir.0.055533-0] [PMID: 24077366]

[24]   Mella C, Suarez-Arrabal MC, Lopez S, *et al.* Innate immune dysfunction is associated with enhanced

disease severity in infants with severe respiratory syncytial virus bronchiolitis. J Infect Dis 2013; 207(4): 564-73.
[http://dx.doi.org/10.1093/infdis/jis721] [PMID: 23204162]

[25] Teijaro JR. Cytokine storms in infectious diseases Semin Immunopathol 2017; 39: 501–503.
[http://dx.doi.org/10.1007/s00281-017-0640-2]

[26] Xi-zhi JG, Thomas PG. New fronts emerge in the influenza cytokine storm. Seminars in immunopathology. Springer 2017; pp. 541-50.

[27] Reghunathan R, Jayapal M, Hsu LY, *et al.* Expression profile of immune response genes in patients with Severe Acute Respiratory Syndrome. BMC Immunol 2005; 6(1): 2.
[http://dx.doi.org/10.1186/1471-2172-6-2] [PMID: 15655079]

[28] Wong CK, Lam CWK, Wu AKL, *et al.* Plasma inflammatory cytokines and chemokines in severe acute respiratory syndrome. Clin Exp Immunol 2004; 136(1): 95-103.
[http://dx.doi.org/10.1111/j.1365-2249.2004.02415.x] [PMID: 15030519]

[29] Di Paolo NC, Shayakhmetov DM. Interleukin 1α and the inflammatory process. Nat Immunol 2016; 17(8): 906-13.
[http://dx.doi.org/10.1038/ni.3503] [PMID: 27434011]

[30] Tate MD, Ong JDH, Dowling JK, *et al.* Reassessing the role of the NLRP3 inflammasome during pathogenic influenza A virus infection *via* temporal inhibition. Sci Rep 2016; 6(1): 27912.
[http://dx.doi.org/10.1038/srep27912] [PMID: 27283237]

[31] Comar CE, Goldstein SA, Li Y, Yount B, Baric RS, Weiss SR. Antagonism of dsRNA-induced innate immune pathways by NS4a and NS4b accessory proteins during MERS coronavirus infection. MBio 2019; 10(2): e00319-19.
[http://dx.doi.org/10.1128/mBio.00319-19] [PMID: 30914508]

[32] Canton J, Fehr AR, Fernandez-Delgado R, *et al.* MERS-CoV 4b protein interferes with the NF-κ--dependent innate immune response during infection. PLoS Pathog 2018; 14(1): e1006838.
[http://dx.doi.org/10.1371/journal.ppat.1006838] [PMID: 29370303]

[33] Gao H, Dong Z, Gong X, *et al.* Effects of various radiation doses on induced T-helper cell differentiation and related cytokine secretion. J Radiat Res (Tokyo) 2018; 59(4): 395-403.
[http://dx.doi.org/10.1093/jrr/rry011] [PMID: 29554285]

[34] Shokri S, Mahmoudvand S, Taherkhani R, Farshadpour F. Modulation of the immune response by Middle East respiratory syndrome coronavirus. J Cell Physiol 2019; 234(3): 2143-51.
[http://dx.doi.org/10.1002/jcp.27155] [PMID: 30146782]

[35] Alcaïs A, Quintana-Murci L, Thaler DS, Schurr E, Abel L, Casanova JL. Life-threatening infectious diseases of childhood: single-gene inborn errors of immunity? Ann N Y Acad Sci 2010; 1214(1): 18-33.
[http://dx.doi.org/10.1111/j.1749-6632.2010.05834.x] [PMID: 21091717]

[36] Shi J, Wen Z, Zhong G, *et al.* Susceptibility of ferrets, cats, dogs, and other domesticated animals to SARS–coronavirus 2. Science 2020; 368(6494): 1016-20.
[http://dx.doi.org/10.1126/science.abb7015] [PMID: 32269068]

[37] Cui J, Han N, Streicker D, *et al.* Evolutionary relationships between bat coronaviruses and their hosts. Emerg Infect Dis 2007; 13(10): 1526-32.
[http://dx.doi.org/10.3201/eid1310.070448] [PMID: 18258002]

[38] Hou Y, Peng C, Yu M, *et al.* Angiotensin-converting enzyme 2 (ACE2) proteins of different bat species confer variable susceptibility to SARS-CoV entry. Arch Virol 2010; 155(10): 1563-9.
[http://dx.doi.org/10.1007/s00705-010-0729-6] [PMID: 20567988]

[39] Cui J, Eden JS, Holmes EC, Wang LF. Adaptive evolution of bat dipeptidyl peptidase 4 (dpp4): implications for the origin and emergence of Middle East respiratory syndrome coronavirus. Virol J 2013; 10(1): 304.

[http://dx.doi.org/10.1186/1743-422X-10-304] [PMID: 24107353]

[40]   Qing E, Hantak MP, Galpalli GG, Gallagher T. Evaluating MERS-CoV entry pathways. MERS Coronavirus. Springer 2020; pp. 9-20.
        [http://dx.doi.org/10.1007/978-1-0716-0211-9_2]

[41]   Park JE, Li K, Barlan A, *et al.* Proteolytic processing of Middle East respiratory syndrome coronavirus spikes expands virus tropism. Proc Natl Acad Sci USA 2016; 113(43): 12262-7.
        [http://dx.doi.org/10.1073/pnas.1608147113] [PMID: 27791014]

[42]   Li K, Wohlford-Lenane CL, Channappanavar R, *et al.* Mouse-adapted MERS coronavirus causes lethal lung disease in human DPP4 knockin mice. Proc Natl Acad Sci USA 2017; 114(15): E3119-28.
        [http://dx.doi.org/10.1073/pnas.1619109114] [PMID: 28348219]

[43]   Walsh D, Mathews MB, Mohr I. Tinkering with translation: protein synthesis in virus-infected cells. Cold Spring Harb Perspect Biol 2013; 5(1): a012351.
        [http://dx.doi.org/10.1101/cshperspect.a012351] [PMID: 23209131]

[44]   Fung TS, Liu DX. Coronavirus infection, ER stress, apoptosis and innate immunity. Front Microbiol 2014; 5: 296.
        [http://dx.doi.org/10.3389/fmicb.2014.00296] [PMID: 24987391]

[45]   Ron D, Walter P. Signal integration in the endoplasmic reticulum unfolded protein response. Nat Rev Mol Cell Biol 2007; 8(7): 519-29.
        [http://dx.doi.org/10.1038/nrm2199] [PMID: 17565364]

[46]   Lazar C, Uta M, Branza-Nichita N. Modulation of the unfolded protein response by the human hepatitis B virus. Front Microbiol 2014; 5: 433.
        [http://dx.doi.org/10.3389/fmicb.2014.00433] [PMID: 25191311]

[47]   Perera N, Miller JL, Zitzmann N. The role of the unfolded protein response in dengue virus pathogenesis. Cell Microbiol 2017; 19(5): e12734.
        [http://dx.doi.org/10.1111/cmi.12734] [PMID: 28207988]

[48]   Carpenter JE, Grose C. Varicella-zoster virus glycoprotein expression differentially induces the unfolded protein response in infected cells. Front Microbiol 2014; 5: 322.
        [http://dx.doi.org/10.3389/fmicb.2014.00322] [PMID: 25071735]

[49]   Versteeg GA, van de Nes PS, Bredenbeek PJ, Spaan WJM. The coronavirus spike protein induces endoplasmic reticulum stress and upregulation of intracellular chemokine mRNA concentrations. J Virol 2007; 81(20): 10981-90.
        [http://dx.doi.org/10.1128/JVI.01033-07] [PMID: 17670839]

[50]   Stertz S, Reichelt M, Spiegel M, *et al.* The intracellular sites of early replication and budding of SARS-coronavirus. Virology 2007; 361(2): 304-15.
        [http://dx.doi.org/10.1016/j.virol.2006.11.027] [PMID: 17210170]

[51]   Reggiori F, Monastyrska I, Verheije MH, *et al.* Coronaviruses Hijack the LC3-I-positive EDEMosomes, ER-derived vesicles exporting short-lived ERAD regulators, for replication. Cell Host Microbe 2010; 7(6): 500-8.
        [http://dx.doi.org/10.1016/j.chom.2010.05.013] [PMID: 20542253]

[52]   Maier HJ, Hawes PC, Cottam EM, *et al.* Infectious bronchitis virus generates spherules from zippered endoplasmic reticulum membranes. MBio 2013; 4(5): e00801-13.
        [http://dx.doi.org/10.1128/mBio.00801-13] [PMID: 24149513]

[53]   Abu-Farha M, Thanaraj TA, Qaddoumi MG, Hashem A, Abubaker J, Al-Mulla F. The role of lipid metabolism in COVID-19 virus infection and as a drug target. Int J Mol Sci 2020; 21(10): 3544.
        [http://dx.doi.org/10.3390/ijms21103544] [PMID: 32429572]

[54]   Zhang J, Lan Y, Sanyal SJB. Membrane heist: coronavirus host membrane remodeling during replication Biochimie 2020; 179: 229-236.
        [http://dx.doi.org/10.1016/j.biochi.2020.10.010]

[55] Knoops K, Kikkert M, Worm SHE, *et al.* SARS-coronavirus replication is supported by a reticulovesicular network of modified endoplasmic reticulum. PLoS Biol 2008; 6(9): e226.
[http://dx.doi.org/10.1371/journal.pbio.0060226] [PMID: 18798692]

[56] Almsherqi ZA, McLachlan CS, Mossop P, Knoops K, Deng Y. Direct template matching reveals a host subcellular membrane gyroid cubic structure that is associated with SARS virus. Redox Rep 2005; 10(3): 167-71.
[http://dx.doi.org/10.1179/135100005X57373] [PMID: 16156956]

[57] Goldsmith CS, Tatti KM, Ksiazek TG, *et al.* Ultrastructural characterization of SARS coronavirus. Emerg Infect Dis 2004; 10(2): 320-6.
[http://dx.doi.org/10.3201/eid1002.030913] [PMID: 15030705]

[58] Oudshoorn D, Rijs K, Limpens RWAL, *et al.* Expression and cleavage of middle east respiratory syndrome coronavirus nsp3-4 polyprotein induce the formation of double-membrane vesicles that mimic those associated with coronaviral RNA replication. MBio 2017; 8(6): e01658-17.
[http://dx.doi.org/10.1128/mBio.01658-17] [PMID: 29162711]

[59] Belouzard S, Millet JK, Licitra BN, Whittaker GR. Mechanisms of coronavirus cell entry mediated by the viral spike protein. Viruses 2012; 4(6): 1011-33.
[http://dx.doi.org/10.3390/v4061011] [PMID: 22816037]

[60] Raj VS, Mou H, Smits SL, *et al.* Dipeptidyl peptidase 4 is a functional receptor for the emerging human coronavirus-EMC. Nature 2013; 495(7440): 251-4.
[http://dx.doi.org/10.1038/nature12005] [PMID: 23486063]

[61] Li F. Structure, function, and evolution of coronavirus spike proteins. Annu Rev Virol 2016; 3(1): 237-61.
[http://dx.doi.org/10.1146/annurev-virology-110615-042301] [PMID: 27578435]

[62] Shirato K, Kawase M, Matsuyama S. Middle East respiratory syndrome coronavirus infection mediated by the transmembrane serine protease TMPRSS2. J Virol 2013; 87(23): 12552-61.
[http://dx.doi.org/10.1128/JVI.01890-13] [PMID: 24027332]

[63] Du L, Yang Y, Zhou Y, Lu L, Li F, Jiang S. MERS-CoV spike protein: a key target for antivirals. Expert Opin Ther Targets 2017; 21(2): 131-43.
[http://dx.doi.org/10.1080/14728222.2017.1271415] [PMID: 27936982]

[64] Burkard C, Verheije MH, Wicht O, *et al.* Coronavirus cell entry occurs through the endo-/lysosomal pathway in a proteolysis-dependent manner. PLoS Pathog 2014; 10(11): e1004502.
[http://dx.doi.org/10.1371/journal.ppat.1004502] [PMID: 25375324]

[65] Bosch BJ, van der Zee R, de Haan CAM, Rottier PJM. The coronavirus spike protein is a class I virus fusion protein: structural and functional characterization of the fusion core complex. J Virol 2003; 77(16): 8801-11.
[http://dx.doi.org/10.1128/JVI.77.16.8801-8811.2003] [PMID: 12885899]

[66] Bosch BJ, Bartelink W, Rottier PJM. Cathepsin L functionally cleaves the severe acute respiratory syndrome coronavirus class I fusion protein upstream of rather than adjacent to the fusion peptide. J Virol 2008; 82(17): 8887-90.
[http://dx.doi.org/10.1128/JVI.00415-08] [PMID: 18562523]

[67] Madu IG, Roth SL, Belouzard S, Whittaker GR. Characterization of a highly conserved domain within the severe acute respiratory syndrome coronavirus spike protein S2 domain with characteristics of a viral fusion peptide. J Virol 2009; 83(15): 7411-21.
[http://dx.doi.org/10.1128/JVI.00079-09] [PMID: 19439480]

[68] Millet JK, Goldstein ME, Labitt RN, Hsu H-L, Daniel S, Whittaker GRJEm. infections, A camel-derived MERS-CoV with a variant spike protein cleavage site and distinct fusion activation properties. Biotechnol Adv 2016; 5: 1-9.

[69] Millet JK, Whittaker GR. Host cell proteases: Critical determinants of coronavirus tropism and

pathogenesis. Virus Res 2015; 202: 120-34.
[http://dx.doi.org/10.1016/j.virusres.2014.11.021] [PMID: 25445340]

[70]   Lai AL, Millet JK, Daniel S, Freed JH, Whittaker GR. The SARS-CoV fusion peptide forms an extended bipartite fusion platform that perturbs membrane order in a calcium-dependent manner. J Mol Biol 2017; 429(24): 3875-92.
[http://dx.doi.org/10.1016/j.jmb.2017.10.017] [PMID: 29056462]

[71]   Chang KW, Sheng Y, Gombold JL. Coronavirus-induced membrane fusion requires the cysteine-rich domain in the spike protein. Virology 2000; 269(1): 212-24.
[http://dx.doi.org/10.1006/viro.2000.0219] [PMID: 10725213]

[72]   Yao Q, Masters PS, Ye R. Negatively charged residues in the endodomain are critical for specific assembly of spike protein into murine coronavirus. Virology 2013; 442(1): 74-81.
[http://dx.doi.org/10.1016/j.virol.2013.04.001] [PMID: 23628137]

[73]   Yang J, Lv J, Wang Y, *et al.* Replication of murine coronavirus requires multiple cysteines in the endodomain of spike protein. Virology 2012; 427(2): 98-106.
[http://dx.doi.org/10.1016/j.virol.2012.02.015] [PMID: 22424735]

[74]   Bosch BJ, de Haan CAM, Smits SL, Rottier PJM. Spike protein assembly into the coronavirion: exploring the limits of its sequence requirements. Virology 2005; 334(2): 306-18.
[http://dx.doi.org/10.1016/j.virol.2005.02.001] [PMID: 15780881]

[75]   Ye R, Montalto-Morrison C, Masters PS. Genetic analysis of determinants for spike glycoprotein assembly into murine coronavirus virions: distinct roles for charge-rich and cysteine-rich regions of the endodomain. J Virol 2004; 78(18): 9904-17.
[http://dx.doi.org/10.1128/JVI.78.18.9904-9917.2004] [PMID: 15331724]

[76]   Gui M, Song W, Zhou H, *et al.* Cryo-electron microscopy structures of the SARS-CoV spike glycoprotein reveal a prerequisite conformational state for receptor binding. Cell Res 2017; 27(1): 119-29.
[http://dx.doi.org/10.1038/cr.2016.152] [PMID: 28008928]

[77]   Walls AC, Tortorici MA, Bosch BJ, *et al.* Cryo-electron microscopy structure of a coronavirus spike glycoprotein trimer. Nature 2016; 531(7592): 114-7.
[http://dx.doi.org/10.1038/nature16988] [PMID: 26855426]

[78]   Yuan Y, Cao D, Zhang Y, *et al.* Cryo-EM structures of MERS-CoV and SARS-CoV spike glycoproteins reveal the dynamic receptor binding domains. Nat Commun 2017; 8(1): 15092.
[http://dx.doi.org/10.1038/ncomms15092] [PMID: 28393837]

[79]   Kindler E, Jónsdóttir HR, Muth D, *et al.* Efficient replication of the novel human betacoronavirus EMC on primary human epithelium highlights its zoonotic potential. MBio 2013; 4(1): e00611-12.
[http://dx.doi.org/10.1128/mBio.00611-12] [PMID: 23422412]

[80]   Zielecki F, Weber M, Eickmann M, *et al.* Human cell tropism and innate immune system interactions of human respiratory coronavirus EMC compared to those of severe acute respiratory syndrome coronavirus. J Virol 2013; 87(9): 5300-4.
[http://dx.doi.org/10.1128/JVI.03496-12] [PMID: 23449793]

[81]   Chan RWY, Chan MCW, Agnihothram S, *et al.* Tropism of and innate immune responses to the novel human betacoronavirus lineage C virus in human ex vivo respiratory organ cultures. J Virol 2013; 87(12): 6604-14.
[http://dx.doi.org/10.1128/JVI.00009-13] [PMID: 23552422]

[82]   Alosaimi B, Hamed ME, Naeem A, *et al.* MERS-CoV infection is associated with downregulation of genes encoding Th1 and Th2 cytokines/chemokines and elevated inflammatory innate immune response in the lower respiratory tract. Cytokine 2020; 126: 154895.
[http://dx.doi.org/10.1016/j.cyto.2019.154895] [PMID: 31706200]

[83]   Nakamura H, Yoshimura K, McElvaney NG, Crystal RG. Neutrophil elastase in respiratory epithelial

lining fluid of individuals with cystic fibrosis induces interleukin-8 gene expression in a human bronchial epithelial cell line. J Clin Invest 1992; 89(5): 1478-84.
[http://dx.doi.org/10.1172/JCI115738] [PMID: 1569186]

[84]   Ito T, Wang Y-H, Liu Y-J. Plasmacytoid dendritic cell precursors/type I interferon-producing cells sense viral infection by Toll-like receptor (TLR) 7 and TLR9. Springer seminars in immunopathology. Springer 2005; pp. 221-9.
[http://dx.doi.org/10.1007/s00281-004-0180-4]

[85]   Diamond MS, Shrestha B, Mehlhop E, Sitati E, Engle M. Innate and adaptive immune responses determine protection against disseminated infection by West Nile encephalitis virus. Viral Immunol 2003; 16(3): 259-78.
[http://dx.doi.org/10.1089/088282403322396082] [PMID: 14583143]

[86]   Faure E, Poissy J, Goffard A, *et al.* Distinct immune response in two MERS-CoV-infected patients: can we go from bench to bedside? PLoS One 2014; 9(2): e88716.
[http://dx.doi.org/10.1371/journal.pone.0088716] [PMID: 24551142]

[87]   Kim ES, Choe PG, Park WB, *et al.* Clinical progression and cytokine profiles of Middle East respiratory syndrome coronavirus infection. J Korean Med Sci 2016; 31(11): 1717-25.
[http://dx.doi.org/10.3346/jkms.2016.31.11.1717] [PMID: 27709848]

[88]   Yu P, Xu Y, Deng W, *et al.* Comparative pathology of rhesus macaque and common marmoset animal models with Middle East respiratory syndrome coronavirus. PLoS One 2017; 12(2): e0172093.
[http://dx.doi.org/10.1371/journal.pone.0172093] [PMID: 28234937]

[89]   Zhao J, Li K, Wohlford-Lenane C, *et al.* Rapid generation of a mouse model for Middle East respiratory syndrome. Proc Natl Acad Sci USA 2014; 111(13): 4970-5.
[http://dx.doi.org/10.1073/pnas.1323279111] [PMID: 24599590]

[90]   Zhao J, Zhao J, Mangalam AK, *et al.* Airway memory CD4+ T cells mediate protective immunity against emerging respiratory coronaviruses. Immunity 2016; 44(6): 1379-91.
[http://dx.doi.org/10.1016/j.immuni.2016.05.006] [PMID: 27287409]

[91]   Wong RSM, Wu A, To KF, *et al.* Haematological manifestations in patients with severe acute respiratory syndrome: retrospective analysis. BMJ 2003; 326(7403): 1358-62.
[http://dx.doi.org/10.1136/bmj.326.7403.1358] [PMID: 12816821]

[92]   Wong C, Lam C, Wu A, *et al.* Plasma inflammatory cytokines and chemokines in severe acute respiratory syndrome. Clinical and Experimental Immunology 2004; 136(1): 95–103,
[http://dx.doi.org/10.1111/j.1365-2249.2004.02415.x]

[93]   Su M, Chen Y, Qi S, Shi D, Feng L, Sun D. A Mini-Review on Cell Cycle Regulation of Coronavirus Infection. Front Vet Sci 2020; 7: 586826.
[http://dx.doi.org/10.3389/fvets.2020.586826] [PMID: 33251267]

[94]   Bacon LD, Hunter DB, Zhang HM, Brand K, Etches R. Retrospective evidence that the MHC (B haplotype) of chickens influences genetic resistance to attenuated infectious bronchitis vaccine strains in chickens. Avian Pathol 2004; 33(6): 605-9.
[http://dx.doi.org/10.1080/03079450400013147] [PMID: 15763730]

[95]   Addie DD, Kennedy LJ, Ryvar R, *et al.* Feline leucocyte antigen class II polymorphism and susceptibility to feline infectious peritonitis. J Feline Med Surg 2004; 6(2): 59-62.
[http://dx.doi.org/10.1016/j.jfms.2003.12.010] [PMID: 15123149]

[96]   O'Brien SJ, Roelke ME, Marker L, *et al.* Genetic basis for species vulnerability in the cheetah. Science 1985; 227(4693): 1428-34.
[http://dx.doi.org/10.1126/science.2983425] [PMID: 2983425]

[97]   Debnath M, Banerjee M, Berk M. Genetic gateways to COVID-19 infection: Implications for risk, severity, and outcomes. FASEB J 2020; 34(7): 8787-95.
[http://dx.doi.org/10.1096/fj.202001115R] [PMID: 32525600]

[98]   Barquera R, Collen E, Di D, *et al.* Binding affinities of 438 HLA proteins to complete proteomes of seven pandemic viruses and distributions of strongest and weakest HLA peptide binders in populations worldwide. HLA 2020; 96(3): 277-98.
[http://dx.doi.org/10.1111/tan.13956] [PMID: 32475052]

[99]   Nguyen A, David JK, Maden SK, *et al.* Human leukocyte antigen susceptibility map for severe acute respiratory syndrome coronavirus. J Virol 2020; 94(13): e00510-20.
[http://dx.doi.org/10.1128/JVI.00510-20] [PMID: 32303592]

[100]   Mihm S. COVID-19: Possible impact of the genetic background in IFNL genes on disease outcomes. J Innate Immun 2020; 12(3): 273-4.
[http://dx.doi.org/10.1159/000508076] [PMID: 32344401]

[101]   Chen LL. The biogenesis and emerging roles of circular RNAs. Nat Rev Mol Cell Biol 2016; 17(4): 205-11.
[http://dx.doi.org/10.1038/nrm.2015.32] [PMID: 26908011]

[102]   Holdt LM, Kohlmaier A, Teupser D, Sciences ML. Molecular roles and function of circular RNAs in eukaryotic cells. Cell Mol Life Sci 2018; 75(6): 1071-98.
[http://dx.doi.org/10.1007/s00018-017-2688-5] [PMID: 29116363]

[103]   Lasda E, Parker R. Circular RNAs: diversity of form and function. RNA 2014; 20(12): 1829-42.
[http://dx.doi.org/10.1261/rna.047126.114] [PMID: 25404635]

[104]   López-Jiménez E, Rojas AM, Andrés-León E. RNA sequencing and prediction tools for circular RNAs analysis. Adv Exp Med Biol 2018; 1087: 17-33.
[http://dx.doi.org/10.1007/978-981-13-1426-1_2] [PMID: 30259354]

[105]   Hansen TB, Jensen TI, Clausen BH, *et al.* Natural RNA circles function as efficient microRNA sponges. Nature 2013; 495(7441): 384-8.
[http://dx.doi.org/10.1038/nature11993] [PMID: 23446346]

[106]   Salmena L, Poliseno L, Tay Y, Kats L, Pandolfi PP. A ceRNA hypothesis: the Rosetta Stone of a hidden RNA language? Cell 2011; 146(3): 353-8.
[http://dx.doi.org/10.1016/j.cell.2011.07.014] [PMID: 21802130]

[107]   Zhang X, Chu H, Wen L, *et al.* Competing endogenous RNA network profiling reveals novel host dependency factors required for MERS-CoV propagation. Emerg Microbes Infect 2020; 9(1): 733-46.
[http://dx.doi.org/10.1080/22221751.2020.1738277] [PMID: 32223537]

[108]   Welsh RM, Waggoner SN. NK cells controlling virus-specific T cells: Rheostats for acute *vs.* persistent infections. Virology 2013; 435(1): 37-45.
[http://dx.doi.org/10.1016/j.virol.2012.10.005] [PMID: 23217614]

[109]   Jordan JA, Guo RF, Yun EC, *et al.* Role of IL-18 in acute lung inflammation. J Immunol 2001; 167(12): 7060-8.
[http://dx.doi.org/10.4049/jimmunol.167.12.7060] [PMID: 11739527]

[110]   Masters PS. The molecular biology of coronaviruses. Adv Virus Res 2006; 66: 193-292.
[http://dx.doi.org/10.1016/S0065-3527(06)66005-3] [PMID: 16877062]

[111]   Almeida MS, Johnson MA, Herrmann T, Geralt M, Wüthrich K. Novel β-barrel fold in the nuclear magnetic resonance structure of the replicase nonstructural protein 1 from the severe acute respiratory syndrome coronavirus. J Virol 2007; 81(7): 3151-61.
[http://dx.doi.org/10.1128/JVI.01939-06] [PMID: 17202208]

[112]   Lokugamage KG, Narayanan K, Huang C, Makino S. Severe acute respiratory syndrome coronavirus protein nsp1 is a novel eukaryotic translation inhibitor that represses multiple steps of translation initiation. J Virol 2012; 86(24): 13598-608.
[http://dx.doi.org/10.1128/JVI.01958-12] [PMID: 23035226]

[113]   Lokugamage KG, Narayanan K, Nakagawa K, *et al.* Middle East respiratory syndrome coronavirus

nsp1 inhibits host gene expression by selectively targeting mRNAs transcribed in the nucleus while sparing mRNAs of cytoplasmic origin. J Virol 2015; 89(21): 10970-81.
[http://dx.doi.org/10.1128/JVI.01352-15] [PMID: 26311885]

[114] Kamitani W, Huang C, Narayanan K, Lokugamage KG, Makino S. A two-pronged strategy to suppress host protein synthesis by SARS coronavirus Nsp1 protein. Nat Struct Mol Biol 2009; 16(11): 1134-40.
[http://dx.doi.org/10.1038/nsmb.1680] [PMID: 19838190]

[115] Huang C, Lokugamage KG, Rozovics JM, Narayanan K, Semler BL, Makino S. SARS coronavirus nsp1 protein induces template-dependent endonucleolytic cleavage of mRNAs: viral mRNAs are resistant to nsp1-induced RNA cleavage. PLoS Pathog 2011; 7(12): e1002433.
[http://dx.doi.org/10.1371/journal.ppat.1002433] [PMID: 22174690]

[116] Terada Y, Kawachi K, Matsuura Y, Kamitani W. MERS coronavirus nsp1 participates in an efficient propagation through a specific interaction with viral RNA. Virology 2017; 511: 95-105.
[http://dx.doi.org/10.1016/j.virol.2017.08.026] [PMID: 28843094]

[117] Raj VS, Smits SL, Provacia LB, *et al.* Adenosine deaminase acts as a natural antagonist for dipeptidyl peptidase 4-mediated entry of the Middle East respiratory syndrome coronavirus. J Virol 2014; 88(3): 1834-8.
[http://dx.doi.org/10.1128/JVI.02935-13] [PMID: 24257613]

[118] Coleman CM, Matthews KL, Goicochea L, Frieman MB. Wild-type and innate immune-deficient mice are not susceptible to the Middle East respiratory syndrome coronavirus. J Gen Virol 2014; 95(2): 408-12.
[http://dx.doi.org/10.1099/vir.0.060640-0] [PMID: 24197535]

[119] Haagmans BL, van den Brand JMA, Provacia LB, *et al.* Asymptomatic Middle East respiratory syndrome coronavirus infection in rabbits. J Virol 2015; 89(11): 6131-5.
[http://dx.doi.org/10.1128/JVI.00661-15] [PMID: 25810539]

[120] Wernery U, Corman VM, Wong EY, *et al.* Acute middle East respiratory syndrome coronavirus infection in livestock Dromedaries, Dubai, 2014, Emerg Infect Dis 2015, 21(6): 1019–1022.
[http://dx.doi.org/10.3201/eid2106.150038]

[121] Munster VJ, de Wit E, Feldmann H. Pneumonia from human coronavirus in a macaque model. N Engl J Med 2013; 368(16): 1560-2.
[http://dx.doi.org/10.1056/NEJMc1215691] [PMID: 23550601]

[122] de Wit E, Rasmussen AL, Falzarano D, *et al.* Middle East respiratory syndrome coronavirus (MERS-CoV) causes transient lower respiratory tract infection in rhesus macaques. Proc Natl Acad Sci USA 2013; 110(41): 16598-603.
[http://dx.doi.org/10.1073/pnas.1310744110] [PMID: 24062443]

[123] Falzarano D, de Wit E, Feldmann F, *et al.* Infection with MERS-CoV causes lethal pneumonia in the common marmoset. PLoS Pathog 2014; 10(8): e1004250.
[http://dx.doi.org/10.1371/journal.ppat.1004250] [PMID: 25144235]

[124] LoPresti M, Beck DB, Duggal P, Cummings DA, Solomon BDJTAJoHG. The role of host genetic factors in coronavirus susceptibility: review of animal and systematic review of human literature Am J Human Genetics 2020; 107(3): 381-402.
[http://dx.doi.org/10.1016/j.ajhg.2020.08.007]

[125] Patarčić I, Gelemanović A, Kirin M, *et al.* The role of host genetic factors in respiratory tract infectious diseases: systematic review, meta-analyses and field synopsis. Sci Rep 2015; 5(1): 16119.
[http://dx.doi.org/10.1038/srep16119] [PMID: 26524966]

CHAPTER 3

History of SARS-CoV-2

Qurat ul Ain Babar[1], **Ayesha Saeed**[1], **Maryam Bashir**[2], **Kamal Niaz**[3], **Muhammad Rafiq**[2], **Muhammad Yasir Waqas**[2], **Muhammad Farrukh Tahir**[4], **Amjad Islam Aqib**[5], **Muhammad Dilawar**[6] and **Muhammad Farrukh Nisar**[2,*]

[1] *Department of Biochemistry, Govt. College University, Faisalabad, Pakistan*

[2] *Department of Physiology and Biochemistry, Faculty of Bio-Sciences, Cholistan University of Veterinary and Animal Sciences (CUVAS), Bahawalpur 63100, Pakistan*

[3] *Department of Toxicology and Pharmacology, Faculty of Bio-Sciences, Cholistan University of Veterinary and Animal Sciences (CUVAS), Bahawalpur 63100, Pakistan*

[4] *Department of Biochemistry, University of Jhang, Jhang 38000, Pakistan*

[5] *Department of Medicine, Cholistan University of Veterinary and Animal Sciences (CUVAS), Bahawalpur 63100, Pakistan*

[6] *Department of Zoology, Cholistan University of Veterinary and Animal Sciences (CUVAS), Bahawalpur 63100, Pakistan*

Abstract: Human CoVs (hCoVs) were discovered in people suffering from the common cold during the early 1960s. This family is comprised of four well-known genera, viz. α-CoV, β-CoV, γ-CoV, and Δ-CoV. Mammals, including humans, pigs, cats, and bats, may be infected by α-CoV and or β-CoV. γ-CoV mainly affects avifauna, whereas Δ-CoVs affect both birds and mammals. The coronavirus (CoV) outbreak has caused great devastation globally. CoVs are positive-sense, non-segmented single-stranded RNA viruses of the order nidovirales and the family Coronaviridae. Deep sequencing examination of lower respiratory tract pathological studies on affected people revealed the presence of a new coronavirus strain, which was termed SARS-CoV-2. Four structural proteins, viz. envelope protein (E), membrane protein (M), nucleocapsid protein (N), and spike protein (S) have also been determined. Following the very initial reports of the novel severe acute respiratory syndrome (SARS) coronavirus back in late 2019 from Wuhan, China, a plethora of research attempts arose on how SARS-CoV-2 made its entry into humans. There is still a difference in ideology for its laboratory escape or the zoonotic spread, but the exact phenomenon is not known yet. Completing a thorough review, the studies suggest that the virus's origin is more complicated than previously known.

Keywords: HCoVs, α-coronavirus, Single-stranded RNA, SARS, Wuhan.

---

[*] **Corresponding author Muhammad Farrukh Nisar:** Department of Physiology and Biochemistry, Faculty of Bio-Sciences, Cholistan University of Veterinary and Animal Sciences (CUVAS), Bahawalpur 63100, Pakistan; Tel: +92-345-7100555; E-mail: mfarrukhnisar@cuvas.edu.pk

Kamal Niaz, Muhammad Sajjad Khan & Muhammad Farrukh Nisar (Eds.)

INTRODUCTION

The coronavirus (CoV) outbreak has caused devastation across the continents. Coronaviruses (CoVs) are positive-sense, non-segmented, single-stranded RNA viruses of the order Nidovirales and the family Coronaviridae [1]. Human CoVs (hCoVs) were first discovered in people suffering from the common cold during the 1960s. This family comprises four well-known genera viz. alpha-coronavirus (α-CoV), beta-coronavirus (β-CoV), gamma-coronavirus (γ-CoV) and delta-coronavirus (Δ-CoV). Mammals, including humans, pigs, cats, and bats, may be infected by α-CoV or β-CoV. γ-CoV mainly affects avifauna, whereas Δ-CoVs affect both birds and mammals. The hCoV-NL63 and hCoV-229E of the genus α-CoV, hCoV HKU1, and hCoV-OC43 of the β-CoV lineage A are commonly implicated in the common cold in immunologically strong adults [2]. Because they spread across species and may infect a variety of animals, these viruses are referred to as zoonotic viruses. CoVs involved in the pathogenesis, such as the Middle East Respiratory Syndrome (MERS) viruses, Severe acute respiratory syndrome (SARS) viruses, and other gastrointestinal or respiratory infections, have been reported in animals and birds [3]. SARS-CoV was first discovered during SARS epidemics in Guangdong province, China, back in early this century [4, 5], while MERS-CoV caused major respiratory illness epidemics in the Middle East during 2012 [6]. These viruses have become pandemic, with SARS causing over 8096 illnesses in 26 countries and over 800 fatalities, while MERS has been found in 2500 documented human infections in 27 countries with 860 deaths (Table **1**) [7, 8]. The outbreak level of CoVs is normally linked with recombination and mutation allowing the generation of new viral strains having greater sensitivity to their newer hosts [9 - 15]. The 2019 novel coronavirus disease (CoVID-19) caused by SARS-CoV-2 was first reported in early December 2019 in Wuhan, Hubei province, China.

Table 1. Cumulative number of cases (Based on WHO 31st December 2003 data).

Areas	Female	Male	Total	Number of Deaths	Date Onset First Probable Case	Date Onset Last Probable Case
Australia	4	2	6	0	26-Feb-03	1-Apr-03
Canada	151	100	251	43	23-Feb-03	12-Jun-03
China	2674	2607	5327	349	16-Nov-02	3-Jun-03
China, Hong Kong Special Administrative Region	977	778	1755	299	15-Feb-03	31-May-03
China, Macao Special Administrative Region	0	1	1	0	5-May-03	5-May-03
China, Taiwan	218	128	346	37	25-Feb-03	15-Jun-03

(Table 1) cont.....

Areas	Female	Male	Total	Number of Deaths	Date Onset First Probable Case	Date Onset Last Probable Case
France	1	6	7	1	21-Mar-03	3-May-03
Germany	4	5	9	0	9-Mar-03	6-May-03
India	0	3	3	0	25-Apr-03	6-May-03
Indonesia	0	2	2	0	6-Apr-03	17-Apr-03
Italy	1	3	4	0	12-Mar-03	20-Apr-03
Kuwait	1	0	1	0	9-Apr-03	9-Apr-03
Malaysia	1	4	5	2	14-Mar-03	22-Apr-03
Mongolia	8	1	9	0	31-Mar-03	6-May-03
New Zealand	1	0	1	0	20-Apr-03	20-Apr-03
Philippines	8	6	14	2	25-Feb-03	5-May-03
Republic of Ireland	0	1	1	0	27-Feb-03	27-Feb-03
Republic of Korea	0	3	3	0	25-Apr-03	10-May-03
Romania	0	1	1	0	19-Mar-03	19-Mar-03
Russian Federation	0	1	1	0	5-May-03	5-May-03
Singapore	161	77	238	33	25-Feb-03	5-May-03
South Africa	0	1	1	1	3-Apr-03	3-Apr-03
Spain	0	1	1	0	26-Mar-03	26-Mar-03
Sweden	3	2	5	0	28-Mar-03	23-Apr-03
Switzerland	0	1	1	0	9-Mar-03	9-Mar-03
Thailand	5	4	9	2	11-Mar-03	27-May-03
United Kingdom	2	2	4	0	1-Mar-03	1-Apr-03
United States	13	14	27	0	24-Feb-03	13-Jul-03
Viet Nam	39	24	63	5	23-Feb-03	14-Apr-03
Total	-	-	**8096**	**774**	-	-

COVID-19 is responsible for serious respiratory infections particularly pneumonia, initially caused by an unknown source depicted by pneumonia-like symptoms and was eventually linked to a seafood market in Wuhan [16]. Deep sequencing examination of lower respiratory tract pathological studies on affected people revealed the presence of a new coronavirus strain, which was termed SARS-CoV-2. In China, the cumulative death toll surpassed 4645 after 84778 diagnoses and hundreds of suspects to date, representing a significant decrease in recent days. Later on, SARS-CoV-2 spread in over 137 countries worldwide and almost in every continent, resulting in about 7,823,289 cases and 431,541 fatalities. According to WHO, initially, the death rate of COVID-19 in China was

2.3% compared to SARS (9.6%) and MERS (34.4%) [17]. The exact number of mortalities caused by COVID-19 is hard to estimate due to the constant hike in cases and deaths worldwide [18]. The scientific, medical, imaging, and potential epidemiologic aspects of such viruses were first documented in clinical trials [19].

SARS-CoV-2 is a single-stranded RNA enveloped β-CoV that causes COVID-19, an acute respiratory disease. The genome of SARS-CoV-2 is nearly 30 kilobases long, and it encodes both structural and non-structural proteins (Fig. **1**). Severe social exclusion has slowed the development of the disease, but a lack of valid drugs means that the most susceptible among us tend to be severely infected with the more severe and fatal pulmonary aspects of COVID-19 [20]. So far, there are no recognized or efficient methods of reducing the effects of COVID-19 pulmonary infection (PI) and the accompanying acute respiratory distress syndrome other than high acuity mechanical ventilation and typical critical care management procedures (ARDS). Accordingly, immediate research and application of the latest technological approaches for the treatment of COVID-19 PI will be required. Local administration of antiviral therapies, in addition to pharmacological and supportive techniques, may represent a potentially key pathway in our defense against SARS-CoV-2.

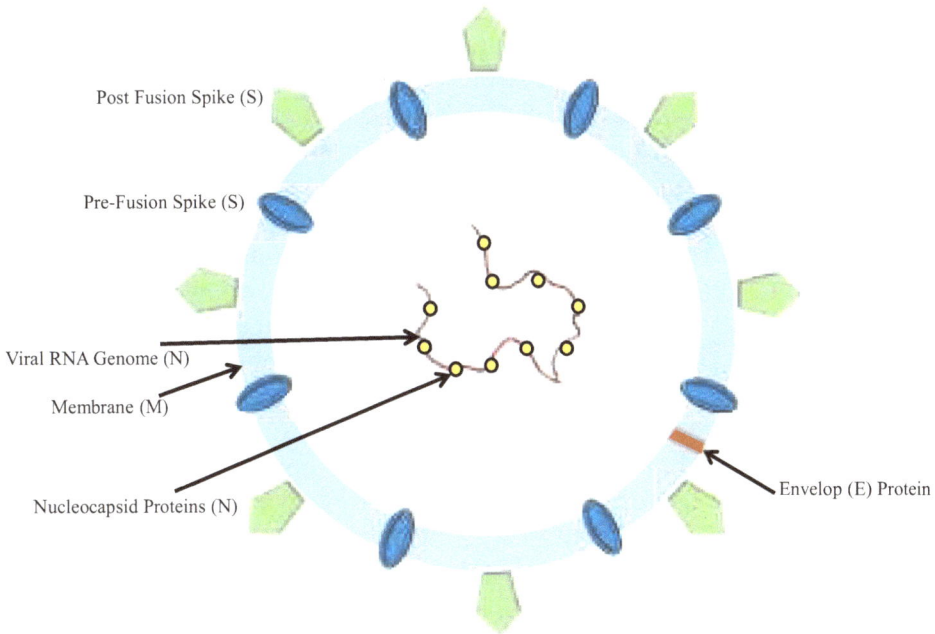

Fig. (1). Structure of the SAR-CoV-2.

SARS-CoV-2 Genesis Theories

At the start of the pandemic, most of the first cases of COVID-19 were linked to the seafood market of Hunan, which was believed to be the root cause of SARS-CoV-2 [21]. However, further research by many Chinese teams called this theory into question. For starters, several of the early instances had no epidemiologic connection to the marketplace [22]. Secondly, intensive screening and testing for SARS-CoV-2 in frozen foods and local animals in the Wuhan area did not produce positive findings [23]. Moreover, coronaviruses that were evolutionarily similar to SARS-CoV-2 were discovered in rhinolophus bats in South Asian nations such as Thailand, Japan, Cambodia, and China, as well as pangolins imported into China from South Asian countries [21, 24]. Furthermore, several minor concentrations of COVID-19 infections in China have been confirmed as the consequence of cold-chain transmission from other regions or contaminated food. Such studies suggest that the virus's origin is more complicated than previously understood [22].

Several ideas regarding the origins of SARS-CoV-2 became viral throughout the global epidemic response, misinforming both the authorities and the public. Certain theories include that the virus is an artificial biological weapon created by genetic changes, unintentional loss of the lab that caused the epidemic, and the virus that scientists unintentionally introduced while on the job. These baseless and deceitful theories have been strongly rejected by the scientific community. Everyone generally accepts that SARS-CoV-2 has a real origin source and was detected either in humans after zoonotic transmission or in an animal host before zoonotic transmission [25, 26]. The "Chinese Academy of Sciences" Wuhan Institute of Virology (WIV) has been conducting a long-term investigation on natural SARS-CoV reservoirs and was one of the first institutes to identify SARS-CoV-2 following the COVID-19 pandemic [27]. Furthermore, in its preserved bat samples retrieved in 2013, WIV detected a viral sequence (RaTG13) with a 96.2% genomic sequence similarity with the SARS-CoV-2 genome [21]. These findings give an essential hint about the genesis of SARS-CoV-2, as well as a basis for understanding the screening of antiviral drugs, developing diagnostic tools, determining the origin of SARS-CoV-2, and developing vaccines. Unfortunately, the WIV was at the center of misleading theories about the origins of the virus, which were not adequately addressed until recent collaborative research was conducted by a team of international experts led by the WHO and Chinese specialists [22, 28].

Global Study of SARS-CoV-2 Origin: China

The expert team has been divided into three sections: i) animal and environment, ii) epidemiology, and iii) molecular research. The specialists collaborated *via* videoconferencing, on-site visits and interviews, and extended considerations. The team spent four weeks reviewing massive quantities of pandemic data and visiting numerous institutions, including the Wuhan National Biosafety Laboratory, the Center for Prevention and Control of Wuhan Diseases, and Wuhan Jinyintan Hospital. They also visited the Hunan seafood market. The researchers conducted interviews with scientists, recovered COVID-19 patients, natives, market managers, local medical personnel, and laboratory workers [22]. The team visited the Wuhan P4 laboratory, which is thought to be the most likely source of the SARS-CoV-2. The Wuhan P4 laboratory is the first to have such facilities in China, and it performs high-level biosafety assessments. The laboratory was designed by French specialists and built by French and Chinese engineers and is approved by the China National Accreditation Service (CNAS) for Conformity Assessment. It was intended to serve as a laboratory for investigating highly classified microorganisms as well as an international partnership research center for emerging infectious illnesses [29]. The China National Health Commission (CNHC) approved all experiments in this laboratory using particular viruses. These two Chinese agencies have strictly monitored all management and administration and have evaluated and analyzed it regularly. Since its beginning at the end of 2017, it has been evaluated four times by CNAS and three times by CNHC. This laboratory is currently authorized to investigate the SARS-CoV-2 2, Xinjiang hemorrhagic fever virus, Nipah virus, and Ebola virus. Through appropriate animal studies and inactivated vaccine production, medication testing, and fundamental research for understanding SARS-CoV-2, this laboratory was crucial in combating the COVID-19 outbreak [30].

The WHO joint team spoke extensively with the scientists, laboratory manager, and employees and applauded the WIV leadership and personnel for their collaboration, honesty, and flexibility. "They preserved a highly rigid and high-quality management system," the team said. "In addition, based on the present facts, we consider the lab leak theory to be exceedingly doubtful," Wuhan stated in a public announcement on February 9, 2021 [31]. The scientists also released new information on the origins of SARS-CoV-2. Among the causes include cold-chain food-borne contamination, direct zoonotic spillover, and intermediate host species. Scientists have indicated that the introduction of the virus *via* an intermediate host species is "the most plausible route. The cold chain is also likely to be transmitted directly or through food. To further understand the origin of

SARS-CoV-2, the researchers propose more studies, including substantial screening of human and animal samples from all across the world, not only in China [32].

Over 70% of new or re-emerging infectious diseases in recent decades have been zoonoses, which have been transferred to humans from their animal reservoirs *via* intermediate hosts. A massive number of undiscovered viruses remain in their natural reservoirs and keep changing, resulting in the emergence of new strains. Many of these viruses may have inherent properties that allow them to traverse species boundaries and cause disease [33]. Rapid global economic growth, such as urbanization, land use, domestication of animals, and intensive agriculture, increases the likelihood of human contact with wildlife, increasing the risk of interspecies transmission of native wild viruses and animals. Long-term and intensive scientific monitoring is the greatest technique for avoiding potential zoonosis. We need to know about undiscovered viruses, estimate the hazards of transmission between species, identify hotspots of human-animal interfaces, and finally develop diagnostic tools to monitor high-risk human and animal populations. With this preventive technique, we can quickly identify and stop the spread of new infections at a preliminary phase, thus preventing the next pandemic. For this purpose, professionals from many disciplines, such as clinical specialists, ecologists, epidemiologists, lawmakers, microbiologists, sociologists, and veterinarians, must collaborate scientifically [34, 35].

SARS-CoV-2 Genomic Evolution

Like SARS-CoV, the SARS-CoV-2 genome is comprised of single-stranded RNA molecules having 82% nucleotide sequence similarity, while 89% sequence similarity with that of SARS-like CoVZXC21 [36]. The SARS-CoV-2 genome (29,891 nucleotide bases) encodes a huge number of (9860) amino acids. The molecular genetic studies revealed about 79% similarity of SARS-CoV-2 with SARS-CoV and 50% with MERS-CoV [37]. The replicase enzyme, spike (S), envelop (E) proteins, membrane (M) proteins, and nucleocapsid (N) are present in the virus particle [36]; however, unlike lineage A β-COVs, SARS-CoV-2 lacks the hemagglutinin-esterase gene. As the COVID-19 outbreak spreads, additional viral genomes are being sequenced. The oldest specimens from Wuhan showed significantly reduced genetic variation, while this rules out general phylogenetic conclusions, this does show that public medical professionals in Wuhan did an excellent job of identifying the initial group of pneumonia patients [38]. However, a pre-outbreak phase of mysterious transmission in humans is not ruled out by this shared ancestry. Although increasing genetic diversity allows for the detection of different phylogenetic groups of SARS-CoV-2 sequences, using genomic comparisons alone, it is difficult to establish if the virus is repairing phenotypically relevant changes as it spreads over the world population, and any such assertions require careful confirmation. Given the immense mutation rates of the RNA virus, it is evident that many additional changes will arise in the viral genome, which will aid in tracking the spread of SARS-CoV-2 [39]. However, when the endemic spreads, our sequencing sample size will probably be so limited in comparison to the total number of patients that it would be difficult to discover individual chains of transmission. When attempting to identify precise transmission events, care must always be maintained. Although coronaviruses are likely to experience reduced mutation rates compared to other RNA viruses due to the possibility of some replay activity due to 30-50 exo-ribonuclease, their long-term genetic recombination rates come from the dispersal of other RNA viruses [40, 41]. This shows that higher viral replication rates within hosts compensate for lower mutation rates. While there is no indication that this ability to mutate would result in dramatic changes in phenotype, as they very rarely change in size in particular outbreaks, it is certainly important to monitor changes in phenotype as the virus is spreading. Any decrease in the number of cases of COVID-19 is very certainly related to growing immunity in humans and the epidemiologic setting instead of alterations in the virus caused by mutations [38, 42].

Evaluation of SARS-CoV-2 Phylogeny and Genomics

Coronaviruses are RNA viruses with a positive strand. They can be found in a wide range of animal species that might or might not induce disease signs in their hosts [43 - 45]. CoV groups are considered to have separated from each other around 2400-3000 BC, and they tend to infect various types of mammals (Fig. **2**). α-CoV and β-CoV are usually found in mammals, but γ-CoV and Δ-CoV are mostly found in birds. However, γ-CoV infects some cetaceans, such as bottlenose dolphins and belugas [46]. The CoVs that have produced recent epidemics and pandemics of illnesses in human populations, including COVID-19, MERS, and SARS, are members of a subclass of β-CoV identified as Sarbecovirus [47]. This CoV family is found in bats as well as other mammals. HCoV-NL63 and HCoV-229E are α-CoV strains among the four commonly identified CoV strains connected to mild symptoms of the common cold in humans, whereas HCoV-HKU1 and HCoV-OC43 are Embecoviruses, a subtype of β-CoV [48]. CoVs are highly prone to recombination [49]. If animals carrying various CoVs come into touch and exchange viruses, recombination between the multiple strains can occur, leading to diversity. Sadly, it appears that similar occurrences in SARS-evolutionary CoV-2's history resulted in the generation of a strong variant able to infect human cells effectively.

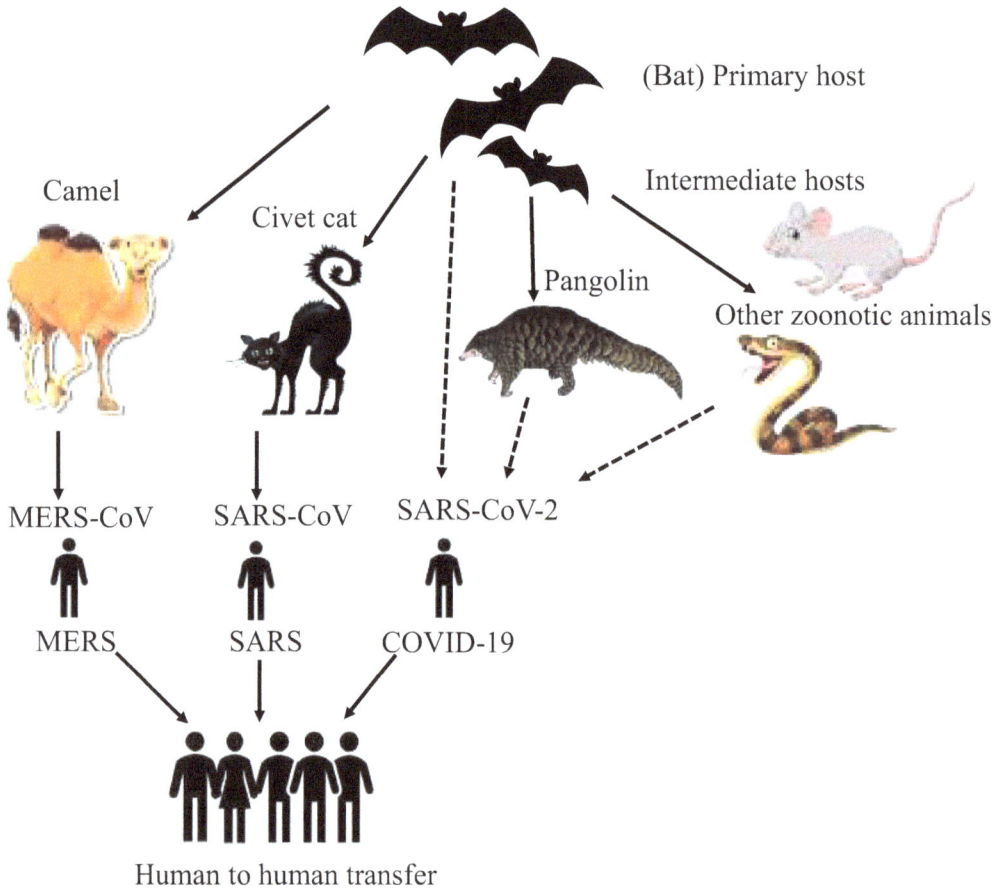

Fig. (2). Origin of various coronaviruses along with intermediary hosts during evolution.

SARS-CoV-2, like other CoVs, has a 30kb genome that encodes four structural proteins: i) E, ii) M, iii) N, and iv) S [50, 51]. In general, the SARS-CoV-2 genome contains some nonstructural open reading frames (ORFs) [51]. Research indicated that more than 60% of all transcriptomes in infected human samples were viral, revealing massive and vital changes in cell biology that occur when human cells are infected. Interestingly, these transcripts contained incomplete transcripts as well as non-canonical fusion transcripts, which had previously been identified in earlier CoV research [52, 53]. While the functional relevance of these transcripts is uncertain, their existence indicates that such a virus is sensitive to a variety of recombination processes inside hosts. A CoV strain discovered in a bat sample from Yunnan province, China, in 2013 is one of the closest known relatives of SARS-CoV-2. This strain is known under the name of "RaTG13". It is widely believed that the genomic sequence of this strain is 96% identical to that of SARS-CoV-2 [50]. A first look showed a similarity of 96% which suggests a tight link between these two virus strains. Given some prior information on how quickly CoV sequences acquire nucleotide changes over time, we can calculate the period between the two strains' most recent common ancestor (tMRCA). SARS-genome CoV-2s are almost completely made up of protein-coding sequences, a feature shared by other coronaviruses [54]. This measure may be used to assess the time of deviation between SARS-CoV-2 and RaTG13 [55]. Recent research examined similar alterations in CoV genomes and calculated equivalent mutation rates ranging from 1.67-4.67×10^{-3}/site/year [56]. More investigations of mutation rates in CoV, including SARS-CoV-2, have yielded comparable results. Numerous studies suggested that the mutation rates in SARS-CoV-2 were 1.19-1.31×10^{-3}/site/year and 1.5-3.3×10^{-3}/site/year,. When these data are compared, the divergence period between RaTG13 and SARS-CoV-2 might be anywhere between 18 and 71.4 years. Divergence times have been estimated using more complex approaches in studies that have yielded comparable results [57]. Specifically, the MRCA of SARS-CoV-2 and RaTG13 was projected to exist in 1969 using a Bayesian phylogenetic technique. RaTG13 and SARSCoV2 are rather distinct in terms of the extremely short periods of viral generation. More CoVs that are significantly more closely related to SARS-CoV-2 are quite likely to exist. Given the wide variety of CoVs seen in bats and other species, comprehensive sequencing of these CoVs must provide a CoV variant more closely related to SARS-CoV-2 [47].

The second point to remember is that while RaTG13 is closely linked to SARS-CoV-2, there is significant fluctuation in sequence homology between these two viruses' genomes, varying between 93.1 to 99.6% [58]. Because of the underlying diversity in mutation rates, some variation across genomic areas is frequently detected in the comparison of genome sequences [59]. Phylogenetic comparison to other CoV variants and reported CoV recombination events, on the other hand, suggest that SARS-CoV-2 underwent complex crossing-over events during its evolution. As a result, the evolutionary history of various genomic segments can vary, and altered parts of the SARS-CoV-2 genome might have significantly different genotypes with CoV strains other than RaTG13 [47].

Studies Indicating Zoonotic Origins of SARS-CoV-2

The α-CoVs HCoV-NL63 and HCoV-229E, as well as the β-CoVs HCoV-HKU1 and HCoV-OC43, are endemic hCoVs, whereas emergent hCoVs include the β-CoVs MERS-CoV, SARS-CoV, and the new SARS-CoV-2. The genomic sequence distances between CoV species are used to characterize them. Members of the viral species SARS-related CoV, which includes SARS-CoV-2 and SARS-CoV, as well as several genetically diverse bat-associated strains, may infect hosts from four distinct animal orders, including primates, pangolins, carnivores, and bats. The wide range of heterospecific bat CoVs and their common ancestral connection to human viruses imply that bats might be possible animal reservoirs for the bulk of HCoVs [60]. In the context of SARS-related CoVs, rhinolophid bats are especially important natural hosts, as evidenced by the wide range of genetically diverse SARS-related CoVs discovered in those bats native to Europe, Africa, and Asia [61]. The direct interaction between bats and humans, which can promote human infection, is more common in the tropics than in temperate climates, including the ingestion of bats as bush meat and the use of bats as traditional medicine [62]. Other species beyond bats, although, have been identified as intermediary hosts and sources of HCoV infection (Fig. **3**) [63]. α-CoVs observed in camels and alpacas, for example, have a common origin with HCoV-229E, but HCoV-OC43 shares a common ancestor with CoVs found in cattle [64]. The developing MERS-CoV is endemic in camels and produces frequent human infections. SARS-CoV was discovered in raccoon dogs and masked palm civets sold in an animal market in Guangdong province, China [65]. Genomic analyses of SARS-CoV sequences from humans and civets revealed 99.6% nucleotide similarity. SARS-related CoVs with a wide genetic diversity were discovered in Chinese horseshoe bats in 2005 [66]. As a result, masked palm civets were most likely intermediate hosts, while horseshoe bats were most likely the SARS-evolutionary CoV's origin. It has been proposed that changes in the SARS-CoV receptor-binding region may have occurred in palm civets, facilitating infection efficiency by boosting binding to the human angiotensin-converting enzyme 2 (hACE2) receptor [67].

Attempts to find probable SARS-CoV-2 intermediary hosts have been unsuccessful thus far. During epidemiological studies on the first cases, the Huanan seafood market in Wuhan was linked to the outbreak's genesis, which was confirmed by SARS-CoV-2-positive samples collected from that market [68]. Retrospective epidemiological research revealed that a former COVID-19 patient had no contact with that seafood market [38]. Therefore, the cause of the pandemic is unknown. So far, the closest known human relatives of SARS-CoV2 are an intermediate horseshoe bat coronavirus from China with nearly 96% nucleotide authenticity and two SARS-related CoVs found in Malayan pangolins with 85.5-92% with nucleotide authenticity of 4%, which is currently averaged over the entire viral genome [67]. Furthermore, phylogenetic investigations of a large subgenomic data set of Chinese bat CoVs show that, like SARS-CoV, SARS-CoV-2 probably evolved in horseshoe bats [69]. However, zoonotic infections of humans with civet-associated SARS-CoV strain were probably due to the genetic similarity of those CoVs, pangolin-, human- and bat-associated SARS-CoV-2 variants are not as strongly linked, and the direct ancestor of SARS-CoV-2 variants infecting people remains unknown [67].

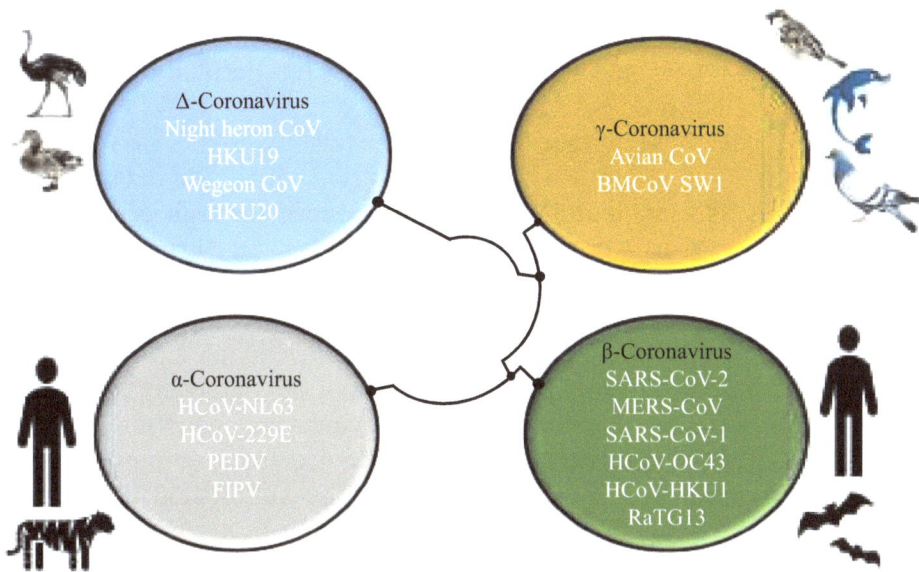

Fig. (3). The evolutionary link of four genera of CoVs with their animal host [44].

Is it Possible that SARS-CoV-2 Got Out of the Lab?

There are examples of laboratory accidents that resulted in discrete illnesses and temporary transmission chains, such as SARS-CoV [70]. Besides the Marburg virus, all recorded laboratory breakouts have been of easily recognized viruses able to infect humans and connected with long-term work in high-titer culture [34]. The sole reported case of a human pandemic produced by science is the A/H1N1 influenza outbreak of 1977, which most probably resulted from an extensive vaccine challenge study. There is no evidence that WIV worked on SARS-CoV-2 or any virus closely enough to be the ancestor before the COVID-19 pandemic. The risk of viral genome sequencing without cell culture exists since viruses are inactivated following RNA extraction, which was regularly conducted at the WIV [71]. No laboratory leaks were reported after sequencing the viral sample. Outbreaks reported in the laboratory have been linked to the working environments of index cases, family members, and the originating laboratory [72]. Despite rigorous surveillance of the first cases during the COVID-19 outbreak, no infections involving WIV laboratory staff have been documented. When tested for SARS-CoV-2 in March 2020, all workers in Dr. Shi Zhengli's lab were found to be seronegative, with the lab presumably following the required biosecurity measures when working on CoV [29, 40]. To be significant during a period of high influenza transmission and other respiratory virus circulation, reports of illnesses triggered by SARS-CoV-2 need to be confirmed. According to epidemiological modeling, the number of potential instances required to result in numerous hospitalized COVID-19 patients before December 2019 is irreconcilable with clinical, genomic, and epidemiological evidence [73]. The WIV has a large collection of bat-derived materials and has effectively cultivated three SARS-CoVs from bats: Rs4874, WIV16, and WIV1 [69]. Notably, all these viruses are connected to SARS/CoV rather than SARS/CoV2. In comparison, RaTG13, a WIV bat virus, has never been grown and only appears as a nucleotide sequence produced through brief sequencing. reads [74]. These viruses were obtained from feces using serial amplification in Vero E6 cells, a method that probably resulted in the deletion of the SARS-CoV-2 cleavage site of furin. As a result, it is exceedingly improbable that these procedures would result in the identification of a SARS/CoV2 progenitor with an intact cleavage site of furin. There is no reported evidence that alternative strategies, such as the development of innovative reverse genetics systems, were utilized at the WIV to replicate infectious SARS-CoVs based on bat sequencing data. Gain of function research (GoFR) would be anticipated to use a proven SARS-CoV genetic backbone or, at the very least, a virus discovered by sequencing. Previous WIV experimental studies employing recombinant CoV utilized a genetic backbone unrelated to SARS-CoV-2 and later finds no trace of genetic markers that would be expected from laboratory tests [40]. Without scientific proof of a SARS-CoV-2-like virus in any preceding WIV publication or research, there is no logical justification to design a new genetic system employing an undiscovered and unproven virus. There is no evidence that the WIV cataloged a virus that is more like SARS-CoV-2 than RaTG13, and there was no need to conduct research on a SARS-CoV-2 -similar virus before the COVID-19 pandemic. SARS-CoV-2 should have been available in a lab before the pandemic in any lab escape scenario, but no evidence is available to support this theory, and no sequencing has been discovered that could have acted as a predecessor. An example of a laboratory leak scenario is unintentional infection during the sequential passage of a SARS-CoV in normal lab animals, for example, mice. The first isolates of SARS-CoV-2, on the other hand, failed to infect wild mice [75]. Although mouse models are important for investigating infection *in vivo* and screening vaccines, in hACE2 transgenic mice, they frequently vary from mild or unusual illnesses [34]. These data contradict the hypothesis that the virus was chosen for its enhanced virulence and mode of transmission *via* repeated transit through vulnerable rats. Although SARS-CoV-2 has now been produced and serially passed through mice, certain alterations in the spike protein, such as N501Y, are required for such adaption in mice [34, 76]. Importantly, N501Y has emerged in numerous SARS-CoV-2 strains of interest in the human population, likely to boost ACE2 binding ability [77]. If attempts to alter a SARS-CoV for study on experimental models resulted in SARS-CoV-2, for effective replication in this approach, it would have most likely acquired alterations like N501Y. The low virulence of SARS-CoV-2 in regularly used laboratory animals, as well as the absence of genomic markers associated with rodent adaptation, implies that SARS-CoV-2 was probably acquired by laboratory workers during disease pathogenesis or GoFR [34].

CONCLUSION

This whole pandemic era is one of history's most severe health crises in recent times. COVID-19, caused by SARS-CoV-2, was first reported in early December 2019 in Wuhan, Hubei Province, China. Proper identification of the origin of SARS-CoV-2 may aid in avoiding any future epidemics of newer and novel coronavirus strains. A huge number of ideas that represent the zoonotic origin of SARS-CoV-2 have been raised. To date, most people agree that β-CoV found in Rhinolophus bats from China based on genetic similarity (genomic SpG dinucleotide patterns) with SARS-CoV-2 is highly accepted and declared as the sole ancestor to date. Moreover, these genomic CpG-dinucleotide patterns suggest that SARS-CoV-2 possibly evolved in a canid gastrointestinal tract before transmission to humans. It is highly suggested to add additional biomarkers to explore any unknown intermediate hosts or tissues.

AUTHOR CONTRIBUTION

QAB, AS, and MB compiled the draft. KN, MR, MYW, and MFN conceptualized this study. QAB, MFT, AIA, and MFN prepared the figures. MR, MYW, KN, and MFN reviewed the draft to its final form.

ACKNOWLEDGEMENTS

The authors acknowledge CUVAS for facilitating in the compilation of the draft.

REFERENCES

[1]　Huang C, Wang Y, Li X, *et al.* Clinical features of patients infected with 2019 novel coronavirus in Wuhan, China. Lancet 2020; 395(10223): 497-506.
[http://dx.doi.org/10.1016/S0140-6736(20)30183-5] [PMID: 31986264]

[2]　Su S, Wong G, Shi W, *et al.* Epidemiology, genetic recombination, and pathogenesis of coronaviruses. Trends Microbiol 2016; 24(6): 490-502.

[http://dx.doi.org/10.1016/j.tim.2016.03.003] [PMID: 27012512]

[3]   Denison MR, Graham RL, Donaldson EF, Eckerle LD, Baric RS. Coronaviruses. RNA Biol 2011; 8(2): 270-9.
       [http://dx.doi.org/10.4161/rna.8.2.15013] [PMID: 21593585]

[4]   Zhong NS, Zheng BJ, Li YM, *et al.* Epidemiology and cause of severe acute respiratory syndrome (SARS) in Guangdong, People's Republic of China, in February, 2003. Lancet 2003; 362(9393): 1353-8.
       [http://dx.doi.org/10.1016/S0140-6736(03)14630-2] [PMID: 14585636]

[5]   Ksiazek TG, Erdman D, Goldsmith CS, *et al.* A novel coronavirus associated with severe acute respiratory syndrome. N Engl J Med 2003; 348(20): 1953-66.
       [http://dx.doi.org/10.1056/NEJMoa030781] [PMID: 12690092]

[6]   Zaki AM, van Boheemen S, Bestebroer TM, Osterhaus ADME, Fouchier RAM. Isolation of a novel coronavirus from a man with pneumonia in Saudi Arabia. N Engl J Med 2012; 367(19): 1814-20.
       [http://dx.doi.org/10.1056/NEJMoa1211721] [PMID: 23075143]

[7]   WHO Summary of probable SARS cases with onset of illness from 1 November 2002 to 31 July 2003.

[8]   Middle East respiratory syndrome coronavirus. MERS-CoV 2019.

[9]   Woo PCY, Wang M, Lau SKP, *et al.* Comparative analysis of twelve genomes of three novel group 2c and group 2d coronaviruses reveals unique group and subgroup features. J Virol 2007; 81(4): 1574-85.
       [http://dx.doi.org/10.1128/JVI.02182-06] [PMID: 17121802]

[10]   Woo PCY, Lau SKP, Yip CCY, *et al.* Comparative analysis of 22 coronavirus HKU1 genomes reveals a novel genotype and evidence of natural recombination in coronavirus HKU1. J Virol 2006; 80(14): 7136-45.
       [http://dx.doi.org/10.1128/JVI.00509-06] [PMID: 16809319]

[11]   Kottier SA, Cavanagh D, Britton P. Experimental evidence of recombination in coronavirus infectious bronchitis virus. Virology 1995; 213(2): 569-80.
       [http://dx.doi.org/10.1006/viro.1995.0029] [PMID: 7491781]

[12]   Lau SKP, Woo PCY, Yip CCY, *et al.* Isolation and characterization of a novel Betacoronavirus subgroup A coronavirus, rabbit coronavirus HKU14, from domestic rabbits. J Virol 2012; 86(10): 5481-96.
       [http://dx.doi.org/10.1128/JVI.06927-11] [PMID: 22398294]

[13]   Lau SKP, Li KSM, Huang Y, *et al.* Ecoepidemiology and complete genome comparison of different strains of severe acute respiratory syndrome-related Rhinolophus bat coronavirus in China reveal bats as a reservoir for acute, self-limiting infection that allows recombination events. J Virol 2010; 84(6): 2808-19.
       [http://dx.doi.org/10.1128/JVI.02219-09] [PMID: 20071579]

[14]   Lau SKP, Lee P, Tsang AKL, *et al.* Molecular epidemiology of human coronavirus OC43 reveals evolution of different genotypes over time and recent emergence of a novel genotype due to natural recombination. J Virol 2011; 85(21): 11325-37.
       [http://dx.doi.org/10.1128/JVI.05512-11] [PMID: 21849456]

[15]   Lau SKP, Poon RWS, Wong BHL, *et al.* Coexistence of different genotypes in the same bat and serological characterization of Rousettus bat coronavirus HKU9 belonging to a novel Betacoronavirus subgroup. J Virol 2010; 84(21): 11385-94.
       [http://dx.doi.org/10.1128/JVI.01121-10] [PMID: 20702646]

[16]   Wuhan; Commission, MH, Report of clustering pneumonia of unknown etiology in Wuhan City. Wuhan Municipal Health Commission 2019.

[17]   Coronavirus Disease 2019 (COVID-19). Situation Summary 2020.

[18]   Hoseinpour Dehkordi A, Alizadeh M, Derakhshan P, Babazadeh P, Jahandideh A. Understanding

epidemic data and statistics: A case study of COVID□19. Journal of medical virology. 2020 Jul; 92(7): 868-82.

[19]   Stadler K, Masignani V, Eickmann M, *et al.* SARS — beginning to understand a new virus. Nat Rev Microbiol 2003; 1(3): 209-18.
[http://dx.doi.org/10.1038/nrmicro775] [PMID: 15035025]

[20]   Stawicki SP. Could tracheo-bronchial ultraviolet C irradiation be a valuable adjunct to the management of severe COVID-19 pulmonary infections? Int J Acad Med 2020. 6(2): p 156-158.
[http://dx.doi.org/10.4103/IJAM.IJAM_19_20]

[21]   Zhou H, Yang J, Zhou C, Chen B, Fang H, Chen S, Zhang X, Wang L, Zhang L. A review of SARS-CoV2: compared with SARS-CoV and MERS-CoV. Frontiers in Medicine. 2021 Dec 7;8: 628370.

[22]   Shi ZL. Immunity, Origins of SARS-CoV-2. Focusing on Science Infect Dis Immun 2021; 1(1): 3–4.
[http://dx.doi.org/10.1097/ID9.0000000000000008]

[23]   Shi Z. Du SRAS et du MERS à la COVID-19: un voyage pour comprendre les coronavirus des chauves-souris. Bulletin de l'Académie Nationale de Médecine 2021; 205(7): 732-6.
[http://dx.doi.org/10.1016/j.banm.2021.05.008]

[24]   Xiao K, Zhai J, Feng Y, *et al.* Isolation and characterization of 2019-nCoV-like coronavirus from Malayan pangolins. Nature 2020; 583(7815): 286-289.
[http://dx.doi.org/10.1038/s41586-020-2313-x]

[25]   Andersen KG, Rambaut A, Lipkin WI, Holmes EC, Garry RF. The proximal origin of SARS-CoV-2. Nat Med 2020; 26(4): 450-2.
[http://dx.doi.org/10.1038/s41591-020-0820-9] [PMID: 32284615]

[26]   Liu S-L, Saif LJ, Weiss SR, Su LJEM. Infections, No credible evidence supporting claims of the laboratory engineering of SARS-CoV-2. 2020; 9(1): 505-7.
[PMID: 31897164]

[27]   Ge XY, Li JL, Yang XL, *et al.* Isolation and characterization of a bat SARS-like coronavirus that uses the ACE2 receptor. Nature 2013; 503(7477): 535-8.
[http://dx.doi.org/10.1038/nature12711] [PMID: 24172901]

[28]   Zheng BJ, Guan Y, Wong KH, *et al.* SARS-related virus predating SARS outbreak, Hong Kong. Emerg Infect Dis 2004; 10(2): 176-8.
[http://dx.doi.org/10.3201/eid1002.030533] [PMID: 15030679]

[29]   Organization, W.H., WHO-convened global study of origins of SARS-CoV-2: China Part. 2021.

[30]   Gallo, R.C., China CDC Weekly: Commentary by Dr. Robert C. Gallo.

[31]   Tosif MM, Najda A, Bains A, *et al.* A comprehensive review on plant-derived mucilage: Characterization, functional properties, applications, and its utilization for nanocarrier fabrication. Polymers (Basel) 2021; 13(7): 1066.
[http://dx.doi.org/10.3390/polym13071066] [PMID: 33800613]

[32]   Koopmans M, Daszak P, Dedkov VG, Dwyer DE, Farag E, Fischer TK, Hayman DT, Leendertz F, Maeda K, Nguyen-Viet H, Watson J. Origins of SARS-CoV-2: window is closing for key scientific studies. Nature. 2021 Aug 26; 596(7873): 482-5.

[33]   Calisher CH, Carroll D, Colwell R, *et al.* Science, not speculation, is essential to determine how SARS-CoV-2 reached humans. Lancet 2021; 398(10296): 209-11.
[http://dx.doi.org/10.1016/S0140-6736(21)01419-7] [PMID: 34237296]

[34]   Holmes EC, Goldstein SA, Rasmussen AL, *et al.* The origins of SARS-CoV-2: A critical review. Cell 2021; 184(19): 4848-56.
[http://dx.doi.org/10.1016/j.cell.2021.08.017] [PMID: 34480864]

[35]   Ludwig, S., Zarbock, A. Coronaviruses and SARS-CoV-2: a brief overview. Anesth Analg 2020;131(1): 93-96.

[http://dx.doi.org/10.1213/ANE.0000000000004845]

[36]   Xu X, Chen P, Wang J, *et al.* Evolution of the novel coronavirus from the ongoing Wuhan outbreak and modeling of its spike protein for risk of human transmission. Sci China Life Sci 2020; 63(3): 457-60.
[http://dx.doi.org/10.1007/s11427-020-1637-5] [PMID: 32009228]

[37]   Mousavizadeh L, Ghasemi S. Genotype and phenotype of COVID-19: Their roles in pathogenesis. J Microbiol Immunol Infect 2021; 54(2): 159-63.
[http://dx.doi.org/10.1016/j.jmii.2020.03.022] [PMID: 32265180]

[38]   Huang C, Wang Y, Li X, *et al.* Clinical features of patients infected with 2019 novel coronavirus in Wuhan, China. Lancet 2020; 395(10223): 497-506.
[http://dx.doi.org/10.1016/S0140-6736(20)30183-5] [PMID: 31986264]

[39]   Grubaugh ND, Ladner JT, Lemey P, *et al.* Tracking virus outbreaks in the twenty-first century. Nat Microbiol 2018; 4(1): 10-9.
[http://dx.doi.org/10.1038/s41564-018-0296-2] [PMID: 30546099]

[40]   Holmes EC, Dudas G, Rambaut A, Andersen KG. The evolution of Ebola virus: Insights from the 2013–2016 epidemic. Nature 2016; 538(7624): 193-200.
[http://dx.doi.org/10.1038/nature19790] [PMID: 27734858]

[41]   Minskaia E, Hertzig T, Gorbalenya AE, *et al.* Discovery of an RNA virus 3′→5′ exoribonuclease that is critically involved in coronavirus RNA synthesis. Proc Natl Acad Sci USA 2006; 103(13): 5108-13.
[http://dx.doi.org/10.1073/pnas.0508200103] [PMID: 16549795]

[42]   Grubaugh ND, Petrone ME, Holmes EC. We shouldn't worry when a virus mutates during disease outbreaks. Nat Microbiol 2020; 5(4): 529-30.
[http://dx.doi.org/10.1038/s41564-020-0690-4] [PMID: 32071422]

[43]   Wertheim JO, Chu DKW, Peiris JSM, Kosakovsky Pond SL, Poon LLM. A case for the ancient origin of coronaviruses. J Virol 2013; 87(12): 7039-45.
[http://dx.doi.org/10.1128/JVI.03273-12] [PMID: 23596293]

[44]   Woo PCY, Lau SKP, Lam CSF, *et al.* Discovery of seven novel Mammalian and avian coronaviruses in the genus deltacoronavirus supports bat coronaviruses as the gene source of alphacoronavirus and betacoronavirus and avian coronaviruses as the gene source of gammacoronavirus and deltacoronavirus. J Virol 2012; 86(7): 3995-4008.
[http://dx.doi.org/10.1128/JVI.06540-11] [PMID: 22278237]

[45]   Jonassen CM, Kofstad T, Larsen IL, *et al.* Molecular identification and characterization of novel coronaviruses infecting graylag geese (Anser anser), feral pigeons (Columbia livia) and mallards (Anas platyrhynchos). J Gen Virol 2005; 86(6): 1597-607.
[http://dx.doi.org/10.1099/vir.0.80927-0] [PMID: 15914837]

[46]   Woo PCY, Lau SKP, Lam CSF, *et al.* Discovery of a novel bottlenose dolphin coronavirus reveals a distinct species of marine mammal coronavirus in Gammacoronavirus. J Virol 2014; 88(2): 1318-31.
[http://dx.doi.org/10.1128/JVI.02351-13] [PMID: 24227844]

[47]   Singh D, Yi SV, Medicine M. On the origin and evolution of SARS-CoV-2. Exp Mol Med 2021; 53(4): 537-47.
[http://dx.doi.org/10.1038/s12276-021-00604-z] [PMID: 33864026]

[48]   Lu R, Zhao X, Li J, *et al.* Genomic characterisation and epidemiology of 2019 novel coronavirus: implications for virus origins and receptor binding. Lancet 2020; 395(10224): 565-74.
[http://dx.doi.org/10.1016/S0140-6736(20)30251-8] [PMID: 32007145]

[49]   Lai MMC, Cavanagh D. The molecular biology of coronaviruses. Adv Virus Res 1997; 48: 1-100.
[http://dx.doi.org/10.1016/S0065-3527(08)60286-9] [PMID: 9233431]

[50]   Zhou P, Yang XL, Wang XG, *et al.* A pneumonia outbreak associated with a new coronavirus of probable bat origin. Nature 2020; 579(7798): 270-3.

[http://dx.doi.org/10.1038/s41586-020-2012-7] [PMID: 32015507]

[51] Kim D, Lee J-Y, Yang J-S, Kim JW, Kim VN, Chang HJC. The architecture of SARS-CoV-2 transcriptome. Cell 2020; 181(4): 914-921. e10.
[http://dx.doi.org/10.1016/j.cell.2020.04.011]

[52] Stewart H, Brown K, Dinan AM, Irigoyen N, Snijder EJ, Firth AE. Transcriptional and translational landscape of equine torovirus. J Virol 2018; 92(17): e00589-18.
[http://dx.doi.org/10.1128/JVI.00589-18] [PMID: 29950409]

[53] Viehweger A, Krautwurst S, Lamkiewicz K, *et al.* Direct RNA nanopore sequencing of full-length coronavirus genomes provides novel insights into structural variants and enables modification analysis. Genome Res 2019; 29(9): 1545-54.
[http://dx.doi.org/10.1101/gr.247064.118] [PMID: 31439691]

[54] Zhao Z, Li H, Wu X, *et al.* Moderate mutation rate in the SARS coronavirus genome and its implications. BMC Evol Biol 2004; 4(1): 21.
[http://dx.doi.org/10.1186/1471-2148-4-21] [PMID: 15222897]

[55] Tang X, Wu C, Li X, *et al.* On the origin and continuing evolution of SARS-CoV-2. Natl Sci Rev 2020; 7(6): 1012-23.
[http://dx.doi.org/10.1093/nsr/nwaa036] [PMID: 34676127]

[56] Zhou, H.; Chen, X.; Hu, T.; *et al.* A novel bat coronavirus reveals natural insertions at the S1/S2 cleavage site of the Spike protein and a possible recombinant origin of HCoV-19. Curr Biol 2020; 30(11): 2196-2203. e3.
[http://dx.doi.org/10.1016/j.cub.2020.05.023]

[57] Boni MF, Lemey P, Jiang X, *et al.* Evolutionary origins of the SARS-CoV-2 sarbecovirus lineage responsible for the COVID-19 pandemic. Nat Microbiol 2020; 5(11): 1408-17.
[http://dx.doi.org/10.1038/s41564-020-0771-4] [PMID: 32724171]

[58] Lam TTY, Jia N, Zhang YW, *et al.* Identifying SARS-CoV-2-related coronaviruses in Malayan pangolins. Nature 2020; 583(7815): 282-5.
[http://dx.doi.org/10.1038/s41586-020-2169-0] [PMID: 32218527]

[59] Elango N, Lee J, Peng Z, Loh YHE, Yi SV. Evolutionary rate variation in Old World monkeys. Biol Lett 2009; 5(3): 405-8.
[http://dx.doi.org/10.1098/rsbl.2008.0712] [PMID: 19324652]

[60] Drexler JF, Corman VM, Drosten C. Ecology, evolution and classification of bat coronaviruses in the aftermath of SARS. Antiviral Res 2014; 101: 45-56.
[http://dx.doi.org/10.1016/j.antiviral.2013.10.013] [PMID: 24184128]

[61] Balboni A, Battilani M, Prosperi S. The SARS-like coronaviruses: the role of bats and evolutionary relationships with SARS coronavirus. Microbiologica-Quarterly Journal of Microbiological Sciences. 2012 Jan 1; 35(1): 1.

[62] Anti P, Owusu M, Agbenyega O, *et al.* Human–bat interactions in rural West Africa. Emerg Infect Dis 2015; 21(8): 1418-21.
[http://dx.doi.org/10.3201/eid2108.142015] [PMID: 26177344]

[63] Corman VM, Eckerle I, Memish ZA, *et al.* Link of a ubiquitous human coronavirus to dromedary camels. Proc Natl Acad Sci USA 2016; 113(35): 9864-9.
[http://dx.doi.org/10.1073/pnas.1604472113] [PMID: 27528677]

[64] Vijgen L, Keyaerts E, Lemey P, *et al.* Evolutionary history of the closely related group 2 coronaviruses: porcine hemagglutinating encephalomyelitis virus, bovine coronavirus, and human coronavirus OC43. J Virol 2006; 80(14): 7270-4.
[http://dx.doi.org/10.1128/JVI.02675-05] [PMID: 16809333]

[65] Kan B, Wang M, Jing H, *et al.* Molecular evolution analysis and geographic investigation of severe acute respiratory syndrome coronavirus-like virus in palm civets at an animal market and on farms. J

Virol 2005; 79(18): 11892-900.
[http://dx.doi.org/10.1128/JVI.79.18.11892-11900.2005] [PMID: 16140765]

[66]   Li W, Shi Z, Yu M, *et al.* Bats are natural reservoirs of SARS-like coronaviruses. Science 2005; 310(5748): 676-9.
[http://dx.doi.org/10.1126/science.1118391] [PMID: 16195424]

[67]   Jo WK, Oliveira-Filho EF, Rasche A, Greenwood AD, Osterrieder K, Drexler JF. Potential zoonotic sources of SARS-CoV-2 infections. Transbound Emerg Dis 2021; 68(4): 1824-34.
[http://dx.doi.org/10.1111/tbed.13872] [PMID: 33034151]

[68]   Zhang Q, Zhang H, Gao J, *et al.* A serological survey of SARS-CoV-2 in cat in Wuhan. Emerg Microbes Infect 2020; 9(1): 2013-9.
[http://dx.doi.org/10.1080/22221751.2020.1817796] [PMID: 32867625]

[69]   Latinne A, Hu B, Olival KJ, *et al.* Origin and cross-species transmission of bat coronaviruses in China. 2020; 11(1): 1-15.
[PMID: 33240407]

[70]   Parry J. Breaches of safety regulations are probable cause of recent SARS outbreak, WHO says. BMJ 2004; 328(7450): 1222.3.
[http://dx.doi.org/10.1136/bmj.328.7450.1222-b] [PMID: 15155496]

[71]   Blow JA, Dohm DJ, Negley DL, Mores CN. Virus inactivation by nucleic acid extraction reagents. J Virol Methods 2004; 119(2): 195-8.
[http://dx.doi.org/10.1016/j.jviromet.2004.03.015] [PMID: 15158603]

[72]   Geddes AM. The history of smallpox. Clin Dermatol 2006; 24(3): 152-7.
[http://dx.doi.org/10.1016/j.clindermatol.2005.11.009] [PMID: 16714195]

[73]   Pekar J, Worobey M, Moshiri N, Scheffler K, Wertheim JO. Timing the SARS-CoV-2 index case in Hubei province. Science 2021; 372(6540): 412-7.
[http://dx.doi.org/10.1126/science.abf8003] [PMID: 33737402]

[74]   Cohen J. American Association for the Advancement of Science. 2020.

[75]   Wan Y, Shang J, Graham R, Baric RS, Li F. Receptor recognition by the novel coronavirus from Wuhan: an analysis based on decade-long structural studies of SARS coronavirus. J Virol 2020; 94(7): e00127-20.
[http://dx.doi.org/10.1128/JVI.00127-20] [PMID: 31996437]

[76]   Gu H, Chen Q, Yang G, *et al.* Adaptation of SARS-CoV-2 in BALB/c mice for testing vaccine efficacy. Science 2020; 369(6511): 1603-7.
[http://dx.doi.org/10.1126/science.abc4730] [PMID: 32732280]

[77]   Starr TN, Greaney AJ, Hilton SK, *et al.* Deep mutational scanning of SARS-CoV-2 receptor binding domain reveals constraints on folding and ACE2 binding. Cell 2020; 182(5): 1295-1310.e20.
[http://dx.doi.org/10.1016/j.cell.2020.08.012] [PMID: 32841599]

CHAPTER 4

Hosts Genetic Diversity of SARS-CoV-2

Kashif Prince[1], Arooj Fatima[2], Sana Tehseen[3], Muhammad Sajjad Khan[4], Muhammad Saeed[5], Firasat Hussain[2], Muhammad Naveed[6], Kashif Rahim[2] and Umair Younas[7,*]

[1] *Department of Medicine, Faculty of Veterinary Science, Cholistan University of Veterinary and Animal Sciences (CUVAS), Bahawalpur 63100, Pakistan*

[2] *Department of Microbiology, Faculty of Veterinary Science, Cholistan University of Veterinary and Animal Sciences (CUVAS), Bahawalpur 63100, Pakistan*

[3] *Department of Botany, Faculty of Science and Technology, Government College Women University, Faisalabad, Pakistan*

[4] *Department of Breeding and Genetics, Faculty of Animal Production and Technology, Cholistan University of Veterinary and Animal Sciences (CUVAS), Bahawalpur 63100, Pakistan*

[5] *Department of Poultry Sciences, Faculty of Animal Production and Technology, Cholistan University of Veterinary and Animal Sciences (CUVAS), Bahawalpur 63100, Pakistan*

[6] *Department of Clinical Pharmacology, School of Pharmacy, Nanjing Medical University, Nanjing 211166, China*

[7] *Department of Livestock Management, Faculty of Animal Production and Technology, Cholistan University of Veterinary and Animal Sciences (CUVAS), Bahawalpur 63100, Pakistan*

Abstract: The coronavirus disease-19 (COVID-19) spread worldwide in no time. Finally, the World Health Organization declared it a pandemic in March 2020. The severe acute respiratory syndrome-coronavirus-2 (SARS-CoV-2) can mutate, and many mutations have been observed worldwide. The severity of symptoms varies from mild to critical cases, and the incubation period ranges from 5-14 days. Various studies have shown that the diversity of SARS-CoV-2 within the hosts is prevalent, and some genomes are more susceptible to the alterations due to mutation. Some of the tissues that exhibited the highest ACE2 expression in different host tissues (humans) were kidneys, thyroid, heart, adipose tissue, small intestine, and testicles. Endothelial cells have also been the site for SARS-CoV-2. Chinese people were the first to be reported with the polymorphism detection for the ACE2 gene. Different variants of the ACE2 gene that are closely linked with hypertension were rs464155, rs4240157, and rs4830542. There has been a close association between ACE2 and TMRSS2 and SARS-COV-2, SARS-CoV-1, and influenza virus. The inducibility of heme oxygenase-1 (HO-1) enzyme to reactive oxygen species is regulated by the GT dinucleotide repeat mutation and polymorphism of the HO-1 gene.

* **Corresponding author Umair Younas:** Department of Livestock Management, Faculty of Animal Production and Technology, Cholistan University of Veterinary and Animal Sciences (CUVAS), Bahawalpur 63100, Pakistan, E-mail: umairyounas@cuvas.edu.pk

Kamal Niaz, Muhammad Sajjad Khan & Muhammad Farrukh Nisar (Eds.)

Keywords: SARS, Coronavirus, ACE2, Mutation, Virus, Genome.

INTRODUCTION

After the first coronavirus case reported in 2019, it has repeatedly modified itself. The new form of coronavirus, *i.e.*, severe acute respiratory syndrome-coronaviru--2 (SARS-CoV-2), has a high capability to mutate itself and has done this to a great extent worldwide [1]. Not only do viruses vary from host to host, but within the host, different types of variants of viruses can be found with various mutations [2]. In 2019, Wuhan, China, reported the first case of coronavirus disease-19 (COVID-19), and it spread all over the world in no time. Finally, the World Health Organization declared the COVID-19 pandemic in March 2020. COVID-19 is a disease affecting the respiratory system, and the symptoms observed in this disease are persistent cough and fatigue [3]. However, a subpopulation of people infected with the virus remains asymptomatic [4]. The severity of symptoms varies from mild to critical cases, and the incubation period also varies from 5-14 days [5, 6]. The ability of coronavirus to proofread (due to nsp-14, *i.e* ., non-structural proteins) is attributed to a decrease in the rate of mutation as compared to other positive-sense ssRNA viruses, but studies have shown the diversity and prevalence of SARS-CoV-2 within the hosts, and some genomes are more susceptible to the alterations due to mutation [7, 8]. Virus isolation and sequencing efforts have led to the cross-examination of the SARS-CoV-2 genome, exhibiting better or more in-depth consideration of the vertical progress of the viral evolution along with its origin and the worldwide pattern of global spread [9, 10]. Researchers have conducted studies to address the ACE2 expression in human tissue samples and analyze the results without considering gender and age factors [11]. Some tissues that exhibited the highest ACE2 expression in different host tissues (humans) were kidneys, thyroid, heart, adipose tissue, small intestine, and testicles. Endothelial cells have also been the site for SARS-CoV-2; therefore, ACE2 expression was noted, thus explaining the possible explanation for the disease affecting various patients' organs at one time [11, 12].

The intermediate level of ACE2 expression was noticed in tissue samples of the liver, esophagus, adrenal gland, lungs, colon, and bladder. In contrast, blood vessels, spleen, bone marrow, muscle, uterus, and brain exhibited the lowest level of ACE2 expression. Given the immune patterns of women and men, the expression of ACE2 was shown to be downregulated and upregulated in the lungs [13]. It was reported that there are vasodilation and antifibrotic effects of angiotensin [14, 15]. In various conditions like heart failure, diabetes, and hypertension, there has been less cardiac expression of ACE2 [16, 17]. Chinese people were the first to be reported with the polymorphism detection for the

ACE2 gene. Different variants of the ACE2 gene that are closely linked with hypertension were rs464155, rs4240157, and rs4830542 [18 - 21]. It was noted that eleven common and rare variants were found to be closely linked with the increased expression of ACE2. These expressions were irregularly distributed for the various population groups [22]. It was noted that in the East-Asian population group, the increased expression of the ACE2 gene was closely related to the ACE2 gene polymorphism (variant 4,646,127), and this finding allows us to understand this vital issue more appropriately [22]. There has been a close association of ACE2 and TMRSS2 with SARS COV-2, SARS CoV-1, and influenza virus to facilitate the virus while entering the infected host cell. The spike protein of SARS CoV-2 is cleaved by TMPRSS2, which is supposed to be an androgen-reactive serine protease enzyme, leading to the activation and entry of the virus [23], as shown in Fig. (**1**). There have been many studies conducted on the polymorphism of single nucleotide in TMPRSS2, as in the case of breast cancer, the high patient endurance is correlated with the rs2276205 (A>G) having a low-frequency allele [24]. Similarly, in the case of prostate cancer, there is a high frequency of TMPRSS2 rs12329760 (C>T) mutation in men with a family history of disease. Additionally, the ERG gene fusion, often associated with prostate cancer, is observed in these cases, suggesting a genetic predisposition to the condition [25, 26].

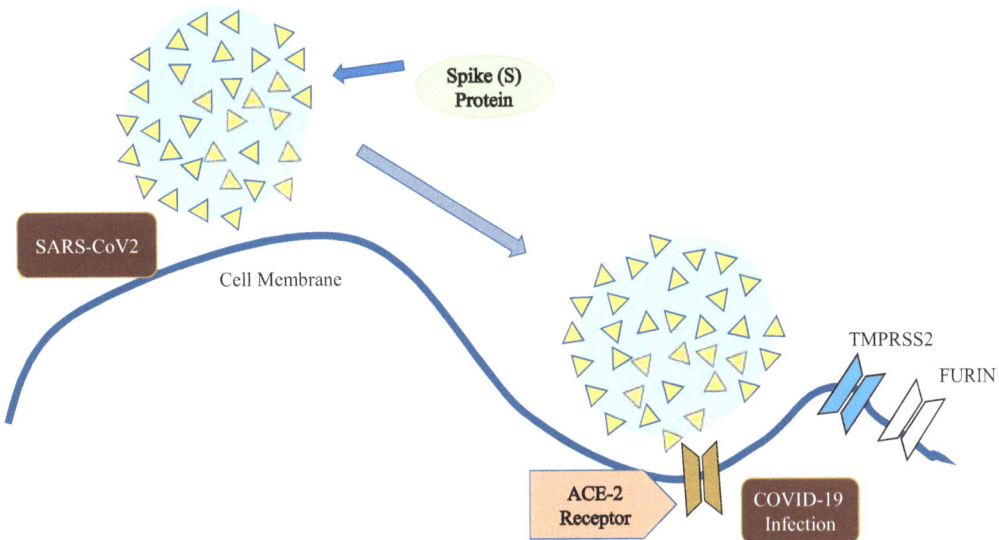

Fig. (1). Demonstration of COVID-19 infection activation: the viral spikes interact with ACE-2 receptors while invading the cell. Spikes are cleaved by TMPRSS2 (membrane protease 2), host cell protease, and furin, activating COVID-19 infection [83].

The inducibility of the heme oxygenase-1 (HO-1) enzyme to reactive oxygen species is regulated by the GT dinucleotide repeat mutation and polymorphism of the HO-1 gene [27 - 33]. Various studies have noted that GT repeats are closely connected with the sensitivity to aortic aneurysms and atherosclerosis coronary artery diseases (cardiovascular endothelium diseases) [27, 30, 31]. Similarly, the HO-1 with reduced expression level in subjects with more GT repeats causes patients to get more affected by the inflammation and decreases endothelial hemostasis [27 - 33]. The RNA editing enzyme has 2 families that are known to take part in the SARS CoV-2 mutational spectrum, which is ADAR, the enzyme causing U>C and A>G mutation (adenosine to inosine changes), and APOBEC (cytosine deaminase enzyme), the enzyme causing C>U transitions [34]. For instance, the C>U transition may be caused by sudden cytosine deamination, whereas the G>U transversion may be elaborated by the oxidation of guanine [35]. The damage in both forms in human cells is considered to be a common mutagenic process [36].

Patterns of within-Host Diversity

Coronavirus has repeatedly modified itself since its first case was reported in 2019 [1]. Not only do viruses vary from host to host, but within the host, different types of variants of viruses can be found with various mutations [1]. In 2019, Wuhan, China, reported the first case of COVID-19, and it spread worldwide in no time. Finally, the World Health Organization declared the COVID-19 pandemic in March 2020. COVID-19 is a disease affecting the respiratory system, and the symptoms that are observed in this disease are persistent cough and fatigue [3]. However, a subpopulation of people infected with the virus remains asymptomatic [26]. The severity of symptoms varies from mild to critical cases, and the incubation period also varies from 5-14 days [22, 24]. This short incubation period helps the virus to spread exponentially within no time. By the end of September 2020, more than thirty-four COVID-19 cases had appeared worldwide [37]. There is a close relationship between SARS-CoV-2 and the *Coronaviridae* family. Over the past two decades, three zoonotic coronaviruses have been known to infect human beings, which are SARS-CoV (2003), MERS-CoV (2012), and SARS-CoV-2 (2019) [38]. There are 13 ORFs (open reading frames) with single-stranded RNA and 29,903 nucleotides [39]. ORF1ab encodes for the non-structural proteins such as RNA-dependent RNA polymerase; other proteins are S proteins (Spike), E gene (Envelop), M gene (Matrix), and N gene (Nucleoprotein), as well as host for accessory genes [40]. Its mechanism of host attachment is quite similar to the SARS-CoV, *i.e* ., on the surface of the virion. The Spike protein attaches to the hACE2 receptor for entry to the host cell by fusion of host and viral envelops [39]. Efforts have been made to isolate and sequence the viral genome and have allowed an understanding of the vertical progress in the virus's structure, its origin point, and the worldwide pattern of spread and outbreak [41, 42]. Such attempts are large-level objections to reverse transcription of the RNA genome in the virus and PCR amplification hybrid capture-based sequencing using oxford nanopore and illumine sequencers [43]. The generated sequences are gathered in the data repositories, *e.g* ., GISAID and SRA (Sequence read archives) [44]. Due to this, platforms like Nextstrain can continuously update and track viral progression and outbreaks to mitigate the diversity of viral genomes among various carriers [45 - 49]. Typically, in epidemiological studies, consensus sequences are employed per patient, and the virus population of a person is taken as a single sequence even if there is minor variation in the virus in that host population [50].

On the other hand, in the case of RNA viruses, the mutation rate is very high due to RNA polymerases, which are more likely to function abnormally, which is the main cause of various virus variants within the same host [51]. The diversity of the viral genome within the same host due to this phenomenon affects disease progression, tissue tropism, transmission risk, transmission heterogeneity, and treatment outcomes in various RNA viruses [52 - 57]. The mutation rate of SARS-CoV-2 is as high as previously observed in SARS-CoV [58, 59].

The capability of the coronavirus to proofread (due to nsp-14, *i.e* ., non-structural proteins) is attributed to a decrease in the rate of mutation compared to other positive-sense ssRNA viruses [8]. Still, studies have shown the diversity and prevalence of SARS-CoV-2 within the hosts, and some genomes are more susceptible to the alterations due to mutations [7, 8]. In one study, the SARS-CoV-E samples were studied in a large cohort of 3939 cases, and 749 samples were observed in an independent validation cohort in Switzerland for intra-host or within-host genetic diversity of SARS-CoV-2 [60]. Genetic diversity across the genome was analyzed, and the diversity across patients was explored. It was observed within the patient that the host viral genetic diversity increased with the patient's age [60, 61]. The older the patient, the more genetically diverse the virus will be (host reference). Heavy tail distribution of diversity per sample was observed, which means much of the diversity was concentrated in the small number of sites and patients. The patient's age is a significant predictor of the diversity of viruses [61]. There has been an increase of 8.6% in the average genetic diversity for every 10 years of increasing age. Age is also associated with disease condition consequences and developing mortality [62]. The more infective strain becomes dominant over time [63]. Subclonal mutations with different variants also show mutation co-existence [64].

Co-Existence of Viral Variants

Virus isolation and sequencing efforts have led to the cross-examination of the SARS-CoV-2 genome, exhibiting better and more in-depth consideration of the vertical progress of the viral evolution, along with its origin and the worldwide pattern of global spread [9, 10, 41]. These efforts and tasks are more likely to rely on reverse transcription of the viral RNA genome and are followed by a hybrid capture base sequence and PCR amplicon [65]. The availability of these sequences is possible in some programs [45] to continuously update and track the viral evolution and spread and give information about viral genetic diversity within the carrier and among the carriers [46 - 49]. At the inter-host level, one sequence per host is considered satisfactory. A summary of each strain is taken, and a few changes are ignored. Still, in the case of RNA viruses, multiple strains can exist within the same host because the RNA polymerases are error-prone and less accurate than the DNA polymerases [51]. This intra-host diversity affects various aspects of RNA viruses, including disease spread, tissue tropism, transmission risks, heterogeneity, and treatment outcomes [52-56]. The mutation rate is very high in SARS-CoV-2, and this mutation is as high as it was observed in the SARS-CoV genome ($0.80-2.38 \times 10^3$ nucleotide substitutions per site per year) [58, 59]. This mutation rate is very high despite the evolution of the proofreading capacity of this virus, which is credited to protein-14, which results in decreased mutations compared to (+) sense sRNA viruses [66 - 68]. Intra-host diversity in clinical cases has been observed in many studies, and genomic regions susceptible to the modifications in the structure of SARS-CoV-2 have been understood [7, 8]. This intra-host diversity can improve the phylogenomic analysis of SARS-CoV-2 [69] and the ability to detect selection pressure [64]. In one study, the SARS-CoV-E samples were studied in a large cohort of 3939 cases, and 749 samples were observed in an independent validation cohort in Switzerland for intra-host or within-host genetic diversity of SARS-CoV-2 [60]. The analyses were made regarding the distribution of genetic diversity across the genome, including small regions and highly diverse bases. The diversity across the patient samples was also estimated [60]. Within the host, diversity was observed to increase with the patient's age. A wide range of genetic variations has been observed across the samples and the genome. Focusing on the positions across the genome, mutation was observed in 4% of samples [60]. The mutation was observed at the start of ORF1ab in the spike S gene and across the Matrix M gene. There were highly diverse individual bases and small regions, particularly in the public data [60].

Analysis of SARS-CoV-2 Nucleotide Variation

Considering the summary of per-gene genetic diversity, it was observed that the average of entropy, along with all the positions of each gene with the same diversity, has been observed in the public cohort, excluding gene M, which possesses much more diversity, whereas, ORF7b do not show any diversity [61]. This diversity was also observed in the Swiss cohort, but larger differences across genes were observed. Approximately half of the samples have clonal or sub-clonal mutations at the 11075 position of the ORF1ab coding for nsp 6 (non-structural protein), a 7-transmembrane helicase containing transmembrane protein [60, 61]. In most circumstances, it was noticed that from the low-frequency deletions, the diversity at this position was derived and was more likely to alter the downstream amino acids and introduce premature stop codons. The deletion was observed at 2.62% on average in samples with mutation [61]. Out of mutated samples, almost 12.5% were shown to include the variant substitution of T > C that happened with an average frequency of 1.75% among those samples. With respect to the reference genome, the phenylalanine amino acid is incorporated by the codon [61]. The outcome of any variation is that it will result in a change in the inserted amino acid, *e.g* ., leucine would be incorporated in the T > C mutation. Near the Phe35, another residue known as Leu37 of nsp-6 was noticed to be substituted by phenylalanine residue in current sequences taken from America, Asia, and Europe [70]. On position 11083, inside the Leu37 codon, there is high entropy, which is affected in 25% of the samples. The phenylalanine residue, as opposed to the Leucine, results from any alteration from reference base G to either C or T. It is also noted that a high average frequency of common deletion is 4.93% and that of thymine bases is 44.65%, leading to a premature stop codon and phenylalanine residue [61].

The D614G amino acid alteration in the spike region is caused by A > G mutation in the genomic position 23403. As a result of these alterations, the virus is strengthened, and this variant has increased dominance in the population over the period [63]. With 36% of samples having mutations relative to their cohort consensus G and 29.7% exhibiting the diversity of distinct variants coexisting, this is the most diverse location in the SARS-CoV-2 genome [60]. The average frequencies of mutations for different bases are 90.4% A, 9.5% G, and 0.1% base deletions. Position 23403 in the Swiss cohort has the second most diverse individual bases [60]. A span of 16 nucleotides in an ORF1ab gene is the most varied area in public and Swiss data [71]. This region is part of non-structural protein 1, which interacts with the 40S and 80S ribosomal subunits to shut down host mRNA translation and protein synthesis. The innate immune response, specifically interferon signaling, is reduced due to the nsp1-induced suppression of translation and protein synthesis [71]. Another diverse genomic region is adjacent at 29187 and 29188 within a single codon in the N gene, forming the nucleoprotein. Bases at these positions are C and A, respectively and this causes the incorporation of alanine residues at position 305 of the nucleoprotein [61]. However, alteration in position 29188 alone does not lead to an alteration at the protein level due to redundancy [72]. Nucleotides from 26780 to 2682, which are 41, are associated with incorporating 15 amino acids from Cys86 to Phe100, forming a section of matrix protein of the transmembrane region. The matrix protein is associated in central assembly with several interacting patterns, including the matrix protein itself, the envelope protein, the nucleoprotein, and the spike protein [73, 74]. On priming, spike protein is split into two subunits, S1 and S2, with the former required for hACE2 recognition and the latter promoting viral entrance into host cells. Another high-entropy area comprises 30 nucleotides within the spike gene, which includes 11 amino acids from Ile664 to Tyr674 in the SARS-CoV-2 S1 subunit [75]. While the majority of the genome is highly conserved, the distribution of total entropy per base has a long tail, resulting in places with extraordinarily high variety. The usage of sequencing equipment, sample processing, and sequencing depth all affect the identification of diversity in each sample [76].

Analysis of Epidemiological Parameters

The disease's epidemiology depends on many factors, among which genetic diversity is one of the leading factors [77]. A study was conducted by Onder *et al.* [78] to test this hypothesis more specifically to determine the relationship of host age, sex, or geographical location to predict the diversity of the virus population. It was found that sex had no ties with genetic diversity, and sex does not predict virus diversity. Conversely, age has a significant relationship with genetic diversity, and total entropy increases by 8.6% each decade. Age has also been associated with strong and worse disease outcomes and death rates [78]. It is also associated with concomitant comorbidities [79]. It is yet unclear whether the diversity increases the infectiousness and disease progression in the case of SARS-CoV-2, as is evident in the case of influenza [54]. Sub-clonal mutation detection is dependent on the depth of sequencing at each site and across the genome; depending on RNA amplification and capture for sequencing, some regions may be less well resolved [63]. The matrix gene (M) is the most diverse and highly diversified. It includes a combination of low-frequency variants that affect a quarter or more of the cohort and uncommon high-frequency sub-clonal mutations that affect about 5% of the cohort [80]. The frequent low-frequency and less common low-frequency genetic variations in SARS-CoV-2 are diverse within and between hosts [46]. The D614G variation appears to be increasing infectivity and becoming increasingly dominant over time [63].

Role of ACE2 Polymorphism

The ACE2 expression from various tissue samples (humans) is provocative due to its identification as a significant and new binding site, whereas SARS-CoV-2 gets entry inside the host cells (human) [81]. Many studies have been carried out recently to detect cell types, with the major expression received from the ACE2 receptor, and they may give a possible explanation for the SARS-CoV-2 targets [82].

Researchers have performed studies to address the ACE2 expression in human tissue samples and analyze the results without considering gender and age factors [83]. Some tissues that exhibited the highest ACE2 expression in different host tissues (humans) were the kidneys, thyroid, heart, adipose tissue, small intestine, and testicles [84]. An intermediate level of ACE2 expression was noticed in the liver, esophagus, adrenal gland, lungs, colon, and bladder tissue samples. In contrast, blood vessels, spleen, bone marrow, muscle, uterus, and brain exhibited the lowest level of ACE2 expression [84]. Because of the immune patterns of women and men, the expression of ACE2 was shown to be downregulated and upregulated in the lungs [13]. The different types of airway epithelial cells, like ciliated nasal epithelium and type II alveolar cells, also exhibited ACE2 expression.

Furthermore, it is largely co-expressed with TMPRSS2 present in the epithelium of the nasal cavity and may explain the massive infectivity by SARS-CoV-2 [85]. The oral cavity mucosa is also used as the target site for localization by ACE2. From the findings of various researchers, it is pretty evident that the underlying mechanism of the oral cavity is a novel SARS-CoV-2 potential target area. Inside the oral mucosa, the ACE2 expression was noted in the lymphocytes [86]. This was why the SARS-CoV-2 attacked the lymphocytes and caused lymphopenia, especially during the severity of the disease [86]. Endothelial cells have also been the site for SARS-CoV-2; therefore, ACE2 expression was noted, thus explaining the disease's possible effect on various patients' organs at one time [11, 87]. As a direct consequence of intervention by an inflammatory response by the host and SARS-CoV-2 action, the initiation of endothelins in different organs is promoted [88].

Furthermore, apoptosis and pyroptosis might have an additional and vital role in endothelial cell injury in patients. Therefore, this may account for the weak performance of the systemic microcirculatory system in different blood vessels as well as clinical consequences in COVID-19 patients [89]. Therefore, various treatment plans are justified during the virus's reproduction for stabilizing endothelium, particularly by ACE inhibitors, cholesterol-lowering drugs, and anti-inflammatory cytokinin drugs [62, 90 - 92]. The patients getting weak from hypertension, obesity, or cardiovascular diseases, co-morbid patients, and others with other endothelial disorders are suitable for this kind of approach [89]. Many variants of ACE2 have been identified in the various database systems. As a consequence of CVD (cardiovascular disease) development and, more importantly, its correlation with hypertension, much attention has been given to the polymorphism of ACE2 during the last decades. ACE2 restricts the negative influence of vasoconstrictor and profibrotic influence of AngII as Ang is formed by the breakdown of AngII as the endothelium of cerebral arteries receives less oxidative stress of AngII [83, 93].

According to a study conducted in India, hypertension patients (246) and normal subjects (274) exhibit the link of rs21068809 (ACE2) with hypertension [94]. Similarly, in African-Americans, polymorphism in ACE has been described to be linked with hypertension [95]. The susceptibility to hypertension with the combined effect of ACE I/D and ACE2G8790A was reported in research on genetic association (Brazilian cohorts) [96]. The infectivity of SARS-CoV-2 is possibly affected by the genetic variation ACE2. The binding of ACE2 receptors is mediated in SARS-CoV by the action of the S2 domain of S protein, whereas post-binding trans-conformational modulation is undergone by the S2 domain, leading to the activating of the fusion to the cell membrane [97]. The shedding activity of the enzyme is significantly weakened by the ACE2 point mutation Leu584AIa, which, conversely, promotes the entrance of the virus inside the host cells [98]. Another study found that viral RBD in the S1 position was adjusted from 270 to 510 (amino acid number) [99]. The soluble form of ACE2 lacks transmembrane, and the cytoplasmic domain prevents the binding of SARS-CoV S protein to ACE2 [100]. The expression of ACE2 was observed for downregulation by the spikes proteins of recombinant SARS-CoV-2 by releasing the sACE2, thereby assisting in the injury of the lungs [101].

The majority of amino acid residues that are important for the binding of ACE2 within the spike S1 domain of SARS-CoV-2; SARS-CoV-2 and SARS-CoV take part in the identity of 76% of such amino acid residues [102]. In another study, the comparison was made by multiple sequence alignment for a large number of amino acid residues of human ACE proteins (n=10); it was noticed that among four various isoforms of ACE2, 100% identity was found in ACE2 sequences. In SARS-CoV-2 infection outcomes, the role of these ACE2 isoforms has been unpredictable [103]. According to the findings, identifications of 32 ACE2 polymorphisms along seven hotspot variables were made among various personals, leading to the understanding that some individuals may show lower to higher susceptibility variation than others [22].

Polymorphism in Viral ACE receptors

Among the different populations of the world, a preliminary study was conducted regarding allele frequency distribution for 1700 polymorphisms of the ACE2 gene. It was noted that eleven common and rare variants were found that were closely linked with increased expression of ACE2 [104]. These expressions were found to be irregularly distributed for the various population groups. It was noted that in the East-Asian population group, the increased expression of the ACE2 gene has been closely related to the ACE2 gene polymorphism (variant 4,646,127), and this finding smoothens the way to understand this vital issue more appropriately [22]. Another similar study validated results by Rao *et al.* [105], which showed that overexpression of ACE2 and allelic frequency of variants are closely associated. The number of proteins was encoded by various ACE2 polymorphisms for the SARS-CoV-2 protein study, and it was observed that there was a difference in compatibility between each variant and the RBD sequence [105]. Most genetic variants showed physical similarity among the majority of the genetic variants. The rs143936283 and rs73635825 are two ACE2 gene alleles that expressed a little binding strength against spike protein of SARS-CoV-2, leading to an understanding of fewer chances of virus binding and chances of infection resistance [106]. It has been seen that the likelihood of some of the ACE2 genetic variants, especially those allocated to join with the spike proteins of SARS-CoV-2, might be connected with adaptable virus-host interaction, in this way probably changing severity and pathogenicity [107]. The genome dataset was extensively analyzed. It was noticed that nine human ACE2 variants (Q102p, T921, T27A, h378R, K26R, N64K, 121V, S19P, and E23K) have the potential to increase the tendency for viral binding against the 17 variants (Q338L, G352V, D509Y, Y83H, F72V, K68E, D355N, M62V, N51S, G326E, D38V, Y50F, E35K, N33I, h34R, K31R, and E37K) of ACE2, protecting from virus entry [108].

Researchers noticed that ACE2 variants (3) found from 5 different Italian centers may be specified (P. Asn720Asp, lys26Arg, and p. Gly211Arg). It was reported that instead of the East Asian population, these ACE2 polymorphisms had been identified in Italy [109]. Since these variants are closely located near the essential sequence of spike proteins binding site in SARS-CoV-2, therefore it may be attributed to the understanding that there might be a modification in the division and viral entry, such as the location of Asn720Asp is only on four AA (amino acids) of TMPRSS2 cleavage site [110]. This may result in a partial explanation for the registration of the increased mortality rate in Italy while making a comparison with China. It is now pretty evident that, practically, ACE3 acts as a receptor for the entry of coronavirus inside the human host cells.

In contrast, some others do not align with the correlation between gene polymorphism and SARS receptivity [111]. According to the findings of other researchers, ACE2 variants are responsible for the expression of differential efficiency in the stimulation of monocytes, natural killer cells (NK), neutrophils, and T helper cells. Therefore, it may be able to increase or reduce the cytokinin storm or inflammatory reaction of AngII. This is a way of helping vasoconstriction and taking part in the improvement of the infection of systemic or topical tissue [112, 113].

Polymorphism Analysis of TMPRSS2 in Relation to COVID-19

There has been a close association of ACE2 and TMRSS2 with SARS COV-2, SARS CoV-1, and influenza virus to facilitate the virus while entering the infected host cell [114]. The spike protein of SARS CoV-2 is cleaved by TMPRSS2, which is supposed to be a androgen-reactive serine protease enzyme, leading to activation and entry of the virus [23]. Many studies have been conducted on the polymorphism of single nucleotides in TMPRSS2. In the case of breast cancer, the high patient endurance is correlated with the rs2276205 (A>G) having a low-frequency allele [24]. Similarly, in the case of prostate cancer, there is a high frequency of TMPRSS2 rs12329760 (C>T) in men with a history of prostate cancer in the family, with the role of ERG gene infusion [25, 26]. In another study, rs2070788 (G>A) and rs383510 (T>C) were found to correlate with the increased lung expression of TMPRSS2, H1N1, and aggressive form of H7N9 [115]. It is reported that about 4% of TMPRSS2 non-identical variants stop codon mutations, whereas harmful mutations account for 59% in the coding region of TMPRSS2 [116].

The coding region of TMPRSS2 carries various harmful variants like p.Gly259Ser, p.Gly432Ala, p.Pro335Leu, p.Gly181Arg, and p. Arg240Cys that have quite a resemblance with somatic alteration found in different types of cancer [83]. It is noted that p.Asp435Tyr has a rare low-frequency allele and is the main site for the binding of TMPRSS2 catalytic residues. It tends to provide metaphors for various genetic infectivity to SARS-CoV-2 along with risk influence in male patients, especially those with tumors [83]. It was reported that TMPRSS2 expression was increased in alveolar epithelial cells type 1 and ciliated cells and also upregulated with increased human age by using a single-cell RNA sequence [117]. The study indicates that there might be a role in the expression of TMPRSS2 relative to the protection of infants and children from SARS-CoV-2. At the same time, it is important to investigate the relationships between age and TMPRSS2 polymorphism with SARS CoV-2 [118].

Genetic Polymorphism of Heme Oxygenase-1 Enzyme and Severity of COVID-19

The GT dinucleotide regulates the inducibility of the HO-1 enzyme to reactive oxygen species repeat mutation and polymorphism of the HO-1 gene [27 - 33]. It is noted that GT repeats have a close connection with the sensitivity to the aortic aneurysm and atherosclerosis coronary artery diseases (cardiovascular endothelium diseases) in various subjects [27, 30, 31, 33]. Similarly, the HO-1 with reduced expression level in subjects with more GT repeats causes patients to get more affected by the inflammation and decreases endothelial hemostasis [10, 28, 32 - 34, 37, 61, 66]. The inflammation is reduced, and cryoprotection increases due to the correlation between the increased inducibility of HO-1 and the short alleles of the GT sequence [33]. It is estimated that longer GT sequences are associated with decreased vessel hemostasis in patients affected by SARS-CoV-2 [119]. There have been poor effects of COVID-19 in obese and diabetic individuals, and the probable reason is that these patients already have high levels of IL-6, and due to insulin resistance and leptin, they are in a proinflammatory state [120, 121].

As a consequence, the negative outcomes of SARS-CoV-2 were expressed in obese patients [121]. Researchers revealed that high-density lipoproteins (HDL) oxidation increases in obesity [122]. Therefore, by the direct action of adipocyte stem cells, the oxidized form of HDL (OX-HDL) resultantly produced inflammatory cytokines [123]. An inflammatory cascading is initiated by the oxidized form of HDL with TNF (tumor necrosis factor), inflammatory cytokines, interleukin-6 (IL-6), and an increased level of AngII considered an indicator/biomarker for cardiovascular diseases at an early stage [122]. This leads to more sensitivity to heart failure in obese patients due to the infection with SARS-CoV-2 [124]. Another study noted that the harmful effects of COVID-19 may be high due to the upregulation of HO-1-derived bilirubin, and the high level of HO-1 assists in increasing this risk [125]. There might be valuable results in the acute form of inflammatory conditions when pharmacological treatment is given in case of upregulation of HO-1 level [125, 126].

Polymorphism of BCL11A

The genetic polymorphism of BCL11A correlates with the overall population to produce fetal hemoglobin. It was later found to cause a modification in the severity of sickle cell diseases and beta-thalassemia. However, it is believed that fetal hemoglobin elevation may help improve the severity of such disorders [127]. To understand the genetic bases for heterogeneity, the genomic base-wide survey was done in a large cohort population of patients with sickle cell disease and beta-thalassemia, whereas a survey was done with 362,129 joint SNPs to explain the correlation between HbF levels and genetic linkage, along with the other traits related to RBSs (red blood cells) [83]. It was reported that among different variants affecting the HbF levels, the SNP rs886868 of BLC11A has been in complete correlation with this trait [128, 129]. Increased HbF (fetal hemoglobin) production was closely associated with this BCL11A variant in beta-thalassemia patients. As for patients with sickle cell anemia, a similar BCL11A variant was partially correlated [128]. Based on these findings, varying BCL11A levels are considered an important factor in improving the potential hemoglobin disorders and the phenotype of beta-thalassemia patients [130]. Under these findings, it might be helpful to understand the molecular mechanism regarding the regulation of fetal globin. Therefore, novel therapeutic decisions and tactics for beta-thalassemia and sickle cell anemia may evolve [131 - 133]. The question of why some patients show quite acute clinical symptoms compared to some who express mild symptoms may be explained. It is imperative to know the part played by genetic polymorphism of the COVID-19 virus in observing the infection severity and the heterogeneity in the predisposition [23, 134].

The Mutational Spectra Reveal Strong Strand Asymmetries

Mutational spectra analysis can help understand the mutational mechanism during a pandemic with the progression in the severity of SARS-CoV-2. It is reported that the major and host variants closely resemble [135]. The spectrum can see two striking characteristics: domination of G>U and C>U, which fluctuates with a large symmetry among minus, plus-strand and within the context of weak extended sequence inferred from C>A/G>U and C>U/G>A ratio, whereas mutations were mapped to plus (reference) strand [136]. Of all the point mutations within the host, the C>U mutations are 47% compared to the G>A mutations, which are 5.9%, whereas the minus-strand accounts for C>U mutations. The G>U mutations account for around 15% of all the mutations in comparison with the C>A mutations (2.2%) [136]. It is observed that the ratio of plus-minus strands for G>U and C>U have been 8.2 and 9.9 folds, respectively. Due to the direct replication errors in mutation, it becomes difficult to explain complex asymmetries [136]. Considering the exact number of -ive to +ive and +ive to -ive replication steps that may have been undergone in any given viral RNA, asymmetries are supposed to be caused by the replication errors subjected to the different error rates of both steps [136].

For instance, a high error rate for C>U exists in both strands in polymerase. It may guess a symmetric number of G>A and C>U plus-strand mutation, whereas C>U would be expressed at balancing rates whenever replicating the minus or the plus strand [137]. It is observed that, theoretically, it would be possible to get a viral population with low G>A mutation at high frequencies within a cell [137, 138]. It is noted that among major variants, there have been the same asymmetries that may work as the fixation of a single genotype and, at the same time, make it an unlikely factor. It is unlikely that the observed asymmetries will be elaborated by replication error if the error rates of RdRp (SARS-CoV-2) are different in both strands [136]. It has been suggested that with plus-strand RNA editing or RNA damage, there may be more consistent strong strand asymmetries in SARS CoV-2. In the infectious genome, the plus strand, which is transferred from replication organelles as compared to the minus strand molecules, resides in the cytoplasm [139]. These are translated and then packaged into the particles so that they are transferred between the hosts and cells. Within the cell, the plus strand is also available in large numbers compared to the minus strand [137].

Therefore, there is the possibility of accumulation of a higher incidence of editing and damage by plus-strand that would lead to the manifestation of strand asymmetries. Considering this hypothesis is true, the dominance of G>U over C>A and C>U over G>A may comprehend that G>U and C>U are the major types of RNA damage or editing, whereas mapping is done to plus-strand [64]. An anti-viral mechanism exists where single-stranded RNA and DNA are subjected to mutagenesis by RNA editing enzymes in human cells [34, 140].

The RNA editing enzyme has 2 families that are known to take part in the SARS CoV-2 mutational spectrum and are ADAR, the enzyme causing U>C and A>G mutation (adenosine to inosine changes), and APOBEC (cytosine deaminase enzyme) causing C>U transitions [34]. The large number of C>U changes in the spectra of SARS CoV-2 might be associated with the lower incidence of U>C and A>G mutations [45]. The mechanism of APOBEC enzyme-induced mutational spectrum is not fully understood. However, a better understanding of APOBEC3A and 3B enzymes is featured in the context of strong sequence in the human cancer cell and may lead to the C>G and C>T variations solely in TpC sites [141]. In comparison, dependence was noticed in the spectrum of SARS-CoV-2. The contribution of RNA editing enzymes in the mutagenesis of SARS CoV-2 has been significant; the damage to the guanine and cytosine within the observed spectrum could be consistent [141].

For instance, the C>U transition may be caused by the sudden cytosine deamination, whereas the G>U transversion could result from the oxidation of guanine [35]. The damage in both forms in human cells is considered to be a common mutagenic process [36]. Regarding the average number of mutations, an approximate estimate within the host viral genome can be derived in a sample, whereas the mutational spectrum has been described [136]. The allelic frequency of a mutation represents the viral RNA fraction molecules carrying a mutation in a sample; researchers may be able to estimate the mean mutation load within the host by observing the allelic frequency of variants in a sample within the host [136]. It is assumed that RNAs originated from the complete viral genome and are surely not always the circumstances, whereas the abundance of sgRNAs is [142, 143]. Such estimates are considered lower bound probably due to the mutations included in both replicates at detectable allele fraction. With a median of 0.37, the 0.72 mutations were found within the host mutation load/viral genome. The mutation rate is estimated at 0.001 mutations/bp/year [144] by phylogenetic studies on SARS CoV-2 or 0.082 mutations per genome per day. Therefore, the consistency of mutation load within the host is expected with the supposed acquisition of mutation within a short time frame of days [145]. Researchers investigated the possible accumulation of *de novo* mutations during infection, and 43 individuals were studied from whom samples were collected at different times [135]. It was noted that there was an increasing trend in the number of variants within the host over time, and the trend was found to be significant [145]. To put this result in a context, the considerable number of variations were observed within the host variants from the samples of the same individuals, although some samples were collected on the same day due to the complexities faced due to the variable sampling method and collected swabs, such as broncho-alveolar lavage and sputum. A high number of variations in the longitudinal samples have been observed in 6/9 hospitalized patients [135].

Data were collected from nine patients using longitudinal samples. On average, the variant frequencies were greater in serial samples collected from one patient compared to the recipient-donor transmission pairs [146]. Throughout infection, the researchers noticed the various instances of fixation of variants. Contrary to that, no change was noticed in the consensus genome sequence, whereas multiple samples were collected from individuals. There is the possibility of the build-up of within-host mutations, which could be used to estimate the time since infection in the future [136].

Genetic Diversity and Evolution through Mutation

The novel coronavirus is spreading throughout the world [48]. The number of infected patients has increased dramatically after the emergence of the virus in the wholesale market of seafood at the end of 2019 [147, 148]. The transmission of the virus through human-to-human contact has been confirmed, and viral load is found to be in saliva [149], broncho-alveolar lavage [148], throat [150], sputum [151], and nasopharyngeal swabs [149]. Among the important mechanisms of viral evolution in nature, nucleotide substitution is important [152]. Various questions have been raised regarding the sudden increase in the severity of SARS-CoV-2. For example, the development of the virus is carried out through genetic diversification. To analyze the genome variation, the complete or partial complete genome of SARS CoV-2 was taken (n=86) from the GISAID. The SARS CoV-2 strain was found in subjects belonging to various regions: one in Vietnam, one in Germany, one in Belgium, one in South Korea, two in Taiwan, two in England, three in Singapore, four in France, five in Japan, five in Australia, eleven in USA, and fifty in China. The analysis of pair-wise nucleotide sequence alignment was done through ClustalX2. Whereas, sequence of the Chinese strain was used as a reference genome [153, 154].

There is a long ORF1ab polyprotein at the 5' end SARS-CoV-2 molecular structure like other beta-coronaviruses, followed by the major structural proteins (n=4), including the matrix protein, small envelope protein, spike surface glycoprotein, and nucleocapsid protein [48]. Three deletions had been noted in the SARS CoV-2 during the genetic analysis in Victoria (Australia), Wisconsin (USA), and Aichi (Japan). Two deletions with 24 nucleotides and 3 nucleotides were noticed in polyprotein ORF1ab, and one deletion of 10 nucleotides was in the 3' of the genome [155]. Ninety-three mutations were observed in nucleotide sequence alignment over the complete SARS CoV-2 genome [48]. Missense mutations (n=42) were noticed in the major structural and non-structural proteins except for the envelope protein.

Similarly, in polyprotein ORF1ab, F367, Y364, and D354 mutations were found in the receptor-binding region of surface glycoprotein in spikes. Spike surface protein may play an important role in host cells for binding receptors and determining the host tropism [156]. This is also the prime focus for neutralizing the antibodies [157]. The conformational changes might be induced by a mutation in the surface spike glycoprotein, leading to a change in antigenicity [158]. However, there is a lack of studies regarding conformational changes in SARS-CoV-2 spike surface protein concerning the involvement of localization of amino acids.

CONCLUSION AND FUTURE PERSPECTIVE

In addition to co-morbid conditions and various risk factors, human genealogy may play an important role in the COVID-19 pandemic caused by SARS-CoV-2, a complex phenomenon. Numerous pieces of evidence point toward SARS-CoV-2 being a systemic condition affecting not only lungs but also the highest ACE2 expression was noted in different host tissues (humans) like kidneys, thyroid, heart, adipose tissue, small intestine, testicles, *etc*. Some genomes are more vulnerable to changes brought on by mutation because of the diversity of SARS-CoV-2 within the hosts. The relationship between genetic variations in the CYP2D6 enzyme system, HO-1 (an anti-inflammatory gene), and ACE2 enzyme has been linked to the clinical course of the disease. Additionally, to the ACE2 polymorphisms, TMPRSS2 gene variation may alter the pathogenesis of the virus by altering how ACE2 and SARS-CoV-2 interact. Novel ways for associating disease severity and susceptibility to host genetics are predicted to emerge with increased data availability and a better understanding of the mechanisms involved in COVID-19 severity.

REFERENCES

[1]   Orooji Y, Sohrabi H, Hemmat N, *et al.* An overview on SARS-CoV-2 (COVID-19) and other human coronaviruses and their detection capability *via* amplification assay, chemical sensing, biosensing, immunosensing, and clinical assays. Nano-Micro Lett 2021; 13(1): 18.
        [http://dx.doi.org/10.1007/s40820-020-00533-y] [PMID: 33163530]

[2]   Luria SE. In Cold Spring Harbor Symposia on Quantitative Biology. Cold Spring Harbor Laboratory Press 1953; Vol. 18: pp. 237-44.

[3]   Menni C, Valdes AM, Freidin MB, *et al.* Loss of smell and taste in combination with other symptoms is a strong predictor of COVID-19 infection. MedRxiv 2020.
        [http://dx.doi.org/10.1101/2020.04.05.20048421]

[4]   Long QX, Tang XJ, Shi QL, *et al.* Clinical and immunological assessment of asymptomatic SARS-CoV-2 infections. Nat Med 2020; 26(8): 1200-4.
        [http://dx.doi.org/10.1038/s41591-020-0965-6] [PMID: 32555424]

[5]   Linton N, Kobayashi T, Yang Y, *et al.* Incubation period and other epidemiological characteristics of 2019 novel coronavirus infections with right truncation: a statistical analysis of publicly available case data. J Clin Med 2020; 9(2): 538.
        [http://dx.doi.org/10.3390/jcm9020538] [PMID: 32079150]

[6]   Lauer SA, Grantz KH, Bi Q, *et al.* Jones, Qulu Zheng, Hannah R Meredith, Andrew S Azman, Nicholas G Reich, and Justin Lessler. The incubation period of coronavirus disease 2019 (covid-19) from publicly reported confirmed cases: estimation and application. Ann Intern Med 2020; 172(9): 577-82.
        [http://dx.doi.org/10.7326/M20-0504] [PMID: 32150748]

[7]   Rose R, Nolan DJ, Moot S, Feehan A. Sissy Cross, Julia Garcia-Diaz, and Susanna L Lamers. Intra-host site-specific polymorphisms of SARS-CoV-2 is consistent across multiple samples and methodologies. MedRxiv 2020.
        [http://dx.doi.org/10.1101/2020.04.24.20078691]

[8]   Karamitros T, Papadopoulou G, Bousali M, Mexias A, Tsiodras S, Mentis A. SARS-CoV-2 exhibits intra-host genomic plasticity and low-frequency polymorphic quasispecies. Genomics 2020; 131: 104585.
        [PMID: 32818852]

[9]   Andersen KG, Rambaut A, Lipkin WI, Holmes EC, Garry RF. The proximal origin of SARS-CoV-2. Nat Med 2020; 26(4): 450-2.
        [http://dx.doi.org/10.1038/s41591-020-0820-9] [PMID: 32284615]

[10]   Xiao K, Zhai J, Feng Y, *et al.* Isolation of SARS-CoV-2-related coronavirus from Malayan pangolins. Nature 2020; 583(7815): 286-9.
        [http://dx.doi.org/10.1038/s41586-020-2313-x] [PMID: 32380510]

[11]   Ferrario CM, Jessup J, Chappell MC, *et al.* Effect of angiotensin-converting enzyme inhibition and angiotensin II receptor blockers on cardiac angiotensin-converting enzyme 2. Circulation 2005; 111(20): 2605-10.
        [http://dx.doi.org/10.1161/CIRCULATIONAHA.104.510461] [PMID: 15897343]

[12]   Vickers NJ. Animal communication: when i'm calling you, will you answer too? Curr Biol 2017; 27(14): R713-5.
[http://dx.doi.org/10.1016/j.cub.2017.05.064] [PMID: 28743020]

[13]   Li MY, Li L, Zhang Y, Wang XS. Expression of the SARS-CoV-2 cell receptor gene ACE2 in a wide variety of human tissues. Infect Dis Poverty 2020; 9(1): 45.
[http://dx.doi.org/10.1186/s40249-020-00662-x] [PMID: 32345362]

[14]   Tallant EA, Clark MA. Molecular mechanisms of inhibition of vascular growth by angiotensin-(1-7). Hypertension 2003; 42(4): 574-9.
[http://dx.doi.org/10.1161/01.HYP.0000090322.55782.30] [PMID: 12953014]

[15]   Crackower M, Sarao R, Oudit GY, *et al.* Angiotensin-converting enzyme 2 is an essential regulator of heart function. 2002; 417(6891): 822-8.
[http://dx.doi.org/10.1038/nature00786]

[16]   Díez-Freire C, Vázquez J, Correa de Adjounian MF, *et al.* ACE2 gene transfer attenuates hypertension-linked pathophysiological changes in the SHR. Physiol Genomics 2006; 27(1): 12-9.
[http://dx.doi.org/10.1152/physiolgenomics.00312.2005] [PMID: 16788004]

[17]   Tikellis C, Pickering R, Tsorotes D, *et al.* Interaction of diabetes and ACE2 in the pathogenesis of cardiovascular disease in experimental diabetes. Clin Sci (Lond) 2012; 123(8): 519-29.
[http://dx.doi.org/10.1042/CS20110668] [PMID: 22616805]

[18]   Liu X, Sheng R, Qin Z. The neuroprotective mechanism of brain ischemic preconditioning. Acta Pharmacol Sin 2009; 30(8): 1071-80.
[http://dx.doi.org/10.1038/aps.2009.105] [PMID: 19617892]

[19]   Chen YY, Liu D, Zhang P, *et al.* Impact of ACE2 gene polymorphism on antihypertensive efficacy of ACE inhibitors. J Hum Hypertens 2016; 30(12): 766-71.
[http://dx.doi.org/10.1038/jhh.2016.24] [PMID: 27121444]

[20]   Luo Y, Liu C, Guan T, *et al.* Association of ACE2 genetic polymorphisms with hypertension-related target organ damages in south Xinjiang. Hypertens Res 2019; 42(5): 681-9.
[http://dx.doi.org/10.1038/s41440-018-0166-6] [PMID: 30542083]

[21]   Niu W, Qi Y, Hou S, Zhou W, Qiu C. Correlation of angiotensin-converting enzyme 2 gene polymorphisms with stage 2 hypertension in Han Chinese. Transl Res 2007; 150(6): 374-80.
[http://dx.doi.org/10.1016/j.trsl.2007.06.002] [PMID: 18022600]

[22]   Cao Y, Li L, Feng Z, *et al.* Comparative genetic analysis of the novel coronavirus (2019-nCoV/SARS-CoV-2) receptor ACE2 in different populations. Cell Discov 2020; 6(1): 11.
[http://dx.doi.org/10.1038/s41421-020-0147-1] [PMID: 32133153]

[23]   Hoffmann M, Kleine-Weber H, Schroeder S, *et al.* SARS-CoV-2 Cell Entry Depends on ACE2 and TMPRSS2 and Is Blocked by a Clinically Proven Protease Inhibitor. Cell 2020; 181: 271.
[http://dx.doi.org/10.1016/j.cell.2020.02.052] [PMID: 32142651]

[24]   Luostari K, Hartikainen JM, Tengström M, *et al.* Type II transmembrane serine protease gene variants associate with breast cancer. PLoS One 2014; 9(7): e102519.
[http://dx.doi.org/10.1371/journal.pone.0102519] [PMID: 25029565]

[25]   FitzGerald LM, Agalliu I, Johnson K, *et al.* Association of TMPRSS2-ERG gene fusion with clinical characteristics and outcomes: results from a population-based study of prostate cancer. BMC Cancer 2008; 8(1): 230.
[http://dx.doi.org/10.1186/1471-2407-8-230] [PMID: 18694509]

[26]   Giri VN, Ruth K, Hughes L, *et al.* Racial differences in prediction of time to prostate cancer diagnosis in a prospective screening cohort of high-risk men: effect of TMPRSS2 Met160Val. BJU Int 2011; 107(3): 466-70.
[http://dx.doi.org/10.1111/j.1464-410X.2010.09522.x] [PMID: 20735386]

[27]   Pechlaner R, Willeit P, Summerer M, *et al.* Heme oxygenase-1 gene promoter microsatellite polymorphism is associated with progressive atherosclerosis and incident cardiovascular disease. Arterioscler Thromb Vasc Biol 2015; 35(1): 229-36.
[http://dx.doi.org/10.1161/ATVBAHA.114.304729] [PMID: 25359861]

[28]   Yamada N, Yamaya M, Okinaga S, *et al.* Microsatellite polymorphism in the heme oxygenase-1 gene promoter is associated with susceptibility to emphysema. Am J Hum Genet 2000; 66(1): 187-95.
[http://dx.doi.org/10.1086/302729] [PMID: 10631150]

[29]   Okamoto I, Krögler J, Endler G, *et al.* A microsatellite polymorphism in the *heme oxygenase -1* gene promoter is associated with risk for melanoma. Int J Cancer 2006; 119(6): 1312-5.
[http://dx.doi.org/10.1002/ijc.21937] [PMID: 16596642]

[30]   Hirai H, Kubo H, Yamaya M, *et al.* Microsatellite polymorphism in heme oxygenase-1 gene promoter is associated with susceptibility to oxidant-induced apoptosis in lymphoblastoid cell lines. Blood 2003; 102(5): 1619-21.
[http://dx.doi.org/10.1182/blood-2002-12-3733] [PMID: 12730098]

[31]   Guénégou A, Leynaert B, Bénessiano J, *et al.* Association of lung function decline with the heme oxygenase-1 gene promoter microsatellite polymorphism in a general population sample. Results from the European Community Respiratory Health Survey (ECRHS), France. J Med Genet 2006; 43(8): e43-3.
[http://dx.doi.org/10.1136/jmg.2005.039743] [PMID: 16882737]

[32]   Exner M, Schillinger M, Minar E, *et al.* Heme oxygenase-1 gene promoter microsatellite polymorphism is associated with restenosis after percutaneous transluminal angioplasty. J Endovasc Ther 2001; 8(5): 433-40.
[http://dx.doi.org/10.1177/152660280100800501] [PMID: 11718398]

[33]   Bao W, Song F, Li X, *et al.* Association between heme oxygenase-1 gene promoter polymorphisms and type 2 diabetes mellitus: a HuGE review and meta-analysis. Am J Epidemiol 2010; 172(6): 631-6.
[http://dx.doi.org/10.1093/aje/kwq162] [PMID: 20682519]

[34]   Di Giorgio S, Martignano F, Torcia MG, Mattiuz G, Conticello SG. Evidence for host-dependent RNA editing in the transcriptome of SARS-CoV-2. Sci Adv 2020; 6(25): eabb5813.
[http://dx.doi.org/10.1126/sciadv.abb5813] [PMID: 32596474]

[35]   Krokan HE, Drabløs F, Slupphaug G. Uracil in DNA – occurrence, consequences and repair. Oncogene 2002; 21(58): 8935-48.
[http://dx.doi.org/10.1038/sj.onc.1205996] [PMID: 12483510]

[36]   Helleday T, Eshtad S, Nik-Zainal S. Mechanisms underlying mutational signatures in human cancers. Nat Rev Genet 2014; 15(9): 585-98.
[http://dx.doi.org/10.1038/nrg3729] [PMID: 24981601]

[37]   Clarke, JM; Majeed, A; Beaney, T. British Medical Journal Publishing Group 2021; Vol. 373.

[38]   Gorbalenya AE, Baker SC, Baric RS, *et al.* The species Severe acute respiratory syndrome-related coronavirus: classifying 2019-nCoV and naming it SARS-CoV-2. Nat Microbiol 2020; 5(4): 536-44.
[http://dx.doi.org/10.1038/s41564-020-0695-z] [PMID: 32123347]

[39]   Wu F, Zhao S, Yu B, *et al.* A new coronavirus associated with human respiratory disease in China. Nature 2020; 579(7798): 265-9.
[http://dx.doi.org/10.1038/s41586-020-2008-3] [PMID: 32015508]

[40]   Letko M, Marzi A, Munster V. Functional assessment of cell entry and receptor usage for SARS-Co-2 and other lineage B betacoronaviruses. Nature microbiology. 2020 Apr; 5(4): 562-9.

[41]   Guan W, Ni Z, Hu Y, *et al.* Clinical characteristics of coronavirus disease 2019 in China. N Engl J Med 2020; 382(18): 1708-20.
[http://dx.doi.org/10.1056/NEJMoa2002032] [PMID: 32109013]

[42]   Xiao K, Zhai J, Feng Y, *et al.* Isolation and characterization of 2019-nCoV-like coronavirus from Malayan pangolins. BioRxiv 2020.
[http://dx.doi.org/10.1101/2020.02.17.951335]

[43]   Xiao M, Liu X, Ji J, *et al.* Multiple approaches for massively parallel sequencing of SARS-CoV-2 genomes directly from clinical samples. Genome Med 2020; 12(1): 57.
[http://dx.doi.org/10.1186/s13073-020-00751-4]

[44]   Shu Y, McCauley J. GISAID: Global initiative on sharing all influenza data–from vision to reality. Eurosurveillance. 2017 Mar 30; 22(13): 30494.

[45]   Hadfield J, Megill C, Bell SM, *et al.* Nextstrain: real-time tracking of pathogen evolution. Bioinformatics 2018; 34(23): 4121-3.
[http://dx.doi.org/10.1093/bioinformatics/bty407] [PMID: 29790939]

[46]   Pachetti M, Marini B, Giudici F, *et al.* Impact of lockdown on Covid-19 case fatality rate and viral mutations spread in 7 countries in Europe and North America. J Transl Med 2020; 18(1): 338.
[http://dx.doi.org/10.1186/s12967-020-02501-x] [PMID: 32878627]

[47]   Jia Y, Shen G, Nguyen S, *et al.* Analysis of the mutation dynamics of SARS-CoV-2 reveals the spread history and emergence of RBD mutant with lower ACE2 binding affinity. BioRxiv 2021; 2020.2004.
[http://dx.doi.org/10.1101/2020.04.09.034942]

[48]   Phan T. Genetic diversity and evolution of SARS-CoV-2. Infect Genet Evol 2020; 81: 104260.
[http://dx.doi.org/10.1016/j.meegid.2020.104260] [PMID: 32092483]

[49]   Alm E, Broberg EK, Connor T, *et al.* Geographical and temporal distribution of SARS-CoV-2 clades in the WHO European Region, January to June 2020. Euro Surveill 2020; 25(32): 2001410.
[http://dx.doi.org/10.2807/1560-7917.ES.2020.25.32.2001410] [PMID: 32794443]

[50]   Lu J, du Plessis L, Liu Z, *et al.* Genomic epidemiology of SARS-CoV-2 in Guangdong province, China. Cell 2020; 181(5): 997-1003.
[http://dx.doi.org/10.1016/j.cell.2020.04.023]

[51]   Lauring AS, Andino R. Quasispecies Theory and the Behavior of RNA Viruses. PLoS Pathog 2010; 6(7): e1001005.
[http://dx.doi.org/10.1371/journal.ppat.1001005]

[52]   Vignuzzi M, Stone JK, Arnold JJ, Cameron CE, Andino R. Quasispecies diversity determines pathogenesis through cooperative interactions in a viral population. Nature 2006; 439(7074): 344-8.
[http://dx.doi.org/10.1038/nature04388] [PMID: 16327776]

[53]   Tsibris AMN, Korber B, Arnaout R, *et al.* Quantitative deep sequencing reveals dynamic HIV-1 escape and large population shifts during CCR5 antagonist therapy *in vivo*. PLoS One 2009; 4(5): e5683.
[http://dx.doi.org/10.1371/journal.pone.0005683] [PMID: 19479085]

[54]   Poon LLM, Song T, Rosenfeld R, *et al.* Quantifying influenza virus diversity and transmission in humans. Nat Genet 2016; 48(2): 195-200.
[http://dx.doi.org/10.1038/ng.3479] [PMID: 26727660]

[55]   Zhang Y, Leitner T, Albert J, Britton T. Inferring transmission heterogeneity using virus genealogies: Estimation and targeted prevention. PLOS Comput Biol 2020; 16(9): e1008122.
[http://dx.doi.org/10.1371/journal.pcbi.1008122] [PMID: 32881984]

[56]   Hu Y, Lu S, Song Z, *et al.* Association between adverse clinical outcome in human disease caused by novel influenza A H7N9 virus and sustained viral shedding and emergence of antiviral resistance. Lancet 2013; 381(9885): 2273-9.
[http://dx.doi.org/10.1016/S0140-6736(13)61125-3] [PMID: 23726392]

[57]   Wensing AM, Calvez V, Ceccherini-Silberstein F, *et al.* 2019 update of the drug resistance mutations in HIV-1. Top Antivir Med 2019; 27(3): 111-21.

[PMID: 31634862]

[58]   Sapoval N, Mahmoud M, Jochum MD, *et al.* Hidden genomic diversity of SARS-CoV-2: implications for qRT-PCR diagnostics and transmission. BioRxiv 2020.
[http://dx.doi.org/10.1101/2020.07.02.184481]

[59]   Zhao Z, Li H, Wu X, *et al.* Moderate mutation rate in the SARS coronavirus genome and its implications. BMC Evol Biol 2004; 4(1): 21.
[http://dx.doi.org/10.1186/1471-2148-4-21] [PMID: 15222897]

[60]   Nadeau S, Beckmann C, Topolsky I, *et al.* Quantifying SARS-CoV-2 spread in Switzerland based on genomic sequencing data. MedRxiv 2020.
[http://dx.doi.org/10.1101/2020.10.14.20212621]

[61]   Kuipers J, Batavia AA, Jablonski KP, *et al.* Within-patient genetic diversity of SARS-CoV-2. BioRxiv 2020.
[http://dx.doi.org/10.1101/2020.10.12.335919]

[62]   Taddei S, Virdis A, Ghiadoni L, Mattei P, Salvetti A. Effects of angiotensin converting enzyme inhibition on endothelium-dependent vasodilatation in essential hypertensive patients. J Hypertens 1998; 16(4): 447-56.
[http://dx.doi.org/10.1097/00004872-199816040-00006] [PMID: 9797190]

[63]   Korber B, Fischer WM, Gnanakaran S, *et al.* Tracking changes in SARS-CoV-2 spike: evidence that D614G increases infectivity of the COVID-19 virus. Cell 2020; 182(4): 812-27.
[http://dx.doi.org/10.1016/j.cell.2020.06.043]

[64]   Graudenzi A, Maspero D, Angaroni F, Piazza R, Ramazzotti D. Mutational signatures and heterogeneous host response revealed *via* large-scale characterization of SARS-CoV-2 genomic diversity. iScience 2021; 24(2): 102116.
[http://dx.doi.org/10.1016/j.isci.2021.102116] [PMID: 33532709]

[65]   Xiao M, Liu X, Ji J, *et al.* Multiple approaches for massively parallel sequencing of SARS-CoV-2 genomes directly from clinical samples. Genome Med 2020; 12(1): 57.
[http://dx.doi.org/10.1186/s13073-020-00751-4] [PMID: 32605661]

[66]   Denison MR, Graham RL, Donaldson EF, Eckerle LD, Baric RS. Coronaviruses. RNA Biol 2011; 8(2): 270-9.
[http://dx.doi.org/10.4161/rna.8.2.15013] [PMID: 21593585]

[67]   Peck KM, Lauring AS. Complexities of viral mutation rates. J Virol 2018; 92(14): e01031-17.
[http://dx.doi.org/10.1128/JVI.01031-17] [PMID: 29720522]

[68]   Romano M, Ruggiero A, Squeglia F, Maga G, Berisio R. A Structural View of SARS-CoV-2 RNA Replication Machinery: RNA Synthesis, Proofreading and Final Capping. Cells 2020; 9(5): 1267.
[http://dx.doi.org/10.3390/cells9051267] [PMID: 32443810]

[69]   Ramazzotti D, Angaroni F, Maspero D, *et al.* Quantification of intra-host genomic diversity of sars-cov-2 allows a high-resolution characterization of viral evolution and reveals functionally convergent variants. BioRxiv 2020.
[http://dx.doi.org/10.1101/2020.04.22.044404]

[70]   Benvenuto D, Angeletti S, Giovanetti M, *et al.* Evolutionary analysis of SARS-CoV-2: how mutation of Non-Structural Protein 6 (NSP6) could affect viral autophagy. J Infect 2020; 81(1): e24-7.
[http://dx.doi.org/10.1016/j.jinf.2020.03.058] [PMID: 32283146]

[71]   Thoms M, Buschauer R, Ameismeier M, *et al.* Structural basis for translational shutdown and immune evasion by the Nsp1 protein of SARS-CoV-2. Science 2020; 369(6508): 1249-55.
[http://dx.doi.org/10.1126/science.abc8665] [PMID: 32680882]

[72]   Ortiz-Prado E, Simbaña-Rivera K, Gómez- Barreno L, *et al.* Clinical, molecular, and epidemiological characterization of the SARS-CoV-2 virus and the Coronavirus Disease 2019 (COVID-19), a comprehensive literature review. Diagn Microbiol Infect Dis 2020; 98(1): 115094.

[http://dx.doi.org/10.1016/j.diagmicrobio.2020.115094] [PMID: 32623267]

[73]   J Alsaadi EA, Jones IM. Membrane binding proteins of coronaviruses. Future Virol 2019; 14(4): 275-86.
[http://dx.doi.org/10.2217/fvl-2018-0144] [PMID: 32201500]

[74]   Arndt AL, Larson BJ, Hogue BG. A conserved domain in the coronavirus membrane protein tail is important for virus assembly. J Virol 2010; 84(21): 11418-28.
[http://dx.doi.org/10.1128/JVI.01131-10] [PMID: 20719948]

[75]   Ou X, Liu Y, Lei X, *et al.* Characterization of spike glycoprotein of SARS-CoV-2 on virus entry and its immune cross-reactivity with SARS-CoV. Nat Commun 2020; 11(1): 1620.
[http://dx.doi.org/10.1038/s41467-020-15562-9] [PMID: 32221306]

[76]   Jadhav A, Zhao L, Liu W, *et al.* Genomic diversity and evolution of quasispecies in newcastle disease virus infections. Viruses 2020; 12(11): 1305.
[http://dx.doi.org/10.3390/v12111305] [PMID: 33202558]

[77]   Hunter DJ. Gene–environment interactions in human diseases. Nat Rev Genet 2005; 6(4): 287-98.
[http://dx.doi.org/10.1038/nrg1578] [PMID: 15803198]

[78]   Onder G, Rezza G, Brusaferro S. Case-fatality rate and characteristics of patients dying in relation to COVID-19 in Italy. JAMA 2020; 323(18): 1775-6.
[http://dx.doi.org/10.1001/jama.2020.4683] [PMID: 32203977]

[79]   Yang J, Zheng Y, Gou X, *et al.* Prevalence of comorbidities in the novel Wuhan coronavirus (COVID-19) infection: a systematic review and meta-analysis. Int J Infect Dis 2020; 94(1): 91-5.
[http://dx.doi.org/10.1016/j.ijid.2020.03.017] [PMID: 32173574]

[80]   Zhao Z, Sokhansanj BA, Malhotra C, Zheng K, Rosen GL. Genetic grouping of SARS-CoV-2 coronavirus sequences using informative subtype markers for pandemic spread visualization. PLOS Comput Biol 2020; 16(9): e1008269.
[http://dx.doi.org/10.1371/journal.pcbi.1008269] [PMID: 32941419]

[81]   Pradhan A, Olsson PE. Sex differences in severity and mortality from COVID-19: are males more vulnerable? Biol Sex Differ 2020; 11(1): 53.
[http://dx.doi.org/10.1186/s13293-020-00330-7] [PMID: 32948238]

[82]   Li M, Chen L, Zhang J, Xiong C, Li X. The SARS-CoV-2 receptor ACE2 expression of maternal-fetal interface and fetal organs by single-cell transcriptome study. PLoS One 2020; 15(4): e0230295.
[http://dx.doi.org/10.1371/journal.pone.0230295] [PMID: 32298273]

[83]   Li MY, Li L, Zhang Y, Wang XS. Expression of the SARS-CoV-2 cell receptor gene ACE2 in a wide variety of human tissues. Infectious diseases of poverty. 2020 Apr 1; 9(02): 23-9.

[84]   Lippi G, Lavie CJ, Henry BM, Sanchis-Gomar F. Do genetic polymorphisms in angiotensin converting enzyme 2 (*ACE2*) gene play a role in coronavirus disease 2019 (COVID-19)? Clin Chem Lab Med 2020; 58(9): 1415-22.
[http://dx.doi.org/10.1515/cclm-2020-0727] [PMID: 32598305]

[85]   Sungnak W, Huang N, Bécavin C, *et al.* SARS-CoV-2 entry factors are highly expressed in nasal epithelial cells together with innate immune genes. Nat Med 2020; 26(5): 681-7.
[http://dx.doi.org/10.1038/s41591-020-0868-6] [PMID: 32327758]

[86]   Xu H, Zhong L, Deng J, *et al.* High expression of ACE2 receptor of 2019-nCoV on the epithelial cells of oral mucosa. Int J Oral Sci 2020; 12(1): 8.
[http://dx.doi.org/10.1038/s41368-020-0074-x] [PMID: 32094336]

[87]   Monteil V, Kwon H, Prado P, *et al.* Inhibition of SARS-CoV-2 infections in engineered human tissues using clinical-grade soluble human ACE2. Int J Oral Sci 2020; 12(1): 1-5.
[http://dx.doi.org/10.1016/j.cell.2020.04.004]

[88]   Hattori Y, Hattori K, Machida T, Matsuda N. Vascular endotheliitis associated with infections: Its

pathogenetic role and therapeutic implication. Biochem Pharmacol 2022; 197: 114909.
[http://dx.doi.org/10.1016/j.bcp.2022.114909] [PMID: 35021044]

[89]   Varga Z, Flammer A, Steiger J, *et al.* Endothelial cell infection and endotheliitis in COVID-19. Lancet 2020; 95(10234): 19-20.
[http://dx.doi.org/10.1016/S0140-6736(20)30937-5]

[90]   Feldmann M, Maini RN, Woody JN, *et al.* Trials of anti-tumour necrosis factor therapy for COVID-19 are urgently needed. Lancet 2020; 395(10234): 1407-9.
[http://dx.doi.org/10.1016/S0140-6736(20)30858-8] [PMID: 32278362]

[91]   Hürlimann D, Forster A, Noll G, *et al.* Anti-tumor necrosis factor-α treatment improves endothelial function in patients with rheumatoid arthritis. Circulation 2002; 106(17): 2184-7.
[http://dx.doi.org/10.1161/01.CIR.0000037521.71373.44] [PMID: 12390945]

[92]   Flammer AJ, Sudano I, Hermann F, *et al.* Angiotensin-converting enzyme inhibition improves vascular function in rheumatoid arthritis. Circulation 2008; 117(17): 2262-9.
[http://dx.doi.org/10.1161/CIRCULATIONAHA.107.734384] [PMID: 18427133]

[93]   Silva RAP, Chu Y, Miller JD, *et al.* Impact of ACE2 deficiency and oxidative stress on cerebrovascular function with aging. Stroke 2012; 43(12): 3358-63.
[http://dx.doi.org/10.1161/STROKEAHA.112.667063] [PMID: 23160880]

[94]   Patnaik M, Pati P, Swain SN, *et al.* Association of angiotensin-converting enzyme and angiotensin-converting enzyme-2 gene polymorphisms with essential hypertension in the population of Odisha, India. Ann Hum Biol 2014; 41(2): 145-52.
[http://dx.doi.org/10.3109/03014460.2013.837195] [PMID: 24112034]

[95]   Duru K, Farrow S, Wang JM, Lockette W, Kurtz T. Frequency of a deletion polymorphism in the gene for angiotensin converting enzyme is increased in African-Americans with hypertension. Am J Hypertens 1994; 7(8): 759-62.
[http://dx.doi.org/10.1093/ajh/7.8.759] [PMID: 7986468]

[96]   Pinheiro DS, Santos RS, Jardim PCBV, *et al.* The combination of ACE I/D and ACE2 G8790A polymorphisms revels susceptibility to hypertension: A genetic association study in Brazilian patients. PLoS One 2019; 14(8): e0221248.
[http://dx.doi.org/10.1371/journal.pone.0221248] [PMID: 31430320]

[97]   Devaux CA, Rolain JM, Raoult D. ACE2 receptor polymorphism: Susceptibility to SARS-CoV-2, hypertension, multi-organ failure, and COVID-19 disease outcome. J Microbiol Immunol Infect 2020; 53(3): 425-35.
[http://dx.doi.org/10.1016/j.jmii.2020.04.015] [PMID: 32414646]

[98]   Xiao F, Zimpelmann J, Agaybi S, Gurley SB, Puente L, Burns KD. Characterization of angiotensin-converting enzyme 2 ectodomain shedding from mouse proximal tubular cells. PLoS One 2014; 9(1): e85958.
[http://dx.doi.org/10.1371/journal.pone.0085958] [PMID: 24454948]

[99]   Babcock GJ, Esshaki DJ, Thomas WD Jr, Ambrosino DM. Amino acids 270 to 510 of the severe acute respiratory syndrome coronavirus spike protein are required for interaction with receptor. J Virol 2004; 78(9): 4552-60.
[http://dx.doi.org/10.1128/JVI.78.9.4552-4560.2004] [PMID: 15078936]

[100] Lambert DW, Yarski M, Warner FJ, *et al.* Tumor necrosis factor-α convertase (ADAM17) mediates regulated ectodomain shedding of the severe-acute respiratory syndrome-coronavirus (SARS-CoV) receptor, angiotensin-converting enzyme-2 (ACE2). J Biol Chem 2005; 280(34): 30113-9.
[http://dx.doi.org/10.1074/jbc.M505111200] [PMID: 15983030]

[101] Glowacka I, Bertram S, Herzog P, *et al.* Differential downregulation of ACE2 by the spike proteins of severe acute respiratory syndrome coronavirus and human coronavirus NL63. J Virol 2010; 84(2): 1198-205.
[http://dx.doi.org/10.1128/JVI.01248-09] [PMID: 19864379]

[102]   Pillay TS. Gene of the month: the 2019-nCoV/SARS-CoV-2 novel coronavirus spike protein. J Clin Pathol 2020; 73(7): 366-9.
        [http://dx.doi.org/10.1136/jclinpath-2020-206658] [PMID: 32376714]

[103]   Scialo F, Daniele A, Amato F, *et al.* ACE2: the major cell entry receptor for SARS-CoV-2. Lung 2020; 198(6): 867-77.
        [http://dx.doi.org/10.1007/s00408-020-00408-4] [PMID: 33170317]

[104]   Choudhary S, Sreenivasulu K, Mitra P, Misra S, Sharma P. Role of genetic variants and gene expression in the susceptibility and severity of COVID-19. Annals of laboratory medicine. 2021 Mar 1; 41(2): 129-38.

[105]   Rao S, Lau A, So HC. Exploring diseases/traits and blood proteins causally related to expression of ACE2, the putative receptor of SARS-CoV-2: a Mendelian randomization analysis highlights tentative relevance of diabetes-related traits. Diabetes Care 2020; 43(7): 1416-26.
        [http://dx.doi.org/10.2337/dc20-0643] [PMID: 32430459]

[106]   Hussain M, Jabeen N, Raza F, *et al.* Structural variations in human ACE2 may influence its binding with SARS-CoV-2 spike protein. J Med Virol 2020; 92(9): 1580-6.
        [http://dx.doi.org/10.1002/jmv.25832] [PMID: 32249956]

[107]   Damas J, Hughes GM, Keough KC, *et al.* Broad host range of SARS-CoV-2 predicted by comparative and structural analysis of ACE2 in vertebrates. Proc Natl Acad Sci USA 2020; 117(36): 22311-22.
        [http://dx.doi.org/10.1073/pnas.2010146117] [PMID: 32826334]

[108]   Stawiski EW, Diwanji D, Suryamohan K, *et al.* Human ACE2 receptor polymorphisms predict SARS-CoV-2 susceptibility. BioRxiv 2020.
        [http://dx.doi.org/10.1101/2020.04.07.024752]

[109]   Goumenou M, Sarigiannis D, Tsatsakis A, *et al.* COVID□19 in Northern Italy: An integrative overview of factors possibly influencing the sharp increase of the outbreak (Review). Mol Med Rep 2020; 22(1): 20-32.
        [http://dx.doi.org/10.3892/mmr.2020.11079] [PMID: 32319647]

[110]   Benetti E, Tita R, Spiga O, *et al.* ACE2 gene variants may underlie interindividual variability and susceptibility to COVID-19 in the Italian population. Eur J Hum Genet 2020; 28(11): 1602-14.
        [http://dx.doi.org/10.1038/s41431-020-0691-z] [PMID: 32681121]

[111]   Chiu RWK, Tang NLS, Hui DSC, *et al.* ACE2 gene polymorphisms do not affect outcome of severe acute respiratory syndrome. Clin Chem 2004; 50(9): 1683-6.
        [http://dx.doi.org/10.1373/clinchem.2004.035436] [PMID: 15331509]

[112]   Liu D, Chen Y, Zhang P, *et al.* Association between circulating levels of ACE2-Ang-(1–7)-MAS axis and ACE2 gene polymorphisms in hypertensive patients. Medicine (Baltimore) 2016; 95(24): e3876.
        [http://dx.doi.org/10.1097/MD.0000000000003876] [PMID: 27310975]

[113]   Yang M, Zhao J, Xing L, Shi L. The association between angiotensin-converting enzyme 2 polymorphisms and essential hypertension risk: A meta-analysis involving 14,122 patients. J Renin Angiotensin Aldosterone Syst 2015; 16(4): 1240-4.
        [http://dx.doi.org/10.1177/1470320314549221] [PMID: 25237167]

[114]   Gadanec LK, McSweeney KR, Qaradakhi T, Ali B, Zulli A, Apostolopoulos V. Can SARS-CoV-2 virus use multiple receptors to enter host cells? Int J Mol Sci 2021; 22(3): 992.
        [http://dx.doi.org/10.3390/ijms22030992] [PMID: 33498183]

[115]   Cheng Z, Zhou J, To KKW, *et al.* Identification of TMPRSS2 as a susceptibility gene for severe 2009 pandemic A (H1N1) influenza and A (H7N9) influenza. J Infect Dis 2015; 212(8): 1214-21.
        [http://dx.doi.org/10.1093/infdis/jiv246] [PMID: 25904605]

[116]   Hou Y, Zhao J, Martin W, *et al.* New insights into genetic susceptibility of COVID-19: an ACE2 and TMPRSS2 polymorphism analysis. BMC Med 2020; 18(1): 216.
        [http://dx.doi.org/10.1186/s12916-020-01673-z] [PMID: 32664879]

[117]   Schuler BA, Habermann AC, Plosa EJ, *et al.* Age-related expression of SARS-CoV-2 priming protease TMPRSS2 in the developing lung. BioRxiv 2020.
[http://dx.doi.org/10.1101/2020.05.22.111187]

[118]   Hashemi SMA, Thijssen M, Hosseini SY, Tabarraei A, Pourkarim MR, Sarvari J. Human gene polymorphisms and their possible impact on the clinical outcome of SARS-CoV-2 infection. Arch Virol 2021; 166(8): 2089-108.
[http://dx.doi.org/10.1007/s00705-021-05070-6] [PMID: 33934196]

[119]   Fakhouri EW, Peterson SJ, Kothari J, Alex R, Shapiro JI, Abraham NG. Genetic polymorphisms complicate COVID-19 therapy: pivotal role of HO-1 in cytokine storm. Antioxidants 2020; 9(7): 636.
[http://dx.doi.org/10.3390/antiox9070636] [PMID: 32708430]

[120]   Zhou Y, Rui L. Leptin signaling and leptin resistance. Front Med 2013; 7(2): 207-22.
[http://dx.doi.org/10.1007/s11684-013-0263-5] [PMID: 23580174]

[121]   Peterson SJ, Dave N, Kothari J. The effects of heme oxygenase upregulation on obesity and the metabolic syndrome. Antioxid Redox Signal 2020; 32(14): 1061-70.
[http://dx.doi.org/10.1089/ars.2019.7954] [PMID: 31880952]

[122]   Peterson SJ, Shapiro JI, Thompson E, *et al.* adipokines, and endothelial dysfunction: a potential biomarker profile for cardiovascular risk in women with obesity. Obesity (Silver Spring) 2019; 27(1): 87-93.
[http://dx.doi.org/10.1002/oby.22354] [PMID: 30569635]

[123]   Peterson SJ, Vanella L, Bialczak A, *et al.* Oxidized HDL and isoprostane exert a potent adipogenic effect on stem cells: where in the lineage? Cell Stem Cells Regen Med 2016; 2(1).
[http://dx.doi.org/10.16966/2472-6990.109] [PMID: 29430566]

[124]   Aghagoli G, Gallo Marin B, Soliman LB, Sellke FW. Cardiac involvement in COVID-19 patients: Risk factors, predictors, and complications: A review. J Card Surg 2020; 35(6): 1302-5.
[http://dx.doi.org/10.1111/jocs.14538] [PMID: 32306491]

[125]   Singh SP, McClung JA, Thompson E, *et al.* Cardioprotective Heme Oxygenase-1-PGC1α Signaling in Epicardial Fat Attenuates Cardiovascular Risk in Humans as in Obese Mice. Obesity (Silver Spring) 2019; 27(10): 1634-43.
[http://dx.doi.org/10.1002/oby.22608] [PMID: 31441604]

[126]   Peterson SJ, Rubinstein R, Faroqui M, *et al.* Positive effects of heme oxygenase upregulation on adiposity and vascular dysfunction: gene targeting *vs.* pharmacologic therapy. Int J Mol Sci 2019; 20(10): 2514.
[http://dx.doi.org/10.3390/ijms20102514] [PMID: 31121826]

[127]   Menzel S, Thein SL. Genetic modifiers of fetal haemoglobin in sickle cell disease. Mol Diagn Ther 2019; 23(2): 235-44.
[http://dx.doi.org/10.1007/s40291-018-0370-8] [PMID: 30478714]

[128]   Pereira C, Relvas L, Bento C, Abade A, Ribeiro ML, Manco L. Polymorphic variations influencing fetal hemoglobin levels: Association study in beta-thalassemia carriers and in normal individuals of Portuguese origin. Blood Cells Mol Dis 2015; 54(4): 315-20.
[http://dx.doi.org/10.1016/j.bcmd.2015.02.001] [PMID: 25842369]

[129]   Sedgewick AE, Timofeev N, Sebastiani P, *et al.* BCL11A is a major HbF quantitative trait locus in three different populations with β-hemoglobinopathies. Blood Cells Mol Dis 2008; 41(3): 255-8.
[http://dx.doi.org/10.1016/j.bcmd.2008.06.007] [PMID: 18691915]

[130]   Galanello R, Origa R. Beta-thalassemia. Orphanet J Rare Dis 2010; 5(1): 11.
[http://dx.doi.org/10.1186/1750-1172-5-11] [PMID: 20492708]

[131]   Menzel S, Garner C, Gut I, *et al.* A QTL influencing F cell production maps to a gene encoding a zinc-finger protein on chromosome 2p15. Nat Genet 2007; 39(10): 1197-9.
[http://dx.doi.org/10.1038/ng2108] [PMID: 17767159]

[132] Lettre G, Sankaran VG, Bezerra MAC, *et al.* DNA polymorphisms at the *BCL11A*, *HBS1L-MYB*, and β- *globin* loci associate with fetal hemoglobin levels and pain crises in sickle cell disease. Proc Natl Acad Sci USA 2008; 105(33): 11869-74.
[http://dx.doi.org/10.1073/pnas.0804799105] [PMID: 18667698]

[133] Uda M, Galanello R, Sanna S, *et al.* Genome-wide association study shows *BCL11A* associated with persistent fetal hemoglobin and amelioration of the phenotype of β-thalassemia. Proc Natl Acad Sci USA 2008; 105(5): 1620-5.
[http://dx.doi.org/10.1073/pnas.0711566105] [PMID: 18245381]

[134] Yan R, Zhang Y, Li Y, Xia L, Guo Y, Zhou Q. Structural basis for the recognition of SARS-CoV-2 by full-length human ACE2. Science 2020; 367(6485): 1444-8.
[http://dx.doi.org/10.1126/science.abb2762] [PMID: 32132184]

[135] Popa A, Genger JW, Nicholson MD, *et al.* Genomic epidemiology of superspreading events in Austria reveals mutational dynamics and transmission properties of SARS-CoV-2. Sci Transl Med 2020; 12(573): eabe2555.
[http://dx.doi.org/10.1126/scitranslmed.abe2555] [PMID: 33229462]

[136] Tonkin-Hill G, Martincorena I, Amato R, *et al.* Patterns of within-host genetic diversity in SARS-CoV-2. eLife 2021; 10: e66857.
[http://dx.doi.org/10.7554/eLife.66857] [PMID: 34387545]

[137] Sawicki SG, Sawicki DL, Siddell SG. A contemporary view of coronavirus transcription. J Virol 2007; 81(1): 20-9.
[http://dx.doi.org/10.1128/JVI.01358-06] [PMID: 16928755]

[138] V'kovski P, Kratzel A, Steiner S, Stalder H, Thiel V. Coronavirus biology and replication: implications for SARS-CoV-2. Nat Rev Microbiol 2021; 19(3): 155-70.
[http://dx.doi.org/10.1038/s41579-020-00468-6] [PMID: 33116300]

[139] Wolff G, Limpens RWAL, Zevenhoven-Dobbe JC, *et al.* A molecular pore spans the double membrane of the coronavirus replication organelle. Science 2020; 369(6509): 1395-8.
[http://dx.doi.org/10.1126/science.abd3629] [PMID: 32763915]

[140] Hoopes JI, Cortez LM, Mertz TM, Malc EP, Mieczkowski PA, Roberts SA. APOBEC3A and APOBEC3B preferentially deaminate the lagging strand template during DNA replication. Cell Rep 2016; 14(6): 1273-82.
[http://dx.doi.org/10.1016/j.celrep.2016.01.021] [PMID: 26832400]

[141] Alexandrov LB, Kim J, Haradhvala NJ, *et al.* The repertoire of mutational signatures in human cancer. Nature 2020; 578(7793): 94-101.
[http://dx.doi.org/10.1038/s41586-020-1943-3] [PMID: 32025018]

[142] Wölfel R, Corman VM, Guggemos W, *et al.* Virological assessment of hospitalized patients with COVID-2019. Nature 2020; 581(7809): 465-9.
[http://dx.doi.org/10.1038/s41586-020-2196-x] [PMID: 32235945]

[143] Perera RAPM, Tso E, Tsang OTY, *et al.* SARS-CoV-2 virus culture and subgenomic RNA for respiratory specimens from patients with mild coronavirus disease. Emerg Infect Dis 2020; 26(11): 2701-4.
[http://dx.doi.org/10.3201/eid2611.203219] [PMID: 32749957]

[144] Fauver JR, Petrone ME, Hodcroft EB, *et al.* Coast-to-coast spread of SARS-CoV-2 during the early epidemic in the United States. Cell 2020; 181(5): 990-6.
[http://dx.doi.org/10.1016/j.cell.2020.04.021]

[145] Liu R, Wu P, Ogrodzki P, *et al.* Genomic epidemiology of SARS-CoV-2 in the UAE reveals novel virus mutation, patterns of co-infection and tissue specific host immune response. Sci Rep 2021; 11(1): 1-14.
[PMID: 33414495]

[146]   Meroni V, Zerrilli E, Genco F, Nocita B, Poletti F, Minoli L. Infection in the immunocompromised host (except HIV). Clin Microbiol Infect 2006; 12: 679-940.

[147]   Velavan TP, Meyer CG. The COVID-19 epidemic. Trop Med Int Health 2020; 25(3): 278-80.
[http://dx.doi.org/10.1111/tmi.13383] [PMID: 32052514]

[148]   Zhu N, Zhang D, Wang W, *et al.* A novel coronavirus from patients with pneumonia in China, 2019. N Engl J Med 2020; 382(8): 727-33.
[http://dx.doi.org/10.1056/NEJMoa2001017] [PMID: 31978945]

[149]   To KKW, Tsang OTY, Yip CCY, *et al.* Consistent detection of 2019 novel coronavirus in saliva. Clin Infect Dis 2020; 71(15): 841-3.
[http://dx.doi.org/10.1093/cid/ciaa149] [PMID: 32047895]

[150]   Bastola A, Sah R, Rodriguez-Morales AJ, *et al.* The first 2019 novel coronavirus case in Nepal. Lancet Infect Dis 2020; 20(3): 279-80.
[http://dx.doi.org/10.1016/S1473-3099(20)30067-0] [PMID: 32057299]

[151]   Lin X, Gong Z, Xiao Z, Xiong J, Fan B, Liu J. Novel coronavirus pneumonia outbreak in 2019: computed tomographic findings in two cases. Korean J Radiol 2020; 21(3): 365-8.
[http://dx.doi.org/10.3348/kjr.2020.0078] [PMID: 32056397]

[152]   Lauring AS, Andino R. Quasispecies theory and the behavior of RNA viruses. PLoS Pathog 2010; 6(7): e1001005.
[http://dx.doi.org/10.1371/journal.ppat.1001005] [PMID: 20661479]

[153]   Saitou N, Nei M. The neighbor-joining method: a new method for reconstructing phylogenetic trees. Mol Biol Evol 1987; 4(4): 406-25.
[PMID: 3447015]

[154]   Stavrinides J, Guttman DS. Mosaic evolution of the severe acute respiratory syndrome coronavirus. J Virol 2004; 78(1): 76-82.
[http://dx.doi.org/10.1128/JVI.78.1.76-82.2004] [PMID: 14671089]

[155]   Chakraborty AK. The 82 GHVMV and 141 KSF deletions in the Nsp1 protein of ORF1ab polyprotein favour the creation of immune-weak SARS-CoV-2. SunText Rev Virol. 2023; 3(2): 137.

[156]   Huang Y, Yang C, Xu X, Xu W, Liu S. Structural and functional properties of SARS-CoV-2 spike protein: potential antivirus drug development for COVID-19. Acta Pharmacol Sin 2020; 41(9): 1141-9.
[http://dx.doi.org/10.1038/s41401-020-0485-4] [PMID: 32747721]

[157]   Ju B, Zhang Q, Ge J, *et al.* Human neutralizing antibodies elicited by SARS-CoV-2 infection. Nature 2020; 584(7819): 115-9.
[http://dx.doi.org/10.1038/s41586-020-2380-z] [PMID: 32454513]

[158]   Singh PK, Kulsum U, Rufai SB, Mudliar SR, Singh S. Mutations in SARS-CoV-2 leading to antigenic variations in spike protein: a challenge in vaccine development. J Lab Physicians 2020; 12(2): 154-60.
[http://dx.doi.org/10.1055/s-0040-1715790] [PMID: 32884216]

CHAPTER 5

Newly Emerging Variants of SARS-CoV-2

Muhammad Safdar[1, *], **Mehmet Ozaslan**[2], **Yasmeen Junejo**[3], **Umair Younas**[4], **Muhammad Zia Ahmad**[5], **Jannat Bibi**[6] and **Sobia Noreen**[7]

[1] *Department of Breeding and Genetics, Cholistan University of Veterinary and Animal Sciences (CUVAS), Bahawalpur 63100, Pakistan*

[2] *Division of Molecular Biology and Genetics, Department of Biology, Gaziantep University, Gaziantep 27000, Turkey*

[3] *Department of Physiology and Biochemistry, Cholistan University of Veterinary and Animal Sciences (CUVAS), Bahawalpur 63100, Pakistan*

[4] *Department of Livestock Management, Cholistan University of Veterinary and Animal Sciences (CUVAS), Bahawalpur 63100, Pakistan*

[5] *Faculty of Social Sciences, University of Sargodha, Sargodha 40100, Punjab, Pakistan*

[6] *Institute for Chinese Olympic Advanced Study, Beijing Sport University, Beijing 100084, China*

[7] *Department of Pharmaceutical Technology, University of Innsbruck, Innsbruck 6020, Austria*

Abstract: Severe acute respiratory syndrome-coronavirus-2 (SARS-CoV-2) virus appeared at the end of 2019 and was subsequently named coronavirus disease-19 (COVID-19). Its worldwide emergence resulted in a large number of infections. Many studies depicted that the information about genomic variations in viruses has important effects on the prognosis and treatment of transmissible diseases. In this chapter, we collected various genomic variants, performed a phylogenetic analysis of recently registered genomes at various databases, and characterized the SARS-CoV-2 operating on silicon tools. Many complete sets of SARS-COV-2 are available in different databases such as GenBank and verified by National Genomics Data Center (NGDC) and National Microbiology Data Center (NMDC) databases. We found various variants, and the most common variants were 3037C>T (ORF1ab), 14408C>T (ORF1ab), 23403A>G (S), 25563G>T (ORF3a), 1059C>T (ORF1ab) and 241C>T (5' UTR) in online data samples. In addition, the complete genome sequence identity of the SARS-COV-2 results was 96.2% similar to that of a bat. These identified variations have increased the frequency of the spread of SARS-CoV-2. This information assists a comprehensive collection that combines genomic characterization, epidemiological and graphical records.

* **Corresponding author Muhammad Safdar:** Department of Breeding and Genetics, Cholistan University of Veterinary and Animal Sciences (CUVAS), Punjab, Bahawalpur 63100, Pakistan; Tel: +92-341-6946240, E-mail: msafdar@cuvas.edu.pk

Kamal Niaz, Muhammad Sajjad Khan & Muhammad Farrukh Nisar (Eds.)

Keywords: Genomic variants, Phylogenetic analysis, SARS-COV-2, ORF3a , epidemiological records .

INTRODUCTION

The World Health Organization (WHO) declared COVID-19 a global pandemic, and this crisis continues to result in millions of deaths worldwide. Furthermore, it has a significant impact on the world economy. Despite the efforts of healthcare workers and scientists worldwide, the number of confirmed cases and deaths continues to rise. As mentioned in the literature, there are currently a limited number of clinically approved vaccines and antiviral medications available to control the spread of the virus [1 - 3]. However, efforts to develop new treatments and vaccines continue, and ongoing vaccination campaigns are underway in many countries to mitigate the impact of the pandemic [1]. This chapter demonstrates the current genome present in the online databases to better understand the variation and genomic characteristics of SARS-CoV-2. It is important to note that the genome is 30 kb, and its structure corresponds to particular features of SARS-CoV and MERS-CoV [2 - 4].

High-quality, complete genome sequences of viral isolates, regardless of their virulence or other unique characteristics, are essential for accurate COVID-19 sequencing and analysis [5]. Therefore, the spread of COVID-19 is expected to persist, with increasing genetic diversity due to seasonal outbreaks. The evolution of its subtype can be revealed through ongoing genome data analysis, and the subtype evolution dynamics will reveal the genome data analysis [6]. Different databases make genomic information of SARS-COV-2 available to the public for research and discovery of new drugs [7]. For data sharing, users must agree to cooperate with all data participants and give appropriate credit. Some countries like China, the Philippines, and Japan have contributed to the success of this initiative, even though they did not share it. WHO supports the rapid release of available coronavirus sequences that provide comprehensive information to the public and researchers through databases. COVID-19 variants and microRNAs are involved in their pathogenesis. However, the role of microRNAs in viral infections is not clear. MicroRNA-mediated gene regulation plays a role in the host's response to different COVID-19 variants. It is necessary to determine the specific microRNAs involved and their functional significance in COVID-19 pathogenesis and its variants.

Therefore, this chapter helps provide comprehensive and instant data that incorporates genomic variants, epidemiology, and clinical features of COVID-19 patients simultaneously [8]. By mining and utilizing the databases and building a statistical framework based on genetic, antigenic, and epidemiological information, more insights are gained into new variants, thereby advancing the potential for preventing and controlling COVID-19 [3, 9, 10]. In this chapter, we focused on discussing the variants between the old and recently sequenced genomes of SARS-CoV-2 and phylogenetic analysis for the origin of this virus.

NGDC and NMDC Databases

We downloaded different available genomes from GenBank and verified them from NGDC and NMDC databases. Previously, some genomes were excluded from the analysis due to excessive variations with gaps. A study utilized the NC_045512 genome sequence as a reference for genomic coordinates to analyze real samples [11]. As a result, the coordinates of the genome should be adjusted for comparison with previous studies [12]. Before conducting the analysis, the genomes were compared and matched to the reference genome. The alignment process used default clearance penalties of 10 and extension penalties of 0.5. The differences were removed compared to NC_045512 to create variants [13]. In this study, the researchers used protein annotations to convert nucleotide-level variants to amino acid codon variants, which were then aligned with the genes [14]. The study also identified nucleotide mutations in the genomes of the coronaviruses. Additionally, a whole-genome-based phylogenetic tree of the coronaviruses was constructed using the maximum-likelihood method with BEAST, and the GTR+I+G nucleotide model of substitution was used. This type of analysis can help researchers understand the genetic relationships between different strains of the virus and how it has evolved. In the phylogenetic trees, it is used to identify COVID-19 variants and understand their origin and relationships with others. By comparing the genetic sequences of different variants, some scientists have determined that the mutations track the spread of the variants worldwide.

Identification of Variants

Many variants were found in different online databases, and some variants were found to be unique (Tables **1** and **2**). Some distinct variants of the genomes, such as missense, synonymous, and non-coding alleles, are shown in Tables **1** and **2**. The variants such as 3037C>T(ORF1ab), 14408C>T (ORF1ab), 23403A>G (S), 25563G>T (ORF3a), 1059C>T (ORF1ab) and 241C>T (5' UTR) [7] were present. Both 3037C>T and 23403A>G (S) are synonymous. Furthermore, 14408C>T causes amino acid modifications such as P4803L in ORF1ab, and 25563G>T causes amino acids to change Q8521H [7]. It is worth noting that the majority of the sub-strains carrying the 14408C>T and 25563G>T variants are found outside of Wuhan, and the most commonly observed base change is C>T. After that, the frequency of the SARS-CoV-2 ORF1ab gene showed that this gene was the most mutated in the viral genome, while E (Envelope) and ORF6 genes were detected as the most stable genes, depending on the available data. Furthermore, the new virus had a genome sequence identity of 96.2% when compared to a bat SARS-related coronavirus (SARSr-CoV; RaTG13) that was discovered in Wuhan, China. However, its genome showed a dissimilarity of about 79% to SARS-CoV and approximately 50% to MERS-CoV. It is important to note that identifying COVID-19 variants is an ongoing process till now, and new variants will emerge over time. Therefore, it is crucial to continue monitoring the spread of the virus and adapting our response as necessary to contain its spread, and the world will continue to cope with it.

SARS-COV-2 Sequence Analysis

Annotation is a critical step in deciphering the genetic information programmed in various organisms. The SARS-CoV genome is relatively small, with a length of less than 30 kilobases. However, some of its coding genes do not conform to the typical features of viral genomes and contain a larger amount of genetic information [15]. The genome also encodes several nonstructural proteins, although information about some of these proteins is lacking [7, 15]. Overall, the number of modifications/changes is determined in the sequenced SARS-CoV-2 sequence data and the evolutionary construction position of the virus. SARS-CoV-2 sequence analysis is used to track the spread of the virus across different geographic regions. By comparing the sequences of viruses from different patients, the scientists construct the tree of the virus and identify clusters of related viruses. Finally, the SARS-CoV-2 sequence analysis is used for the epidemiology of COVID-19 and for developing effective strategies to control its spread worldwide.

ORFs Genes Variants

SARS-CoV-2 virus contains several open reading frames (ORFs) encoding various genes. Some of these genes and variants are associated with them, such as spike (S) protein. So, variants in the S protein gene, particularly N501Y and E484K, are related to transmissibility and potential immune evasion. Another one is the nucleocapsid (N) protein that plays a role in virus replication and is also the target of some diagnostic tests. The variants in the N protein gene, including P80R, are identified in some cases of re-infection. An RNA-dependent RNA polymerase (RdRp) protein is the target of some antiviral drugs.

The variants in the RdRp gene, including P323L, are identified in drug-resistance cases. In addition, ORF1a and ORF1b are involved in virus replication and assembly in the host. These variants in the ORFs are associated with changes in viral pathogenicity. In the case of ORF3a, it encodes a protein that plays a role in viral entry and immune evasion. The variants in this ORF, including Q57H, were associated with increased transmissibility. Therefore, the identification and characterization of these genes and variants are associated with SARS-CoV-2, which are crucial for understanding the transmission of COVID-19 and for developing effective treatments and vaccines. Furthermore, several studies have highlighted the significance of ORF genes in the pathogenesis of the novel coronavirus disease [15 - 18]. So, in this chapter, a large number of variants are presented (Tables **1** and **2**). The genome analysis revealed that a significant number of genomes did not show any variations, except for some missing base pairs at the start and end. However, there were some distinct variants observed in the remaining genomes, which included missense, synonymous, and non-coding alleles. These variants are documented and presented in Tables **1** and **2**, which may be useful in understanding the genetic diversity and evolution of the coronaviruses. The most common variants were 3037C>T (ORF1ab), 14408C>T (ORF1ab), 23403A>G (S), 25563G>T (ORF3a), 1059C>T (ORF1ab), and 241C>T (5' UTR) [7]. Both 3037C>T and 23403A>G (S) are called synonymous. It should be noted that 14408C>T, which is a change of amino acids such as P4803L in ORF1ab, and 25563G>T cause amino acids to change Q8521H [7]. Notably, most 14408C>T and 25563G>T variant sub-strains are found outside Wuhan, China. As far as base changes are considered, the most often observed one is C>T [7]. It appears that due to coronaviruses being single-stranded RNA viruses, the study did not combine C>T and G>A mutations. This is likely because these mutations occur in different contexts and may have different functional consequences. The study has also taken into account the strong bias towards base transition mutations *versus* base transversion mutations that have been observed in its genome [31]. This information is important in understanding the molecular biology of SARS-COV-2 and its potential impact on public health. Also, in this chapter, the frequency of the SARS-CoV-2 ORF1ab gene showed that this gene was the most mutated in the viral genome, while E (Envelope) and ORF6 genes were detected as the most stable genes, depending on the available data [32]. The novel virus has a whole-genome sequence collected in Wuhan, China. However, its similarity to the genomes of SARS-CoV is only about 79%, and to those of MERS-CoV, it is about 50% [19, 33]. Viral evolution in nature is primarily driven by nucleotide substitution and recombination, which are thought to be the main mechanisms behind the emergence of new viruses [19, 33]. The rapid spread of SARS-CoV-2 has led researchers to investigate whether the virus's evolution is driven by mutations [20, 33]. Understanding the rate and types of mutations that occur in the virus can provide insight into how it spreads, how it interacts with host cells, and how it can potentially be treated or prevented. Identifying and tracking mutations in the virus can also help in the development of diagnostic tests, vaccines, and treatments. Therefore, studying the evolution of SARS-CoV-2 is crucial in mitigating its impact on public health.

Table 1. Mutation list that is identified in the genomes of SARS-CoV-2 [7].

Accession No.	Locations	Variations	Genes	Results	Mutations
MT308702	APR/2020-USA:NC	1059C>T	ORF1ab	-	Synonymous
MT308702	APR/2020-USA:NC	3037C>T	ORF1ab	-	Synonymous
MT308702	APR/2020-USA:NC	14408C>T	ORF1ab	P4803L	Missense
MT308702	APR/2020-USA:NC	23403A>G	S	-	Synonymous
MT308702	APR/2020-USA:NC	25563G>T	ORF3a	Q8521H	Missense
MT308703	APR/2020-USA:NC	490T>A	ORF1ab	D75E	Missense
MT308703	APR/2020-USA:NC	3177C>T	ORF1ab	P971L	Missense
MT308703	APR/2020-USA:NC	8782C>T	ORF1ab	-	Synonymous
MT308703	APR/2020-USA:NC	15960C>T	ORF1ab	-	Synonymous
MT308703	APR/2020-USA:NC	18736T>C	ORF1ab	F6245L	Missense
MT308703	APR/2020-USA:NC	19684G>T	ORF1ab	-	Synonymous
MT308703	APR/2020-USA:NC	26729T>C	M	-	Synonymous
MT308703	APR/2020-USA:NC	27635C>T	ORF7a	-	Synonymous
MT308703	APR/2020-USA:NC	28077G>C	ORF8	V62L	Missense
MT308704	APR/2020-USA:NC	833T>C	ORF1ab	L278P	Missense
MT308704	APR/2020-USA:NC	3037C>T	ORF1ab	-	Synonymous
MT308704	APR/2020-USA:NC	14408C>T	ORF1ab	P4803L	Missense
MT308704	APR/2020-USA:NC	23403A>G	S	-	Synonymous
MT308704	APR/2020-USA:NC	25563G>T	ORF3a	Q8521H	Missense
MT308704	APR/2020-USA:NC	27964C>T	ORF8	H9321Y	Missense
MT350253	APR/2020-USA:VA	3037C>T	ORF1ab	-	Synonymous
MT350253	APR/2020-USA:VA	14408C>T	ORF1ab	P4803L	Missense
MT350253	APR/2020-USA:VA	23403A>G	S	-	Synonymous

Table 2. Genomes of SARS-CoV-2 contain variations (mutations) in non-coding region [7].

Accession No.	Locations	Variations (Mutation)	Non-coding Region
MT308702	APR/2020-USA:NC	241C>T	5UTR
MT308703	APR/2020-USA:NC	29700A>G	3UTR
MT308704	APR/2020-USA:NC	241C>T	5UTR
MT350254	APR/2020-USA:VA	241C>T	5UTR
MT350255	APR/2020-USA:VA	241C>T	5UTR
MT350256	APR/2020-USA:VA	241C>T	5UTR
MT350257	APR/2020-USA:VA	241C>T	5UTR
MT350257	APR/2020-USA:VA	29733C>T	3UTR
MT358644	01/APR/2020-USA:WA	31A>T	5UTR
MT358644	01/APR/2020-USA:WA	34A>T	5UTR
MT358644	01/APR/2020-USA:WA	35A>T	5UTR
MT358644	01/APR/2020-USA:WA	36C>T	5UTR
MT358644	01/APR/2020-USA:WA	241C>T	5UTR
MT358743	01/APR/2020-USA:WA	241C>T	5UTR
MT358744	01/APR/2020-USA:WA	241C>T	5UTR
MT345882	31/MAR/2020-USA:WA	36C>T	5UTR
MT345883	31/MAR/2020-USA:WA	36C>T	5UTR
MT345883	31/MAR/2020-USA:WA	241C>T	5UTR
MT358645	31/MAR/2020-USA:WA	241C>G	5UTR
MT358646	31/MAR/2020-USA:WA	36C>T	5UTR
MT358646	31/MAR/2020-USA:WA	241C>T	5UTR
MT358647	31/MAR/2020-USA:WA	34A>T	5UTR
MT358647	31/MAR/2020-USA:WA	35A>T	5UTR
MT358647	31/MAR/2020-USA:WA	36C>T	5UTR
MT358647	31/MAR/2020-USA:WA	241C>T	5UTR

It is also important to know that the replicase enzyme comprises two polyproteins, such as ORF1a and ORF1ab, which undergo cleavage by three viral proteases to form 12 nonstructural proteins [18, 21]. The ORF1ab polyprotein comprises nsps 1-3 proteins, which are considered the most significant region among coronaviruses [22]. Many researchers have investigated that genomic databases contain information about the association of ORFs with COVID-19, specifically the 8782C>T (ORF1ab) and 28144T>C (ORF8) mutations [3, 12, 16, 23]. As a result, dividing the biological role of the specific ORF1ab protein in SARS-CoV-

2 would have clinical relevance. However, a motif VLVVL (amino acid 75-79) was found in the Orf8b protein of SARS-CoV, which may activate intracellular stress pathways and downregulate the target receptors [3, 21]. Therefore, investigating the role of the orf8 protein in COVID-19 is crucial, especially when considering ORF10, a short peptide consisting of 38 amino acids. A study demonstrated that the disease is associated with ORF10, which has no similar proteins in the NCBI database [7, 12]. This distinct protein has the potential to detect infections faster than PCR-based methods [12], but further characterization is necessary to investigate the detailed pattern for further use.

NSP3 Gene Variants

The NSP3 gene is a significant point of contrast and a putative protein in SARS-CoV [24, 25], suggesting a crucial association between nsp3 and the onset of coronavirus infection [26]. Moreover, additional research has revealed that nsp3 comprises a papain-like protease, which is essential for SARS-CoV infection [27 - 29]. Furthermore, Sawicki *et al.* sequenced ORF1 from a vast amount of laboratory-established data [30]. Many researchers reported point transformations from non-synonymous substitutions in NSPs 4, 5, 10, 12, 14, and 16 in ORF1a and ORF1ab [7, 18, 30]. Specifically, seven of the eight reported mutations in MHV have an impact on amino acid residues that are associated with SARS-CoV [30]. This was the reason for determining such genomic variants in SARS-COV-2 genomes. Taken together, this chapter fully supports and will be used as an effective way for the development of treatment and vaccine production for COVID-19.

Other Variants of SARS-CoV-2 in the World

Multiple variants emerged due to genetic changes in the spike proteins, causing concern for the global immunization campaign. The first significant genetic change in SARS-CoV-2 spike proteins (D614 to G614) resulted in greater speed and infectious loads but not improved clinical outcomes [34]. Most of the COVID-19 vaccines are targeted at receptor binding protein (RBD) for the original spike protein of Wuhan-Hu-1. This part of the virus is always subject to immunological pressure for vaccine neutralization to mutate, escape, or decrease [35]. This resulted in the development of a few significant variants, including B117 (UK), B1351 (South Africa), P1 (Brazilian), and B16172 (India), which boosted the dissemination and infection rate of SARS CoV-2 in individuals [36]. Additionally, the novel virus shared 96.2% similarity in its genome sequence with a bat SARS-related coronavirus (SARSr-CoV; RaTG13) identified in Wuhan, China. Nevertheless, the comparison revealed that it had a dissimilarity of around 79% to SARS-CoV and approximately 50% to MERS-CoV in their respective genomes [37 - 39]. It is worth knowing that some of these variants have been identified in Pakistani citizens, highlighting the importance of continued monitoring and surveillance of the virus's evolution to prevent its spread and control its impact on public health. The primary cause of this transmission could be unscreened commercial flights and no examination upon arrival in Pakistan from other countries, resulting in the quick introduction of variants of concern in Pakistan.

CONCLUSION

The emergence of new variants of COVID-19 has elevated concerns about their potential impact on the global pandemic. Multiple variants, such as alpha, beta, gamma, and delta, were identified and further analyzed. The analysis of genomic signatures shows a robust correlation between the sample collection time, sample location, and the accumulation of genetic diversity. The most common variants were 3037C>T(ORF1ab), 14408C>T (ORF1ab), 23403A>G (S), 25563G>T (ORF3a), 1059C>T (ORF1ab), and 241C>T (5' UTR) [7]. These genomic and proteomic mutations in SARS-CoV-2 may impact its severity and transmission. However, it is important to continue monitoring the situation related to them closely and adapting our response as necessary for the body's conditions. This includes ongoing surveillance of the spread of the virus, the emergence of new variants, and the development of new vaccines and treatments that better target these deadly variants. The emergence of new variants is a major cause, and it will remain vigilant for the spread of COVID-19. Therefore, in this chapter, collecting information about the genomics of this virus and sharing the data with the whole world will be useful for developing a cure and possible achievement of the vaccine against COVID-19.

REFERENCES

[1] Ozaslan M, Safdar M, Kilic IH, Khailany RA. Practical Measures to Prevent COVID-19: A Mini-Review. J Biol Sci 2020; 20: 100-2.
[http://dx.doi.org/10.3923/jbs.2020.100.102]

[2] de Wit E, van Doremalen N, Falzarano D, Munster VJ. SARS and MERS: recent insights into emerging coronaviruses. Nat Rev Microbiol 2016; 14(8): 523-34.
[http://dx.doi.org/10.1038/nrmicro.2016.81] [PMID: 27344959]

[3] Luk HKH, Li X, Fung J, Lau SKP, Woo PCY. Molecular epidemiology, evolution and phylogeny of SARS coronavirus. Infect Genet Evol 2019; 71: 21-30.
[http://dx.doi.org/10.1016/j.meegid.2019.03.001] [PMID: 30844511]

[4] Schoeman D, Fielding BC. Coronavirus envelope protein: current knowledge. Virol J 2019; 16(1): 69.
[http://dx.doi.org/10.1186/s12985-019-1182-0] [PMID: 31133031]

[5] Churko JM, Mantalas GL, Snyder MP, Wu JC. Overview of high throughput sequencing technologies to elucidate molecular pathways in cardiovascular diseases. Circ Res 2013; 112(12): 1613-23.
[http://dx.doi.org/10.1161/CIRCRESAHA.113.300939] [PMID: 23743227]

[6]   McHardy AC, Adams B. The role of genomics in tracking the evolution of influenza A virus. PLoS Pathog 2009; 5(10): e1000566.
[http://dx.doi.org/10.1371/journal.ppat.1000566] [PMID: 19855818]

[7]   Khailany RA, Safdar M, Ozaslan M. Genomic characterization of a novel SARS-CoV-2. Gene Rep 2020; 19: 100682.
[http://dx.doi.org/10.1016/j.genrep.2020.100682] [PMID: 32300673]

[8]   Payne DC, Biggs HM, Al-Abdallat MM, *et al.*, Multihospital outbreak of a Middle East respiratory syndrome coronavirus deletion variant, Jordan: a molecular, serologic, and epidemiologic investigation. Open forum Infectious Diseases. US: Oxford University Press 2018; 5: p. (5)ofy095.

[9]   Ge XY, Li JL, Yang XL, *et al.* Isolation and characterization of a bat SARS-like coronavirus that uses the ACE2 receptor. Nature 2013; 503(7477): 535-8.
[http://dx.doi.org/10.1038/nature12711] [PMID: 24172901]

[10]   Yang XL, Hu B, Wang B, *et al.* Isolation and Characterization of a Novel Bat Coronavirus Closely Related to the Direct Progenitor of Severe Acute Respiratory Syndrome Coronavirus. J Virol 2016; 90(6): 3253-6.
[http://dx.doi.org/10.1128/JVI.02582-15] [PMID: 26719272]

[11]   Lu R, Zhao X, Li J, *et al.* Genomic characterisation and epidemiology of 2019 novel coronavirus: implications for virus origins and receptor binding. Lancet 2020; 395(10224): 565-74.
[http://dx.doi.org/10.1016/S0140-6736(20)30251-8] [PMID: 32007145]

[12]   Koyama T. Platt D. & Parida. L. Variant analysis of COVID-19 genomes. Bull World Health Organ 2020.
[http://dx.doi.org/10.2471/BLT.20.253591]

[13]   Rice P, Longden I, Bleasby A. EMBOSS: The European Molecular Biology Open Software Suite. Trends Genet 2000; 16(6): 276-7.
[http://dx.doi.org/10.1016/S0168-9525(00)02024-2] [PMID: 10827456]

[14]   Arvestad, . alv: a console-based viewer for molecular sequence alignments. Journal of Open Source Software. 2018; 3: 955.
[http://dx.doi.org/10.21105/joss.00955]

[15]   Xu J, Hu J, Wang J, *et al.* Genome organization of the SARS-CoV. Genomics Proteomics Bioinformatics 2003; 1(3): 226-35.
[http://dx.doi.org/10.1016/S1672-0229(03)01028-3] [PMID: 15629035]

[16]   Kirchdoerfer RN, Ward AB. Structure of the SARS-CoV nsp12 polymerase bound to nsp7 and nsp8 co-factors. Nat Commun 2019; 10(1): 2342.
[http://dx.doi.org/10.1038/s41467-019-10280-3] [PMID: 31138817]

[17]   van der Meer Y, van Tol H, Krijnse Locker J, Snijder EJ. ORF1a-encoded replicase subunits are involved in the membrane association of the arterivirus replication complex. J Virol 1998; 72(8): 6689-98.
[http://dx.doi.org/10.1128/JVI.72.8.6689-6698.1998] [PMID: 9658116]

[18]   Graham RL, Sparks JS, Eckerle LD, Sims AC, Denison MR. SARS coronavirus replicase proteins in pathogenesis. Virus Res 2008; 133(1): 88-100.
[http://dx.doi.org/10.1016/j.virusres.2007.02.017] [PMID: 17397959]

[19]   Rehman S, Shafique L, Ihsan A, Liu Q. Evolutionary Trajectory for the Emergence of Novel Coronavirus SARS-CoV-2. Pathogens 2020; 9(3): 240.
[http://dx.doi.org/10.3390/pathogens9030240] [PMID: 32210130]

[20]   Phan T. Genetic diversity and evolution of SARS-CoV-2. Infect Genet Evol 2020; 81(July): 104260.
[http://dx.doi.org/10.1016/j.meegid.2020.104260] [PMID: 32092483]

[21]   Shi CS, Nabar NR, Huang NN, Kehrl JH. SARS-Coronavirus Open Reading Frame-8b triggers

intracellular stress pathways and activates NLRP3 inflammasomes. Cell Death Discov 2019; 5(1): 101.
[http://dx.doi.org/10.1038/s41420-019-0181-7] [PMID: 31231549]

[22]   Woo PCY, Huang Y, Lau SKP, Yuen KY. Coronavirus genomics and bioinformatics analysis. Viruses 2010; 2(8): 1804-20.
[http://dx.doi.org/10.3390/v2081803] [PMID: 21994708]

[23]   Yin C. Genotyping coronavirus SARS-CoV-2: methods and implications. Genomics. 2020 Sep 1; 112(5): 3588-96.

[24]   Putics Á, Filipowicz W, Hall J, Gorbalenya AE, Ziebuhr J. ADP-ribose-1"-monophosphatase: a conserved coronavirus enzyme that is dispensable for viral replication in tissue culture. J Virol 2005; 79(20): 12721-31.
[http://dx.doi.org/10.1128/JVI.79.20.12721-12731.2005] [PMID: 16188975]

[25]   Snijder EJ, Bredenbeek PJ, Dobbe JC, *et al.* Unique and conserved features of genome and proteome of SARS-coronavirus, an early split-off from the coronavirus group 2 lineage. J Mol Biol 2003; 331(5): 991-1004.
[http://dx.doi.org/10.1016/S0022-2836(03)00865-9] [PMID: 12927536]

[26]   Hurst KR, Koetzner CA, Masters PS. Characterization of a critical interaction between the coronavirus nucleocapsid protein and nonstructural protein 3 of the viral replicase-transcriptase complex. J Virol 2013; 87(16): 9159-72.
[http://dx.doi.org/10.1128/JVI.01275-13] [PMID: 23760243]

[27]   Lindner HA, Fotouhi-Ardakani N, Lytvyn V, Lachance P, Sulea T, Ménard R. The papain-like protease from the severe acute respiratory syndrome coronavirus is a deubiquitinating enzyme. J Virol 2005; 79(24): 15199-208.
[http://dx.doi.org/10.1128/JVI.79.24.15199-15208.2005] [PMID: 16306591]

[28]   Niemeyer D, Mösbauer K, Klein EM, *et al.* The papain-like protease determines a virulence trait that varies among members of the SARS-coronavirus species. PLoS Pathog 2018; 14(9): e1007296.
[http://dx.doi.org/10.1371/journal.ppat.1007296] [PMID: 30248143]

[29]   Hurst KR, Koetzner CA, Masters PS. Characterization of a critical interaction between the coronavirus nucleocapsid protein and nonstructural protein 3 of the viral replicase-transcriptase complex. J Virol 2013; 87(16): 9159-72.
[http://dx.doi.org/10.1128/JVI.01275-13] [PMID: 23760243]

[30]   Sawicki SG, Sawicki DL, Younker D, *et al.* Functional and genetic analysis of coronavirus replicase-transcriptase proteins. PLoS Pathog 2005; 1(4): e39.
[http://dx.doi.org/10.1371/journal.ppat.0010039] [PMID: 16341254]

[31]   Lyons DM, Lauring AS. Evidence for the Selective Basis of Transition-to-Transversion Substitution Bias in Two RNA Viruses. Mol Biol Evol 2017; 34(12): 3205-15.
[http://dx.doi.org/10.1093/molbev/msx251] [PMID: 29029187]

[32]   Tang X, Wu C, Li X, *et al.* On the origin and continuing evolution of SARS-CoV-2. Natl Sci Rev 2020; 7(6): 1012-23.
[http://dx.doi.org/10.1093/nsr/nwaa036] [PMID: 34676127]

[33]   Makkoch J, Suwannakarn K, Payungporn S, *et al.* Whole genome characterization, phylogenetic and genome signature analysis of human pandemic H1N1 virus in Thailand, 2009-2012. PLoS One 2012; 7(12): e51275.
[http://dx.doi.org/10.1371/journal.pone.0051275] [PMID: 23251479]

[34]   Ozono S, Zhang Y, Ode H, *et al.* SARS-CoV-2 D614G spike mutation increases entry efficiency with enhanced ACE2-binding affinity. Nat Commun 2021; 12(1): 848.
[http://dx.doi.org/10.1038/s41467-021-21118-2] [PMID: 33558493]

[35]   Ahmad L. Implication of SARS-CoV-2 Immune Escape Spike Variants on Secondary and Vaccine Breakthrough Infections. Front Immunol 2021; 12: 742167.

[http://dx.doi.org/10.3389/fimmu.2021.742167] [PMID: 34804022]

[36]   Khan A, Hanif M, Ahmed A, Syed S, Ghazali S, Khanani R. SARS-CoV-2 UK, South African and Brazilian Variants in Karachi- Pakistan. Front Mol Biosci 2021; 8: 724208.
[http://dx.doi.org/10.3389/fmolb.2021.724208] [PMID: 34760923]

[37]   Deng X, Garcia-Knight MA, Khalid MM, *et al.* Transmission, infectivity, and antibody neutralization of an emerging SARS-CoV-2 variant in California carrying a L452R spike protein mutation. MedRxiv 2021.
[http://dx.doi.org/10.1101/2021.03.07.21252647]

[38]   Jangra S, Ye C, Rathnasinghe R, *et al.* SARS-CoV-2 spike E484K mutation reduces antibody neutralisation. Lancet Microbe 2021; 2(7): e283-4.
[http://dx.doi.org/10.1016/S2666-5247(21)00068-9]

[39]   Garcia-Beltran WF, Lam EC, St Denis K, *et al.* Multiple SARS-CoV-2 variants escape neutralization by vaccine-induced humoral immunity. Cell 2021; 184(9): 2372-2383.e9.
[http://dx.doi.org/10.1016/j.cell.2021.03.013] [PMID: 33743213]

CHAPTER 6

Genetic Architecture of Host Proteins Involved in SARS-CoV-2

Abdullah[1], Muhammad Ibrar[2] and **Fazlullah Khan[3,*]**

[1] *Department of Pharmacy, University of Malakand, Chakdara Dir Lower, KP, Pakistan*

[2] *Department of Allied and Health Sciences, Iqra National University Swat Campus, Swat, Pakistan*

[3] *Department of Pharmacy, Faculty of Pharmacy, Capital University of Science and Technology (CUST), Islamabad, Pakistan*

Abstract: Proteins are the functional units of the cell that allow viruses to reproduce inside host cells. Proteins are essential for a cell's proper operation. Gene variations can reveal potential new therapeutic targets. Examining the innate immune system, coagulation, and other host proteins about the severity or mortality of COVID-19 reveals potentially changeable maladaptive host responses. Proteins are considered to be the high prevalent biological group of pharmacological factors, and high-throughput proteomics methods are quickly being employed to find prospective target molecules for innovative development of new drugs and repurposing studies. Researching the naturally occurring variations in the human gene sequence that code for therapeutic targets can also show how treatments work and ensure that people are safe. Researchers can create novel or repurposed therapeutics by examining the host protein's genetic makeup that interacts with SARS-CoV-2 or supports host responses to COVID-19.

Keywords: COVID-19, RNA viruses, Ritonavir, Nucleocapsid, Spike proteins.

INTRODUCTION

During December 2019, many cases of respiratory infections due to unknown reasons were reported in Wuhan city, spreading rapidly to other countries. The infectious virus was isolated, identified, and named 2019 novel coronavirus, and the condition was diagnosed as coronavirus disease-2019 [1, 2]. The virus has a more substantial transmission capacity, and the rapid increase in confirmed COVID-19 cases makes control and prevention extremely challenging. Novel pathological conditions caused by RNA viruses with genetic recombination, mutation, and cross-species transmission are considered a critical health chall-

---
* **Corresponding author Fazlullah Khan:** Department of Pharmacy, Faculty of Pharmacy, Capital University of Science and Technology (CUST), Islamabad, Pakistan; Tel: +92-3469433155, E-mail: fazlullahdr@gmail.com

Kamal Niaz, Muhammad Sajjad Khan & Muhammad Farrukh Nisar (Eds.)

enge worldwide, exemplified by COVID-19 [3]. Researchers struggle to search for possible strategies to control disease and develop therapies for prevention in the future. Currently, there is an intense need to find specific targets for treating the disease and develop new treatment strategies or repurpose existing drugs. Finding agents might prevent vulnerable persons from contracting COVID-19 and successfully treat people with severe COVID-19 symptoms [4 - 6].

It is critical to comprehend the genetic makeup of pharmacological targets to determine the genetic connections between molecular targets and illnesses [7, 8]. Human drug targets' human gene sequence variations can be employed to directly assist therapeutic mechanisms and guarantee human safety. Major pharmaceutical companies have implemented this strategy to find and validate therapeutic targets for a range of non-communicable disorders as well as for drug repurposing. Recently, extensive research has been done on the genomes and plasma based on aptamer-proteome data of over ten thousand people who had not been exposed to COVID-19. Understanding the genetic structure of 179 host proteins that are important to SARS-CoV-2 was the goal of these investigations. These results emphasise the possibility of using genetic variations as tools to confirm therapeutic targets in newly emerging genome-wide association studies [1] on COVID-19 [9, 10].

SARS-CoV-2 Relevant Proteins

A single-stranded RNA virus (SSRV) called SARS-CoV-2 has a genome that is about 30 kb in size. It has fourteen open reading frames (ORFs), which can be used to encode several different proteins. The nucleocapsid (N) protein, the spike (S) protein, the membrane (M), and the envelope (E) protein are the four primary structural proteins of the virus [11].

Spike Proteins

Many experiments have been performed to target the S protein of SARS-CoV-2, which is found on the virus's outer coat and is necessary for viral entry into host cells. The ability of the S protein's spike protein to trigger antiviral antibodies has made it a key target for the development of a SARS-CoV-2 vaccine. S protein-targeting antibodies can prevent the virus from infecting and replicating in the host cell [12]. The spike protein is the most antigenic part of any viral protein and is responsible for inducing humoral immunological reactions [13] and the production of neutralizing antibodies, both of which result in protective immunity against viral infections. As a result, the spike protein has been chosen as a crucial target for SARS-CoV-2 immunization [14, 15]. Around 35 of the 47 vaccine candidates currently undergoing clinical testing use spike proteins and different technological platforms. The full-length S protein (FLSP), the receptor-binding protein (RBD) domain, the S1 subunit, the S2 subunit, the N-terminal domain (NTD), and the membrane fusion peptide (FP) are a few examples of the S protein's possible antigens [16].

The Nucleocapsid Protein

The N protein, which is found in the viral envelope, is essential for forming the helical nucleocapsid during virion assembly by wrapping the RNA. In comparison to the other four human coronaviruses, a recent study suggests that the SARS-CoV-2 N protein (S2N protein) demonstrates a higher level of conservation with SAS-CoV and MERS-CoV. It is interesting to note that compared to the S protein, the S2N protein appears to trigger a higher humoral and cellular immune response against SARS-CoV-2 [17].

Membrane Protein (M Protein)

The coronavirus M protein, which is principally in charge of starting the virus budding process, is situated in the virus envelope between S proteins and minor amounts of the E protein and is essential for virus assembly [18]. The M protein interacts with several additional SPs during viral assembly, including the N protein, E protein, and S protein [19]. Significant CD4+ and CD8+ T cell-mediated immune responses against the S2M protein have been found in virus-infected and recovered patients in recent investigations. Notably, S2M was highly recognized, and significant reactivity was seen [20]. Previous research has demonstrated the immunogenicity of the SARS-CoV M protein by demonstrating that synthetic peptides derived from immunodominant epitopes triggered potent antibody-induced immune responses in immunized rabbits [21]. The envelope protein and Nsp3 protein, which include numerous functional domains and play significant roles in helping viral pathogenesis, are two other proteins that require attention in addition to the M protein.

Local Genetic Architecture of Protein Targets

About 220 DNA sequence variations that affect 97 proteins in trans have been found using a total of 106 aptamers. Seven of these proteins were recognized and demonstrated by multiple aptamer pairs or triplets [22]. Thirty six of the 96 proteins were identified, and 15 of these previously identified proteins interact with proteins that are encoded in the genome of SARS-CoV-2 (such as COMT, PLOD2, DCTPP1, SDF2, ERO1LB, GLA, ERLEC1, MFGE8, EIF4E2, IL17RA, MARK3, FKBP7, PTGES2, PLAT, and COL6A1) and are targets for currently available drugs [23]. In addition, 16 proteins, including PLG, IL2RA, F2, F5, F8, F9, F10, CD14, FGB, IL6ST, IL1R1, IL2RB, VWF IL6R, SERPINE1, and

SERPINC1, have been found to encode biomarkers associated with COVID-19 prognosis and severity [24].

A Tiered System for *Trans*-pQTL

Proteins are crucial elements in biological processes that have an impact on both health and sickness, making them interesting drug development targets [25]. Findings from GWAS that investigate the connections between single-nucleotide polymorphisms (SNPs) and disease are important to integrate with those related to genetic variants associated with protein levels, or pQTLs, to gain a better understanding of the causal role of proteome in the disease. A detailed examination of the genetic causes of SARS-CoV-2 is required because it is still one of the world's leading killers. We can learn a lot about this condition by analyzing the pQTL variants linked to COVID-19 in GWAS, determining causation, and investigating the functions of genes and proteins in COVID-19 pathogenesis [25]. Based on how closely they are related to the target gene, expression QTLs, or eQTLs, can be categorized into cis and trans groups. Trans-eQTLs are found elsewhere and indirectly control gene expression, whereas cis-eQTLs occur at the same site as the gene [26]. 220 Cis-acting DNA sequence variants that influence 97 protein-coding genes were found in a recent investigation of 98 aptamers. Of these, 27 showed signs of horizontal pleiotropy, with associations in trans for only one or no aptamers. According to these results, some of these variants may be utilized as tools for genetically forecasting protein levels in separate cohorts, which would make determining causality easier [27].

Host Factors Related to Candidate Proteins

Examining host variables and illuminating the variability in plasma concentrations of aptamers that target high-priority candidate proteins need the use of a variance decomposition approach. Notably, genetic hits that code for proteins that interact with Nsp7 of the virus, which displays a high level of interaction among SARS-CoV-1, SARS-CoV-2, and MERS-CoV, are enriched. For instance, Nsp7 from these 3 viruses interacts functionally with PGES2 (encoded by PTGES2). It was discovered that several dependencies were unique to SARS-CoV-2, such as IL17RA's interaction with SARS-CoV-2 ORF8. Additionally, it was discovered that SIGMAR1 interacts with Nsp6 and TOMM70 interacts with ORF9b, which are shared interactors between SARS-CoV-2 and SARS-CoV-1. According to reports, SARS-CoV-1 and SARS-CoV-2 ORF9b are localized to the mitochondria both during overexpression and in cells carrying SARS-CoV-2. Both the SARS-CoV-1 and SARS-CoV-2 interaction maps have identified TOMM70, a mitochondrial outer membrane protein, as a high-confidence interactor of ORF9b, making it a host-dependency factor for these viruses [28].

Integration of Gene Expression Data

The expression of the genes that code for proteins in distinct tissues is one of several factors that affect the amount of proteins in plasma. Predicted gene expression data from the GTEx project were integrated across five tissues, including the liver, whole blood, heart, and lung, to determine if pQTLs also function as gene expression QTLs [29, 30]. In 31 instances, the protein-encoding gene model in at least one tissue was the most persuasive. As reported by prior studies, the anticipated gene expression of the protein-encoding gene at 65 loci was substantially related to various tissue specificity [31, 32]. Notably, at least three tissues consistently showed a correlation between the anticipated gene expression of druggable targets such as EIF4E2, FKBP7, IL17RA, EROLB1, and SERPINC1 and the corresponding protein levels in plasma for RAB2A, C1RL, POR, KDELC2, ACADM, and AES. Furthermore, the plasma concentrations of SERPINA10, SAA1, and SAA2 were connected to the gene expression in the lung [22].

Cross-Platform Comparison

A study was conducted to evaluate the consistency of detected pQTLs across platforms because protein alternating variations (PAV) can change binding epitopes and affect cross-platform comparisons. Olink's polyclonal antibody-based proximity extension assays were utilized to evaluate 33 protein targets across 12 panels, utilizing data from 485 Fenland research participants. The resulting estimates of 29 cis- and 96 trans-pQTLs were compared using a reciprocal look-up. Results revealed a substantial correlation ($r = 0.75$) between 29 cis-pQTLs and a weaker correlation ($r = 0.54$) for trans-pQTLs, showing excellent concordance across platforms for this particular set of proteins [22]. For 2 of the 33 protein targets, the investigation also discovered inconsistent lead cis-pQTLs. Specifically, despite a strong and well-developed signal cis for the Olink measure, the main cis-pQTL for GDF-15 from SomaScan (rs75347775) was not substantially linked with GDF-15 levels evaluated utilizing the Olink [33].

Analysis of Drug Target

The pQTLs for 105 COVID-19-related proteins were identified, 75 with a minimum of one cis-pQTL, already known to be druggable or the targets for existing drugs [34]. The cis-pQTLs may be used to target these proteins used for COVID-19 treatment. Alleles, during meiosis, are allocated randomly and inherited independent of exposure to the virus. Therefore, it represents the effect of lifelong higher or lower levels of plasma protein, which makes a person susceptible or protected against severe symptoms of COVID-19. One target that is responsible for biosynthesis of prostaglandin, prostaglandin E synthase 2

(PGES2), was identified through host-virus protein interaction analysis. NSAIDs inhibit PG synthesis, however currently the evidence is weak, and there may be chances that the use of NSAIDs may cause the symptoms to worsen in COVID-19 patients [35].

Similarly, two pQTL targets (catechol O-methyl transferase and alpha-galactosidase-A) have been identified that interact with the host-virus protein. Catechol O-methyl transferase targets Parkinsonism (entacapone), while in Fabry's disease, a lysosomal disorder that is treated by migalastat, the levels of alpha-galactosidase-A are deficient. Migalastat acts to stabilize some mutant forms of alpha-galactosidase-A [22]. About 24 druggable protein targets currently have no licensed medicines. These complement cascade components include Complement factor H, component C8, C2 and C8 gamma chain [22].

Clinical Outcomes with Cis-pQTLs

To assess the potential negative effects and phenotypic repercussions of the cis-pQTLs, three systematic approaches were used. Firstly, it was investigated whether any of the 220 cis-pQTLs or proxies in high LD ($r^2 > 0.8$) have been documented in the GWAS Catalogue, and it was found that some of the cis-pQTLs lead at F2 were verified drug targets genetically linked to corresponding indications, such as venous thrombosis (rs1799963), rheumatoid arthritis (IL6R), and coronary artery disease (PLG) [36 - 38]. Second, all 106 aptamers in the cis-GRS were examined for connections with 633 ICD-10 coded outcomes in the UK Biobank to see if elevated plasma protein levels are related to disease risk. Significant correlations between the thrombin-cis-GRS and a high risk of thrombophlebitis and pulmonary embolism were found [39]. Last but not least, it was mentioned that the proteins used by viruses (SMOC1, IL-6, or MARK3 receptors) can elevate the number of cells related to innate immunity, leading to hyper-inflammatory or hypercoagulation disorders [22].

Coagulation Factors and the *ABO* Locus

Two genetic regions that raise the probability of respiratory failure in patients with COVID-19 were found by a GWAS investigation [1]. The lead ABO signal was responsible for respiratory failure, and a group of ten aptamers targeting SVEP1, plasminogen, factor VIII, Van Willebrand factor, ferritin, heme oxygenase 1, PLOD2, and CD14 shared a genetic signal (regional probability: 0.88; rs941137) that was in high LD (r2=0.85) [22]. Another study discovered seven proteins that were prominently linked with the lead variant (rs11385942) at 3p21.31 but not with the lead signal (rs657152) at the ABO locus (factor VIII, sulfhydryl oxidase 2 (QSOX2), von Willebrand factor, SVEP1, and heme oxygenase 1), which was found to be inversely associated.

Webserver

The in-depth investigation of potential proteins (one cis- pQTL at least) is facilitated by creating an online Web (https://omicscience.org/apps/covidpgwas/). It furnishes instinctive genetic findings representation that includes statistics for protein targets and genome regions of interest and the opportunity for customized look-ups. Moreover, it provides relative information on each protein target and links to the database, such as Reactome or UniProt, available drug information, drugs in development stages, and the characterization of related SNPs. Additionally, it permits SNP query across proteins to evaluate the selectivity and discover co-associated protein targets [22].

CONCLUSION

Searching the specific proteins and genetic architecture of host proteins and studying the mechanism involved in SARS-CoV-2 can play a key role in the rapid identification and clinical classification of proper targets against novel infecting agents. It is possible to argue that SARS-CoV-2 has affected and propagated in those who have no immunity; it has not yet been exposed to the type of immune pressure that shaped the evolution of endemic viruses. Its evolutionary potential is uncertain. As a result, we must continue to monitor genetic alterations to track their dissemination and detect antigenic shifts swiftly if they are possessed. It is also critical to remember that it is seen as a slow genetic drift, which is typical of a virus having a stable genome, and to keep these and other SARS-CoV-2 genetic diversity findings in context, especially when conveying them to the general population.

REFERENCES

[1]   Severe COVID-19 GWAS Group; David Ellinghaus D, Degenhardt F, Bujanda L, Buti M, Albillos A, Invernizzi P *et al..* Genomewide association study of severe COVID-19 with respiratory failure. N Engl J Med 2020; 383(16): 1522-34.
        [http://dx.doi.org/10.1056/NEJMoa2020283]

[2]   Lillie PJ, Samson A, Li A, *et al.* Novel coronavirus disease (Covid-19): The first two patients in the UK with person to person transmission. J Infect 2020; 80(5): 578-606.
        [http://dx.doi.org/10.1016/j.jinf.2020.02.020] [PMID: 32119884]

[3]   Ghale-Noie ZN, Salmaninejad A, Bergquist R, Mollazadeh S, Hoseini B, Sahebkar A. Genetic Aspects and Immune Responses in Covid-19: Important Organ Involvement. Identification of Biomarkers, New Treatments, and Vaccines for COVID-19. Springer 2021; pp. 3-22.
        [http://dx.doi.org/10.1007/978-3-030-71697-4_1]

[4]   Zhang L, Yan X, Fan Q, *et al.* D-dimer levels on admission to predict in-hospital mortality in patients with Covid-19. J Thromb Haemost 2020; 18(6): 1324-9.
        [http://dx.doi.org/10.1111/jth.14859] [PMID: 32306492]

[5]   Violi F, Pastori D, Cangemi R, Pignatelli P, Loffredo L. Hypercoagulation and antithrombotic treatment in coronavirus 2019: a new challenge. Thromb Haemost 2020; 120(6): 949-56.
        [http://dx.doi.org/10.1055/s-0040-1710317] [PMID: 32349133]

[6]   Messner CB, Demichev V, Wendisch D, *et al.* Clinical classifiers of COVID-19 infection from novel ultra-high-throughput proteomics. MedRxiv 2020.
[http://dx.doi.org/10.1101/2020.04.27.20081810]

[7]   Nelson MR, Tipney H, Painter JL, *et al.* The support of human genetic evidence for approved drug indications. Nat Genet 2015; 47(8): 856-60.
[http://dx.doi.org/10.1038/ng.3314] [PMID: 26121088]

[8]   King EA, Davis JW, Degner JF. Are drug targets with genetic support twice as likely to be approved? Revised estimates of the impact of genetic support for drug mechanisms on the probability of drug approval. PLoS Genet 2019; 15(12): e1008489.
[http://dx.doi.org/10.1371/journal.pgen.1008489] [PMID: 31830040]

[9]   Pairo-Castineira E, Clohisey S, Klaric L, *et al.* Genetic mechanisms of critical illness in COVID-19. Nature 2021; 591(7848): 92-8.
[http://dx.doi.org/10.1038/s41586-020-03065-y] [PMID: 33307546]

[10]   Youssef JG, Zahiruddin F, Al-Saadi M, *et al.* Brief Report: Rapid Clinical Recovery from Critical COVID-19 with Respiratory Failure in a Lung Transplant Patient Treated with Intravenous Vasoactive Intestinal Peptide. Crit Care Explor 2022; 4(1): e0607.
[http://dx.doi.org/10.1097/CCE.0000000000000607]

[11]   Malik JA, Mulla AH, Farooqi T, Pottoo FH, Anwar S, Rengasamy KRR. Targets and strategies for vaccine development against SARS-CoV-2. Biomed Pharmacother 2021; 137: 111254.
[http://dx.doi.org/10.1016/j.biopha.2021.111254] [PMID: 33550049]

[12]   Walls AC, Park Y-J, Tortorici MA, Wall A, McGuire AT, Veesler D. Structure, function, and antigenicity of the SARS-CoV-2 spike glycoprotein. Cell 2020; 181: 281-292.
[http://dx.doi.org/10.1016/j.cell.2020.02.058]

[13]   Korkmaz S, Radovits T, Barnucz E, *et al.* Pharmacological activation of soluble guanylate cyclase protects the heart against ischemic injury. Circulation 2009; 120(8): 677-86.
[http://dx.doi.org/10.1161/CIRCULATIONAHA.109.870774] [PMID: 19667237]

[14]   Salvatori G, Luberto L, Maffei M, *et al.* SARS-CoV-2 SPIKE PROTEIN: an optimal immunological target for vaccines. J Transl Med 2020; 18(1): 222.
[http://dx.doi.org/10.1186/s12967-020-02392-y] [PMID: 32493510]

[15]   Wang K, Chen W, Zhou Y-S, *et al.* SARS-CoV-2 invades host cells *via* a novel route: CD147-spike protein. BioRxiv 2020.
[http://dx.doi.org/10.1101/2020.03.14.988345]

[16]   Zhang J, Zeng H, Gu J, Li H, Zheng L, Zou Q. Progress and prospects on vaccine development against SARS-CoV-2. Vaccines (Basel) 2020; 8(2): 153.
[http://dx.doi.org/10.3390/vaccines8020153] [PMID: 32235387]

[17]   Ong E, Wang H, Wong MU, Seetharaman M, Valdez N, He Y. Vaxign-ML: supervised machine learning reverse vaccinology model for improved prediction of bacterial protective antigens. Bioinformatics 2020; 36(10): 3185-91.
[http://dx.doi.org/10.1093/bioinformatics/btaa119] [PMID: 32096826]

[18]   Neuman BW, Kiss G, Kunding AH, *et al.* A structural analysis of M protein in coronavirus assembly and morphology. J Struct Biol 2011; 174(1): 11-22.
[http://dx.doi.org/10.1016/j.jsb.2010.11.021] [PMID: 21130884]

[19]   J Alsaadi EA, Jones IM. Membrane binding proteins of coronaviruses. Future Virol 2019; 14(4): 275-86.
[http://dx.doi.org/10.2217/fvl-2018-0144] [PMID: 32201500]

[20]   Grifoni A, Weiskopf D, Ramirez SI, *et al.* Targets of T cell responses to SARS-CoV-2 coronavirus in humans with COVID-19 disease and unexposed individuals. Cell 2020; 181(7): 1489-1501.e15.
[http://dx.doi.org/10.1016/j.cell.2020.05.015]

[21] He Y, Zhou Y, Wu H, *et al.* Identification of immunodominant sites on the spike protein of severe acute respiratory syndrome (SARS) coronavirus: implication for developing SARS diagnostics and vaccines. J Immunol 2004; 173(6): 4050-7.
[http://dx.doi.org/10.4049/jimmunol.173.6.4050] [PMID: 15356154]

[22] Pietzner M, Wheeler E, Carrasco-Zanini J, *et al.* Genetic architecture of host proteins involved in SARS-CoV-2 infection. bioRxiv [Preprint] 2020; 1: 2020.07.01.182709.
[http://dx.doi.org/10.1101/2020.07.01.182709]

[23] Gordon DE, Jang GM, Bouhaddou M, *et al.* A SARS-CoV-2 protein interaction map reveals targets for drug repurposing. Nature 2020; 583(7816): 459-68.
[http://dx.doi.org/10.1038/s41586-020-2286-9]

[24] Messner CB, Demichev V, Wendisch D, *et al.* Ultra-high-throughput clinical proteomics reveals classifiers of COVID-19 infection. Cell Syst 2020; 11(1): 11-24.e4.
[http://dx.doi.org/10.1016/j.cels.2020.05.012]

[25] Yao C, Chen G, Song C, *et al.* Genome-wide mapping of plasma protein QTLs identifies putatively causal genes and pathways for cardiovascular disease. Nat Commun 2018; 9: 1-11.
[http://dx.doi.org/10.1038/s41467-018-05512-x]

[26] Bryois J, Buil A, Evans DM, *et al.* Cis and trans effects of human genomic variants on gene expression. PLoS Genet 2014; 10(7): e1004461.
[http://dx.doi.org/10.1371/journal.pgen.1004461] [PMID: 25010687]

[27] Pietzner M, Wheeler E, Carrasco-Zanini J, *et al.* Genetic architecture of host proteins involved in SARS-CoV-2 infection. Nat Commun 2020; 11(1): 6397.
[http://dx.doi.org/10.1038/s41467-020-19996-z] [PMID: 33328453]

[28] Gordon DE, Hiatt J, Bouhaddou M, *et al.* Comparative host-coronavirus protein interaction networks reveal pan-viral disease mechanisms. Science 2020; 370(6521): eabe9403.
[http://dx.doi.org/10.1126/science.abe9403] [PMID: 33060197]

[29] G.C.J. Science, The Genotype-Tissue Expression (GTEx) pilot analysis: Multitissue gene regulation in humans. Science 2015; 348(6235): 648-660..
[http://dx.doi.org/10.1126/science.1262110]

[30] Gamazon ER, Segrè AV, van de Bunt M, *et al.* Using an atlas of gene regulation across 44 human tissues to inform complex disease-and trait-associated variation. Nat Genet 2018; 50(7): 956-67.
[http://dx.doi.org/10.1038/s41588-018-0154-4]

[31] Sun BB, Maranville JC, Peters JE, *et al.* Genomic atlas of the human plasma proteome. Nature 2018; 558(7708): 73-9.
[http://dx.doi.org/10.1038/s41586-018-0175-2]

[32] Suhre K, Arnold M, Bhagwat AM, *et al.* Connecting genetic risk to disease end points through the human blood plasma proteome. Nat Commun 2017; 8: 14357.
[http://dx.doi.org/10.1038/ncomms14357]

[33] Folkersen L, Fauman E, Sabater-Lleal M, *et al.* Mapping of 79 loci for 83 plasma protein biomarkers in cardiovascular disease. PLoS Genet 2017; 13(4): e1006706.
[http://dx.doi.org/10.1371/journal.pgen.1006706]

[34] Finan C, Gaulton A, Kruger FA, *et al.* The druggable genome and support for target identification and validation in drug development. Sci Transl Med 2017; 9(383): eaag1166.
[http://dx.doi.org/10.1126/scitranslmed.aag1166]

[35] Little P. Non-steroidal anti-inflammatory drugs and covid-19. In: British Medical Journal Publishing Group. 2020.

[36] Klarin D, Busenkell E, Judy R, *et al.* Genome-wide association analysis of venous thromboembolism identifies new risk loci and genetic overlap with arterial vascular disease. Nat Genet 2019; 51(11):

1574-9.
[http://dx.doi.org/10.1038/s41588-019-0519-3]

[37]   Okada Y, Wu D, Trynka G, *et al.* Genetics of rheumatoid arthritis contributes to biology and drug discovery. Nature 2014; 506(7488): 376-81.
[http://dx.doi.org/10.1038/nature12873]

[38]   Nikpay M, Goel A, Won H-H, *et al.* A comprehensive 1000 Genomes–based genome-wide association meta-analysis of coronary artery disease. Nat Genet 2015; 47(10): 1121-30.
[http://dx.doi.org/10.1038/ng.3396]

[39]   Hemani G, Zheng J, Elsworth B, *et al.* The MR-Base platform supports systematic causal inference across the human phenome. Elife 2018; 7: e34408.
[http://dx.doi.org/10.7554/eLife.34408]

CHAPTER 7

Landscape of Host Genetic Factors Correlating with SARS-CoV-2

Ihtisham Ulhaq[1], Abdul Basit[2], Firasat Hussain[3], Muhammad Humayun[1], Umair Younas[4], Sartaj Ali[1], Amjad Islam Aqib[5] and Kashif Rahim[3,*]

[1] *Department of Biosciences, COMSATS University, Islamabad, Pakistan*

[2] *Department of Microbiology, University of Jhang, Jhang 38000, Pakistan*

[3] *Department of Microbiology, Cholistan University of Veterinary and Animal Sciences (CUVAS), Bahawalpur 63100, Pakistan*

[4] *Department of Livestock Management, Cholistan University of Veterinary and Animal Sciences (CUVAS), Bahawalpur 63100, Pakistan*

[5] *Department of Medicine, Faculty of Veterinary Science, Cholistan University of Veterinary and Animal Sciences (CUVAS), Bahawalpur 63100, Pakistan*

Abstract: The researchers revealed a novel coronavirus in the Chinese population on 7th January 2020, named severe acute respiratory syndrome coronavirus-2 (SARS-CoV-2). The previous coronaviruses proved merely the tip of the iceberg after the emergence of the recently identified SARS-CoV-2. The potential of pandemic status significantly revealed the concealed capabilities of virulence and contagiousness of the betacoronaviruses group. This book chapter discusses the landscape of host genetic factors correlating with SARS-CoV-2. All SARS-CoV-2 genes code for the structural and non-structural proteins that have distinct interactions with host proteins. NSP13 is associated with centrosome and insulin signals in humans, NSP5 is associated with the ATPases of host cells, and NSP9 is associated with the nuclear pore's host proteins. The ORF8ab and ORF8b avoid the host immune responses and inhibit the signaling cascade of INF-β. Cytokine storm is associated with TLR2, FOXO1, and MYC genes of SARS-CoV-2 that further cause host cell death during infection. STAT1, IFIH1, IRF9, OAS1-3, and PML are associated with the immune response to SARS-CoV-2 infection, particularly the production of type I interferon. The SARS-CoV-2 entry is affected by the TMEM106B gene, and this gene can prevent virus-induced cell death. Replication of SARS-CoV-2 reduces due to deletions in TMEM106B and VAC14 genes. Genetic variants also influence the host susceptibility in the major histocompatibility complex antigen loci (HLA). The susceptibility of COVID-19 is considerably associated with the genetic variation in HLA and plays a significant role in identifying populations at higher risk.

* **Corresponding author Kashif Rahim:** Department of Microbiology, Cholistan University of Veterinary and Animal Sciences (CUVAS), Bahawalpur 63100, Pakistan, E-mail: kashifrahim@cuvas.edu.pk

Kamal Niaz, Muhammad Sajjad Khan & Muhammad Farrukh Nisar (Eds.)

Keywords: SARS-CoV-2, COVID-19, Host, Genetic factors, GWAS, TWAS, HLA, Virus-host interactions.

INTRODUCTION

At the end of December 2019, Chinese people were diagnosed with a respiratory tract infection of an unidentified etiology in Wuhan, Hubei Province [1]. Initially, physicians considered it pneumonia due to the clinical conditions of the patients. During laboratory investigations, a novel coronavirus was identified from throat samples of hospital-admitted patients through Real-time PCR (Polymerase Chain Reaction) and next-generation sequencing [2]. Therefore, a new coronavirus was ascertained on 7th January 2020 and given the name novel coronavirus 2019 by WHO (World Health Organization) [3]. ICTV (International Committee on Taxonomy of Viruses) later named it SARS-CoV-2 (severe acute respiratory syndrome coronavirus-2) as it was genetically parallel to the previous SARS coronavirus that emerged in 2002 [4]. The person infected with SARS-CoV-2 had the symptoms of coughing, sneezing, fatigue, difficulty breathing, and sometimes diarrhea, while the disease was named COVID-19 (Coronavirus Disease 2019) officially by WHO [5]. The acknowledgment of the *Coronaviridae* family comes about by ICTV (The International Committee on Taxonomy of Viruses), which works on viral nomenclature and classification [6]. Coronaviruses are respiratory pathogens belonging to the family of *Coronaviridae*. Coronaviruses have the largest genome size among RNA viruses with a positive sense [7]. Coronaviruses have a non-segmented genome covered in an envelope. The order Nidovirales includes the largest family, *Coronaviridae,* which is divided into two subfamilies: *Orthocoronavirinae and Torobirinae* [8]. *Orthocoronavirinae* is classified into four genera: alpha, beta, gamma, and delta. Each of these genera targets different animal species for infections. Alphacoronavirus and betacoronavirus have broad host tropism as they infect birds, animals, and humans, while deltacoronavirus and gammacoronavirus infect only birds [9]. Betacoronaviruses infect various animals. Host tropism is broad and has zoonotic potential but is frequently reported in humans, bats, and camels [10 - 13]. The size of the betacoronavirus genome is 26-32kb, while the overall virus size is about 60-140nm [14, 15]. The recently identified SARS-CoV-2 (severe acute respiratory syndrome coronavirus-2) genome contains 29844 to 29891 coding nucleotides, lacking the hemagglutinin-esterase gene [16]. The virus's genome is covered in a capsid whose symmetry is helical and constructed from structural proteins. The genome and capsid have collectively been termed the nucleocapsid. Further, the nucleocapsid is wrapped by a membrane, an envelope assembled by lipids and proteins [17]. These membranous structures prevent the environmental factor's influence on the virus and ensure its safety in unfavorable conditions [18]. Moreover, spikes protrude from the envelope made of glycoproteins, making the virus appear like a crown. Based on this morphology, it has been named coronavirus by ICTV [19]. Furthermore, the glycoproteins in spikes are essential for viral structural proteins (VSP). Additionally, they play a role in the virus's binding to the susceptible host cell and entering genetic material [20]. There are two domains in spike glycoproteins with different roles; one is associated with the viral envelope, and the other is part of the receptor-binding portion [21]. SARS-CoV-2 is phylogenetically similar to SARS-CoV, and there is a higher similarity in the receptor-binding domain and S gene of both SARS coronaviruses, indicating their capability for human-to-human transmission [22]. Genetic analysis of RBD in the S gene revealed that new mutations would deviate from the host range and cellular tropism of SARS-CoV-2 [23 - 26]. The enzyme RNA-dependent RNA polymerases in RNA viruses triggered the mutations and frequently made genetic recombinations [27 - 30] that ultimately caused an evolution in SARS-CoV-2. Single nucleotide polymorphisms (SNPs) identified two major subtypes of SARS-CoV-2 as L and S; the subtype L is more destructive and contagious [31]. The mutations and genetic recombinations make the virus more lethal and are strongly associated with disease severity and mortality rate [31]. All the functional characteristics of SARS-CoV-2, such as transmission, pathogenesis, response to host defenses, and receptor affinity, are altered due to the high mutation rate that leads to genetic diversity [31]. Full-length genome analysis of SARS-CoV-2 showed that the protein profile of the SARS-CoV-2 has a strong association with the human host proteins [32]. This book chapter aims to analyze the SARS-CoV-2 –host interactions on genetic level genome-wide associated studies (GWAS), transcriptome-wide associated studies (TWAS), regional human leukocyte antigen (HLA) associations, the role of pro and anti-viral genes, and cross trait associations, as shown in Fig. (**1**).

Genome-Wide Associated Studies (GWAS)

After a few weeks of COVID-19 emergence in December 2019, on January 24, 2020, the first genome of SARS-CoV-2 was sequenced [33]. Moreover, it had 75–80% genetic similarity to SARS-CoV [34, 35]. Besides, SARS-CoV and SARS-CoV-2 have genetic similarities with bat-derived SARS-related coronavirus and RaTG13 [36]. The size of the betacoronavirus genome is 26-32kb, while the overall virus size is about 60-140nm [37, 38]. The recently identified SARS-CoV-2 (severe acute respiratory syndrome coronavirus-2) genome contains 29844 to 29891 coding nucleotides, lacking the hemagglutinin-esterase gene [39]. The virus's genome is roofed in a capsid whose symmetry is helical and constructed from structural proteins. The genome and capsid have collectively been termed the nucleocapsid.

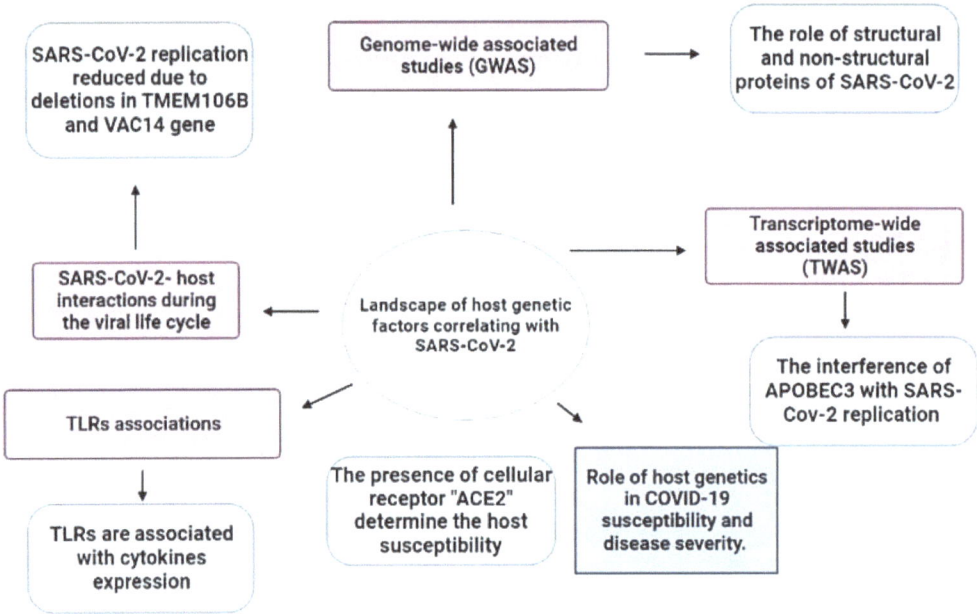

Fig. (1). Schematic illustration of the whole chapter.

Further, the nucleocapsid is wrapped by a membrane, an envelope assembled by lipids and proteins [40]. All these membranous structures prevent the environmental factors' influence on the virus and ensure its safety in unfavorable conditions [41]. Moreover, spikes protrude from the envelope made of glycoproteins, making the virus appear like a crown [42]. The 16 non-structural proteins are encoded by SARS-CoV-2 and associated with viral pathogenesis and replication. Envelope (E), nucleocapsid (N), membrane (M), and spike (S) glycoprotein are the structural proteins of SARS-CoV-2 that are phenotypically associated with the virus and important for subtyping of the virus. In addition to that, these proteins are also important for therapeutics and nine other accessory factors [43, 44]. All the functional characteristics of SARS-CoV-2, such as transmission, pathogenesis, response to host defenses, and receptor affinity, are altered due to the high mutation rate that leads to genetic diversity [45]. Full-length genome analysis of SARS-CoV-2 showed that the protein profile of the SARS-CoV-2 has a strong association with the human host proteins [22]. All genes code for the structural and non-structural proteins and have individual interactions with host proteins [22]. NSP13 is associated with centrosomes and insulin signals in humans, NSP5 is associated with ATPases of the host cell, and NSP9 is associated with the host proteins of the nuclear pore. N proteins are associated with host RNA processing. ORF10 influences the CUL2 gene of humans, leading to any secondary abnormalities in the host [22].

Moreover, an accessory gene known as "ORF8" is only found in SARS-CoV and SARS-CoV-2, while the other sarbecoviruses lack this gene. During the life cycle of SARS-CoV-2, functional flexibility is provided by the proteins of ORF8 according to the conditions. It is a significant constituent of immunity [46]. The ORF8ab and ORF8b avoid the host immune responses by acting as an interferon (IFN) opponent, and the signaling cascade of INF-β is inhibited in the initial steps [47, 48]. Moreover, interferon is degraded by both the ORFs of SARS-CoV-2 by physical interaction with interferon regulatory factor 3 [49]. The nucleocapsid proteins ORF6 and ORF8 of SARS-CoV-2 are also reported to avoid innate immunity responses. All of these were reported to inhibit the signaling pathway of interferon type-1 at the promoter site [50]. So far, various studies have reported the key role of ORFs and angiotensin-converting enzyme 2 (ACE2) genes in the functionality of SARS-CoV-2 from entry until it causes infection [51, 52]. Papain–like protease enzymes encoded by NSP3 have a considerable role in viral infection [53]. A genome-wide association study (GWAS) conducted in Italy and Spain analyzed single nucleotide polymorphisms that revealed that Leucine Zipper Transcription Factor Like 1 (LZTFL1) encodes Solute Carrier Family 6 Member 20 (SLC6A20), which functionally interacts with cellular receptor "ACE2" of SARS-CoV-2 [54, 55]. However, the expression of SLC6A20 is increased in SNP rs11385942, but on the other hand, it is associated with a reduction in CXCR6 expression [56].

Transcriptome-wide Associated Studies (TWAS)

Transcriptome-wide analysis studies help understand SARS-CoV-2 pathogenesis and other events during interaction with the host. Various hosts, including humans and cell culture studies, have reported the transcriptional changes induced by SARS-CoV-2 infection [57 - 59]. Moreover, transcriptional changes are reported from the various humans infected with COVID-19 in blood samples [57], bronchoalveolar lavage fluid [60], and nasopharyngeal samples [61]. The host immune system can alter the mechanisms of sensing viral antigens and produce anti-viral responses as they are intracellular parasites and largely dependent on the host [62]. A powerful anti-viral response re-triggered by endogenous deaminase came from the editing of DNA and RNA [62].

Moreover, deaminase is also responsible for the diversity in the mRNA. There are two families of deaminase found in mammals, the editing enzyme, catalytic polypeptide, and adenines of double-stranded DNA converted into inosines by ADARs [63, 64], while APOBECs cause the deamination of cytosines into uracils in single-stranded DNA and RNA [65, 66]. The host transcripts are edited by ADARs, which leads to the modulation of cellular response in viral infections. In addition to that, viral RNA is hypermutated directly by ADARs, which influence the immune response [67]. APOBECs target the DNA in the middle of the genome [68]. APOBECs use two mechanisms: hypermutation and a non-enzymatic pathway, which is associated with reverse transcription of the viral genome [69, 70]. *In vitro*, the interference of APOBEC3 proteins with the replication of coronaviruses replication is not understood clearly [71]. However, viral infectivity is strongly increased by the demoralization of these host mechanisms that ultimately upsurge the evolutionary potential of the virus [72 - 74].

Moreover, higher mortality rates due to SARS-CoV-2 infection are associated with significant transcriptional changes that lead to excitation and unrestrained immune response from the host [75]. On the other hand, it is also reported that neutrophils are enriched by transcription, suggesting that transcription changes play an important role in the SARS-CoV-2 clearance [3]. Previously, transcriptome analysis reported that the expression of host genes strongly modulates the pathogenicity of SARS-CoV and MERS-CoV [75]. Moreover, transcriptome-wide analysis studies also help determine the host's tissue tropism. Besides the lungs, the SARS-CoV-2 receptor ACE2 is also expressed in kidneys in renal tubules [76] but is most significantly expressed in proximal tubules according to transcriptome-wide analysis studies [77]. Recently, the transcriptomic profile of the host revealed that the activation of leukocyte, humoral, neutrophil, and myeloid cells is significantly associated with SARS-CoV [78].

Several host genes, including STAT1, IFIH1, IRF9, OAS1-3, and PML, are highly associated with the immune response to SARS-CoV-2 infection, particularly the production of type I interferon. Additionally, miRNA is involved in the anti-viral response. Cytokine storm is associated with TLR2, FOXO1, and MYC genes of SARS-CoV-2 that further cause host cell death during infection [78]. The datasets of lung transcriptomes have been analyzed recently, showing that patients with background diseases such as hypertension, diabetes, and chronic obstructive pulmonary disease have a comparatively higher expression rate of ACE2 [79].

Role of Host Genetics in COVID-19 Susceptibility and Disease Severity

To encounter a wide range of pathogens, particularly viral infections, primarily innate immunity is triggered, which is the first line of defense. Viral infections induce various interferons, such as alpha, beta, and lambda interferons, which further trigger adaptive immunity by activating hundreds of antiviral proteins [80]. The presence determines the host's susceptibility to the cellular receptor of SARS-CoV-2, which is ACE2. So far, 31 human tissues, including the testis and seminal vesicle, have been reported to code genes responsible for ACE2 expression [81]. Among 31 tissues, ACE2 is moderately expressed in the lungs. Before this study, SARS-CoV-2 was detected in the stool of SARS-CoV-2 infected patients, indicating that ACE2 was also expressed in the tissues of the gastrointestinal tract [82]. Similarly, cardiac injury has been reported in the SARS-CoV-2 infected patients [83]. A variety of predominant symptoms in the SARS-CoV-2 infection indicate that it has the potential to enter various tissues by using the cellular receptor ACE2 [81]. However, the expression levels of the ACE2 gene remain the same among males and females, and no significant difference was observed in the age-wise analysis [81]. The expression of ACE2/AT2R is influenced by the inhalation of nicotine or by smoking, affecting several organs, including the lungs, brain, and heart, and leading to the disruption of the renin-angiotensin system balance [81]. Interestingly, a difference found in the protein expression of ACE2 and its mRNA pattern indicated that the mapping of mRNA is affected by some factors, such as post-translational modification [81]. Neutrophilia and lymphopenia have been reported consistently in COVID-19 patients, particularly those suffering from severe complications of COVID-19. Moreover, the expression of lambda interferons and CD4+ T cell counts decreased significantly, and in addition to that, memory T cells were also reduced [84 - 86]. Several interleukins, such as (IL)-1β, IL-6, and IL-8, which are plasma pro-inflammatory cytokines, are also reported to increase along with tumor necrosis factors in the disease severity associated with cytokine storm [87, 88]. Additionally, T cell exhaustion markers, programmed cell death protein-1, and Tim-3 were reported to be elevated in SARS-CoV-2 infection, while in healthy individuals, they remain normal and play a key role in protecting the host from COVID-19 severity [89, 90]. Clonal expansion of CD8+ T cells was reported to increase in mild SARS-CoV-2 cases and decrease in severe cases [91]. In some cases, younger individuals also developed severe COVID-19, although absence of co-morbidities was noted. Later, it was discovered that it is due to inborn errors of immunity that the course of SARS-CoV-2 infection was altered [80]. Dysregulation or embellished immune responses due to any genetic variant contributed to the SARS-CoV-2 infection severity and, in most cases, developed life-threatening clinical manifestations as well [80]. It has been proposed that innate immunity responses are destabilized due to deficient type I interferon production in SARS-CoV-2 infection that takes infection towards severity [80]. Previously, in SARS-CoV epidemics, it had been noted that infection susceptibility and severity were associated with single nucleotide polymorphisms (SNPs) in the IFN-inducible genes OAS1 and MX1 [92, 93]. Interestingly, the replication of SARS-CoV was reported to inhibit the administration of type I IFN *in vivo* [94] and *in vitro* [95]. The above data claimed the significance of the type I interferon pathway in the innate immune response to SARS-CoV infection, and it has been proposed that genetic mutations in their genes can be the reason for SARS-CoV-2 infection severity [80]. Consequently, it is worth considering that clinical outcomes may be influenced by mutations of the PRRs and immune signaling pathways involved in the recognition of SARS-CoV-2, including RIG-I, MDA5, TLR3, and downstream IRF3 and IRF7, as well as molecules involved in effector function of type I and III IFN, such as IFNAR1/2 or the Janus kinase (JAK)-signal transducer and activator of transcription (STAT) signaling pathways. Recently, it has been found that initiation of the complement system plays a key role in the pathogenesis of SARS-CoV-2 lung pathology [96, 97]. However, targeting complement protein 5 to inhibit the terminal complement pathway can help in the prevention of SARS-CoV-2 infection and can contribute to the development of therapeutics against SARS-CoV-2 infection [98]. Still, certain other pathways remain to be explored to evaluate the complement system contribution in SARS-CoV-2 infection. The influence of primary immunodeficiencies linked with antibody deficiencies is not clarified fully in SARS-CoV-2 infection outcomes. However, the common variable immunodeficiency and agammaglobulinemia profiles have been compared with SARS-CoV-2-infected individuals [99]. Agammaglobulinemia has been reported to reduce disease severity, but it increases when low levels of agammaglobulinemia are accompanied by immune dysregulation due to any common variable immunodeficiencies disease [100]. Similarly, T-cell deficiency, abnormal B immune cells, immune dysregulation, and potentially excessive production of IL-6 contributed to the SARS-CoV-2 pathogenesis and disease severity [110]. Based on insight into immunopathogenesis and pathology during COVID-19, potential susceptibility genes may be involved in mechanisms of immune dysregulation, auto-inflammation, or autoimmunity, thus involving the gain-of-function or loss of inhibition of various genes and pathways in cytokine and TLR signaling cascades, especially those affecting IL-1 and IL6 synthesis and production [101 - 103]. Moreover, host susceptibility is also influenced by genetic variants in the major histocompatibility complex antigen loci (HLA) [104], and very few studies have evaluated the HLA haplotypes' influence on SARS-CoV-2 infection susceptibility and severity. There are some inexplicable differences in the SARS-CoV-2 infection severity and mortality rates identified by HLA haplotypes throughout the world across different populations [105 - 109]. Previously, in Taiwan, the identification of HLA-B- 4601 was found to have an association with SARS-CoV infection. A genetic approach should be used to analyze the role of inflammation, immunopathology, and associated genes, including NLRP1, NLRP3, CASP1, and MEFV, in the pathogenesis of SARS-CoV-2 and disease severity [80]. All these genes are involved in encoding proteins responsible for inflammatory pathways [110]. Mutations in these genes may decrease individual susceptibility. Moreover, the receptor "ACE2" used by

SARS-CoV-2 during entry plays a key role in the host susceptibility and resistance. Recently, genetic polymorphism of ACE2 has been reported in various cases, which fluctuate the host susceptibility and resistance patterns by altering virus-host interactions [111]. Besides ACE2, the TMPRSS2 gene is also reported with the same activity [112].

TLRs Association

Immunity and infections are significantly accompanied by particular sensory proteins linked with the innate immune, also known as TLRs, and critically associated with cytokine expression by triggering signalling pathways [113]. However, the cytokine storm that is a widespread phenomenon in the infection of SARS-CoV-2 is significantly triggered by TLR signals. The individuals lacking TLRs, particularly adaptor TRIF, TLR3, and TLR4, are more susceptible to infection by SARS coronavirus [114]. The host susceptibility to SARS-CoV is greatly influenced by allelic variation in Ticam2 proteins linked with toll-like receptor adaptors [115]. It has been reported that genetic variation of TLR genes strongly influences TLR molecules' expression, and its distribution, patterns, expression rate, and efficacies are different among various populations.

Moreover, the immunological redundancy of the host is different with different TLRs, which indicates that patterns of immune responses are different [116]. TLR genes suggest important interactions between SARS-CoV infection and host antiviral pathways, which can be a crucial genetic determinant in the analysis of COVID-19 susceptibility and disease outcomes. Moreover, there is a strong association between SARS coronavirus infection and its receptor ACE2. The transcriptional activity of the ACE2 gene is significantly altered by the presence of potentially functional variants in the X chromosome [114]. Interestingly, it has been found that the allele present in the coding region of ACE2 shows frequency variation [117]. rs758278442 and rs759134032 SNPs, located in the protective variants (K31R and Y83H) of the ACE2 gene, show a relatively higher frequency of a mutant allele in the Asian population as compared to other populations of the world, such as Europeans and Americans. The less susceptibility of the host to SARS-CoV-2 infection might be associated with the ACE2 variants [118]. Moreover, the expression of ACE2 genes is crucial in the SARS-CoV-2 infection outcomes as well as host susceptibility, especially in hypertension and diabetes mellitus patients. In addition to this, it plays a significant role in inflammatory processes [119]. The expression of cytokines is up-regulated by a genetic deficiency of ACE2 that leads to vascular inflammation [120].

Virus-host Interactions During the Viral Life Cycle

Various studies have illuminated the interactions between SARS-CoV-2 and the host during the virus's life cycle. A wide-ranging interactome has been revealed between their genes during various phases of the SARS-CoV-2 life cycle and infection [121, 122]. These studies have provided relationships among host and viral genes that give insights into identifying vaccine design and anti-viral or host-directed treatment strategies [123]. Various heparan sulfate biosynthetic genes, such as UGDH, FAM20B, B4GALT7, EXT2, and B3GALT6, are required by SARS-CoV-2 for efficient infection [124]. The transcriptional program of NRF2 induces an anti-viral environment in the cell that protects SARS-CoV-2. Moreover, the agonists of NRF2 were reported to produce antiviral responses in cell culture and suggested the target of novel therapeutics [125, 126]. Various variants of host exocyst genes have been identified associated with the binding of secretory vesicles to the cell membrane. This system has been supposed to be involved in the facilitation of SARS-CoV-2 trafficking during entry and egress [123]. TMEM106B is a poorly characterized protein gene of lysosomal transmembrane associated with frontotemporal dementia. However, lysosome trafficking is reported to have defects due to deletions in TMEM106B. Moreover, the levels of lysosome enzymes were also reduced due to deletions in these regions [127]. The SARS-CoV-2 entry is affected by the TMEM106B gene, and virus-induced cell death can be prevented by this gene [122]. SCAP is a gene that encodes for a protein that acts as a sterol sensing domain, which has been reported to interact with viral proteins. In *in vitro* studies, it was found that deletions in these genes, including ACE2, reduced RNA levels of SARS-CoV-2 [122]. It was found that cholesterol levels are positively influenced by the regulation of SCAP activity as a result of interaction between host and viral proteins. Remarkably, using cholesterol-reducer statins reduced the symptoms of coronavirus disease in 2019 patients in various cases [128, 129]. Systematically, according to the genetic studies and pharmacological experiments, it was concluded that the efficient entry of SARS-CoV-2 required cellular cholesterol. Moreover, replication of SARS-CoV-2 was reduced due to deletions in TMEM106B and VAC14. Additionally, in the absence of PI3K genes or any other endosomal genes, the SARS-CoV-2 was unable to cause infection efficiently [121]. Overwhelmingly, these comprehensive genetic studies revealed that the host genes play major functional roles in the SARS-CoV-2 infection. This new human pathogenic coronavirus belongs to lineage B betacoronaviruses according to the RNA sequence of its genome revealed by interpreting RNA [130]. Various genetic determinants have been reported to have an association with resistance and susceptibility. The genotyping of various patients infected with SARS-CoV suggests that the following genes, CD14, MBL2, IFN gamma, CCL5, CD209, OAS1, and MX1, have a genetic susceptibility to infection of SARS-CoV [131 - 137]. The manifestation of

COVID-19 disease fluctuates and varies according to the patient's immune state. Usually, infection is characterized by a typical severe acute respiratory syndrome, but in some cases, it also causes death [138]. It is implied that the susceptibility of humans is different, and it is important to understand the basis of these variations in susceptibilities associated with different clinical manifestations. The susceptibility of individuals is highly associated with human genetics, and genetic variants and their frequencies cause the deviation in the patient vulnerability, which further decides the clinical condition of viral infection in patients [138]. The overall viral pathogenesis and infection sequences from the entrance to the exit are greatly accompanied by the human genes responsible for receptors, co-receptors of the virus, and the enzymes involved in modifying receptors [139]. All these genes are closely related to the susceptibility of humans to viral infection. Besides these genes, some other genes are also accountable for the disease severity and outcomes, such as genes expressed in virus sensing, anti-viral immunity, and antiviral factors [138]. A recent study used monozygotic and dizygotic twins for the symptomatic study of COVID-19 and revealed that patients' clinical conditions are highly associated with genetic factors [140]. There is a 76% sequence similarity in the spike proteins of SARS-CoV and SARS-Co-2. ACE2 plays a considerable role in the infection by providing entry to the SARS-CoV inside the host cell [141]. ACE2 is the human receptor that provides an entry site to SARS-CoV-2 [142]. Moreover, different routes are used by SARS-CoV-2 depending on the level of TMPRSS2 on target cells and the mutation rate of S proteins of the virus, particularly in the polybasic S1/S2 [143]. A human enzyme activates the spike proteins of SARS-CoV-2, also called TMPRSS2 (Human transmembrane protease serine 2) [143]. The plasma membrane provides a site for S SARS-CoV-2 cleavage through TMPRSS2. However, it can also take place on endolysosomes by cathepsins. The requirement of cathepsin is mostly ablated in case of sufficient levels of TMPRSS2 due to its overexpression. So, cathepsins are not the crucial host factor in SARS-CoV-2 infection [144]. The expressions of TMPRSS2 are usually high in the respiratory tract, especially in nasal and lung epithelial cells, which are the primary targets of SARS-CoV-2 [145]. On the other hand, TMPRSS2 levels are fluctuated among different hosts and, in many cases, do not present inadequately due to low expressions, as reported in A549 and VeroE6 cells. Thus, in such a scenario, SARS-CoV-2 preferentially relied on cathepsins for entry [146]. During the initial stage, the proteases of the host cell are utilized by SARS-CoV-2 to cleave the spike proteins into two parts, N-terminal and C-terminal, which are involved in the recognition of receptors and entry into the cell, respectively. Moreover, furin or furin-like enzymes are further required to cleave the C-terminal at furin sites before entry into the cell [147]. Furin sites are also cleaved by plasmin [148], and the individuals in which plasmin is expressed in higher concentrations are more susceptible to COVID-19 [149]. Additionally, trypsin and TMPRSS11a (airway proteases) enzymes are also associated with cleaving the S protein of SARS-Co-2 [143]. A total of 17 genetic variants are revealed in humans in the coding regions of the ACE2 gene by computational prediction methods performed for the analysis of protein structure [138]. It is indicated that the higher expressions of furin genes also increase the susceptibility of humans to SARS-CoV-2 infection besides the expression of ACE2. The genotyping studies on hospitalized COVID-19 patients revealed that the higher expressions of airway protease plasmin genes increased the infection chances and severe disease outcomes [150]. Moreover, the population with higher expression of the HLA-B*46:01 (Human Leukocyte Antigen) allele is at higher risk for COVID-19 infection, which was also reported in the previous SARS coronavirus epidemic that emerged in 2002 [151]. Moreover, in the airway epithelium, the expression of a gene is modified by T2 cytokines and remodeled in the epithelial, resulting in mucus metaplasia [152 - 154]. Microbial infections, particularly caused by respiratory viruses, are strong regulators and modulators of genes present in the respiratory epithelium and influence the expressions of those genes that are also involved in the triggering of immune responses [155 - 158]. The genes of cyclophilins are one of the most important genetic determinants in response to viral infections. These proteins are associated with the folding coronaviruses and host proteins that significantly favor the propagation of the virus [159]. The nucleocapsid of SARS coronaviruses directly interacts with cyclophilin A [160] and merges with purified prions [161].

Pro-viral and Anti-viral Genes

The pro-viral and antiviral genes provide more insights into understanding the SARS-CoV-2 pathogenesis, development of therapeutics, and vaccine design. Various studies have been performed to evaluate the screening of identified pro-viral genes, such as ACE2 and CTSL, that assist in regulating SARS-CoV-2 infection [162 - 164]. In one study, 25 pro-viral and antiviral genes were evaluated with individual sgRNAs in an arrayed format, and additionally, small molecule antagonists molecules were also identified that protect the host in SARS-CoV-2 infection [165]. Recently, a novel function of high mobility group box protein 1 (HMGB1) has been identified in the susceptibility of SARS-CoV-2 infection [165]. HMGB1 is a pleiotropic protein that regulates the chromatin in the nucleus by binding nucleosomes and transporting the DNA. It also acts as a sentinel, protects non-self-nucleic acids, and secretes alarming responses to viral infections [166 - 168]. In the past, anti-HMGB1 therapies were reported to reduce the severity of the viral infection in the case of influenza A and respiratory syncytial virus in animal models [169, 170].

Moreover, pro-inflammatory functions are inhibited in the case of adenovirus infection by binding protein VII to HMGB1 [171]. The interactions between HMGB1 SARS-CoV-2 on a molecular level are essential features that need to be clarified to provide prevention and treatment strategies. The transforming growth factors (TGF-β and SWI/SNF chromatin remodeling complex components pathway) are associated with pro-viral pathways. Activin SMAD3, 1RB, and SMAD4 can be used to speculate that the TGF-β signaling pathway, through Activin 1RB, SMAD3, and SMAD4, might alter the architecture of chromatin by SWI/SNF-driven changes to chromatin architecture that ultimately lead to prompting an expression of a pro-viral gene [165]. The SMAD3 was reported to bind with previous SARS-CoV nucleoprotein, preventing the interactions of SMAD3/SMAD4, which leads to downstream of TGF-β signaling and virus-induced apoptosis [172]. The phenotypes of SARS-CoV-2 infection vary, ranging from asymptomatic to severe and even death. However, all these fluctuations are linked to the health status of the infected individuals [173, 174]. The genetic profiles and pathways of all these individuals need to be clarified to interpret the variation in clinical manifestations of the infected individuals [165], *e.g.*, the SARS-CoV-2 infection patterns and pathogenesis are more severe in smokers as ACE2 gene expression is higher in them, leading to the worsening of infection outcomes [175]. It is indicated that chromatin and the genes that modify histones are associated with the expression of various pro-viral genes, which control the ACE2 and other viral interacting genes [180]. Previously, it has been reported that SMARCA4 regulates the expression of ACE2 in cardiac endothelial cells under stress conditions [176]. A significant target of SARS-CoV-2 in the susceptible host is alveolar epithelial cells, which are found to be proliferated by SMARCA4 and provide protection against pulmonary fibrosis [177, 178].

Regional HLA Associations

Human leukocyte antigen genes are found in the major histocompatibility complex (MHC) on the short arm of chromosome 6, one of the most complex genetic systems. Several classical transmembrane proteins such as A, B, C, DR, DQ, and DP are encoded by HLA genes, which are predominantly associated with the presentation of antigens on the surface of cells that further trigger anti-viral response [179]. The alleles of HLA influence T cell immune response by presenting a variety of peptide fragments from the invading pathogens [180]. Previously, genetic variants of HLA were reported to influence host susceptibility and resistance patterns in various viral infectious diseases such as SARS [181], MERS [182], influenzas [183], dengue [184], and hepatitis B [185]. Moreover, various other factors influence host susceptibility and resistance patterns, such as individual age [186], gender [187], and obesity [188], and are also reported to be associated with the severity of SARS-CoV-2 infection [189]. COVID-19 has affected all types of human populations worldwide, but various individuals noticed high susceptibility, and the disease progressed severely and even caused deaths. The vital question that needs to be answered quickly is the risk analysis of highly susceptible individuals that could be acquired or genetic factors. However, among genetic factors, the prevalence of HLA alleles can predict individual susceptibility. In human DNA, the most polymorphic region is the HLA locus. The proteins of HLA play a considerable role in establishing human immunity by controlling a variety of destined epitopes [190, 191]. The human leukocyte antigen (HLA) has the potential role of recognizing any foreign antigens by T cells. In establishing adaptive immune responses to viral antigens, the key role is played by HLA to which viral antigen is presented by APC cells and direct presentation of HLA I to cytotoxic CD8 T cells [192]. The human population's infectious pathologies and autoimmune diseases are highly associated with genetic polymorphism. Previously, various infections such as the human hepatitis C virus, human immunodeficiency virus, papillomavirus (HPV), and human hepatitis B virus have increased their pathogenicity by HLA-specific subtypes.

Therefore, the susceptibility to viral infections is strongly influenced by HLA [193 - 196]. The susceptibility of COVID-19 and disease severity is considerably associated with the genetic variation in HLA and significantly identifies populations at higher risk for COVID-19 disease [192]. The haplotypes and HLA-specific alleles can be suitable parameters and give a clue about the highly susceptible population of COVID-19 [197]. Across the country, HLA can be the most suitable marker in evaluating COVID-19 susceptibility in epidemic tendencies across the country. However, HLA association with COVID-19 susceptibility and epidemic situations can have similar patterns across different countries, as clearly explained by HLA polymorphisms [192]. It has been reported that HLA haplotypes/alleles are associated with more potent immune responses to viral infections. Several polymorphisms have been reported to influence the SARS virus susceptibility, including HLA-B*07:03, HLA-Cw*08:01, HLADRB1*12:02, and HLA-B*46:01 [198 - 200]. On the other hand, various allelotypes, such as HLA-A*02:01, HLA-DR*03:01, and HLA-Cw*15:02, were protective against SARS infection, as shown in Table **1** [202].

Table 1. Host HLA allelic interactions with SARS-CoV-2 infection.

Human Leukocyte Antigens	Association with SARS-CoV-2 Infection	References
HLA-B*07:03, HLA-Cw*08:01, HLADRB1*12:02, HLA-B*46:01	Increase the susceptibility	[198 - 200]
HLA-A*02:01, HLA-DR*03:01, and HLA-Cw*15:02	Provide protection	[202]

(Table 1) cont.....

Human Leukocyte Antigens	Association with SARS-CoV-2 Infection	References
Alleles of HLA	Help in the development of protective antibodies against SARS-CoV-2 infection	[204 - 209]
HLA-A HLA-C allele HLA-C*01 and/or HLA-B*44 HLA-C*01 and B*44 alleles	Have the potential to present the antigens of SARS-CoV-2 significantly Have the minimum ability to present SARS-CoV-2 antigens Have association with inflammatory autoimmune diseases in SARS-CoV-2 infection and inappropriate immunological reaction Can significantly help in the understanding of disease transmission and physio-pathogenesis	[192] [192] [222 - 226] [227]

However, the anchorage of different HLA proteins is mediated by compromising the motifs of specific amino-acidic [202, 203]. In vaccine development, SARS-CoV-2 consequential epitopes of B and T cells and their association with alleles of HLA can play a significant role. In addition to that, it can also help develop protective antibodies [204 - 209]. A study on HLA conducted in Italy found single alleles and haplotypes with significant differences [210]. It has been found that the HLA-A allele has the potential to present the antigens of SARS-CoV-2 significantly, while the HLA-C allele has the minimum ability to present SARS-CoV-2 antigens, according to the results tools used for the prediction of binding affinity of SARS-CoV-2 [192]. Various alleles such as HLA-A*02:01, HLA-B*08:01, HLAC*07:01, and HLA-B*18:01 have been reported to have the potential to present peptides of SARS-CoV-2 [211]. The ability of peptides to bind HLA proteins strongly relies on alleles [202, 203].

Moreover, HLA molecules of class I/II have a considerable role in human immunity, and it indicates the individual susceptibility to COVID-19 infection and plays a crucial role in the immune responses toward viruses [212]. HLA alleles are correlated with the morbidity and lethality of COVID-19 disease as these are strongly associated with eliciting the immunity of humans [213]. Various alleles such as HLA-C*01C*03, B*08, A*25, B*44, B*51, and B*15:01 are positively correlated with the incidence rate of COVID-19. However, according to a study conducted in Italy, various other alleles showed negative correlations, such as HLA-B*18, B*14, and B*49 [214]. Remarkably, the incidence of COVID-19 is not influenced by any single allele. People with a different HLA profile may have completely different immunity, and while encountering the same antigens, they may trigger different T-cell-mediated immune-responses [215 - 221]. HLA-B*01 and/or HLA-B*44 are usually found in healthy people, and individuals with HLA-B*08 and LA-A*25 are at higher risk for COVID-19 infection as they lack immune-dominant virus-derived epitope peptides and cannot trigger sufficient immune responses [214]. The pathogen may spread efficiently to various organs from oropharyngeal mucosae in such a scenario.

Moreover, HLA-C*01 and/or HLA-B*44 were also reported to associate inflammatory autoimmune diseases with SARS-CoV-2 infection and inappropriate immunological reactions [222 - 226]. HLA-C*01 and HLA-B*44 are the potential molecular determinants. Meanwhile, evaluating the risk of individuals and the class I and II HLA genotyping in COVID-19 patients provides a basis to identify the individuals at higher risk for cytokine storms. Consequently, vaccination is a must for such a population [227]. The avenues of HLA-C*01 and B*44 alleles can significantly help understand disease transmission and physio-pathogenesis that may play a significant role in the management of COVID-19 disease, vaccination, and other preventive strategies in terms of clinical management [227].

Significance of SARS-CoV-2 and Host Interactions in the Development of Host-Directed Therapies

The economic stability and security of human health are considerably troubled by infectious diseases as they cause one-fourth of mortalities worldwide. With the development of the advanced healthcare system, viral infections continue to grow significantly [228]. The recent outbreak of SARS-COV-2 infection appeared to be a highly pathogenic and life-threatening infection with high mortality rates that affected almost every country in the world [229]. The current scenario strongly recommends developing antiviral drugs, vaccines, or alternative therapies for this deadly infectious disease. In the absence of specific antiviral drugs and vaccines, host-directed therapies are the best treatment strategy frequently used against viral infections [230]. Emerging viral infections are one of the most common health issues worldwide that have become a headache for researchers. Fundamentally, viral replication requires specific host factors to ensure its survivability, and these host factors are identified and targeted during the development of host-directed therapy to control the virus replication [231]. Scientists are looking to use the same approach in treating SARS-CoV-2 as this approach has also been used against previous human pathogenic coronaviruses such as SARS and MERS by blocking cellular pathways. According to the existing literature, all those genetic factors used by coronaviruses' replication indirectly favor their replication [232]. The SARS-CoV-2 has emerged without premeditated epidemiological studies and therapeutic options that lead to devastating mortalities worldwide.

The researchers failed to develop specific anti-viral drugs and vaccines to treat SARS-CoV-2 infection. However, various FDA-approved drugs have been used to treat SARS-CoV-2 infection indirectly [233]. In the absence of specific anti-viral drugs, scientists depend on host-directed therapies that target the host genes and proteins associated with the entry of SARS-CoV-2 or have a role in the replication cycle. In this context, various drugs have shown promising activity, including genistein, androgen receptor antagonist enzalutamide, and estrogen-related compound estradiol, which have been reported to downregulate TMPRSS2. TMPRSS2 is a host protein used by spike proteins of SARS-CoV-2 to penetrate inside the host cell. These approaches have proved fruitful in reducing disease severity and symptoms of COVID-19 patients [234]. Moreover, transcription factors and microRNAs are the most important regulators that control gene expression during transcription and after transcription. Viruses are obligate cellular parasites that completely depend on host genes and down-regulate the expression of host genes during transcription or after transcription in the cellular compartments [230]. In host genes, the prevention of assembly of enzyme RNA polymerase II can lead to the blockage of SARS-CoV-2 transcription [234]. Transcription factors control gene regulation during transcription, while microRNAs do so after transcription. The cross-talk of miRNA–TF can provide helpful information for therapeutic purposes during viral infections. Viral infections can influence the expression level of miRNAs. In developing novel therapeutic agents against viral infections, the modulation of particular TFs' interactions of miRNA–TF is thoroughly explored and understood [230]. According to one gene regulatory study, it was identified that the *HMOX1* and *SCRAB1* genes are influenced by STAT1 and STAT2, leading to interaction with NPS7 and ORF3a SARS-CoV-2 [230]. The SARS-CoV-2 infection reported upregulating the expression of TFs, indicating their role in anti-viral immunity. Recently, genome-wide studies have been conducted to analyze the interaction of miRNAs and TFs, revealing the 2,197 miRNAs pursuing host genes interactions with the proteins of SARS-CoV-2.

Among 2,197, 38 miRNAs are reported to target approximately 150 genes in the host associated with immune responses against viruses. Fascinatingly, six anti-viral miRNAs, namely, hsa-miR-1-3p, hsa-miR-17-5p, hsa-miR-199a-3p, hsa-miR-429, hsa-miR-15a-5p, and hsa-miR-20a-5p, are reported to be down-regulated post-infection in various viral respiratory diseases infecting the lungs while expressed highly in normal cases. Recently, miRNAs, hsa-mir-9-5p, target the 3' UTR of ACE2 [234], and other miRNAs, hsa-mir-27b-3p, are associated with the signaling of ACE2 [234]. Therefore, ACE2 is strongly influenced by miRNA hsa-mir-27b-3p, leading to a strong correlation. Conclusively, host-directed therapies are beneficial as they allow pre-existing drugs to be repurposed and deliver broad-spectrum inhibition against various viral infections. In comparison with anti-viral treatment, host-directed therapies are more commonly used for rapidly mutating viruses, particularly for SARS-CoV-2. Several SARS-

CoV-2 genes code for the structural and non-structural proteins that have distinct interactions with host proteins, as shown in Fig. (**2**).

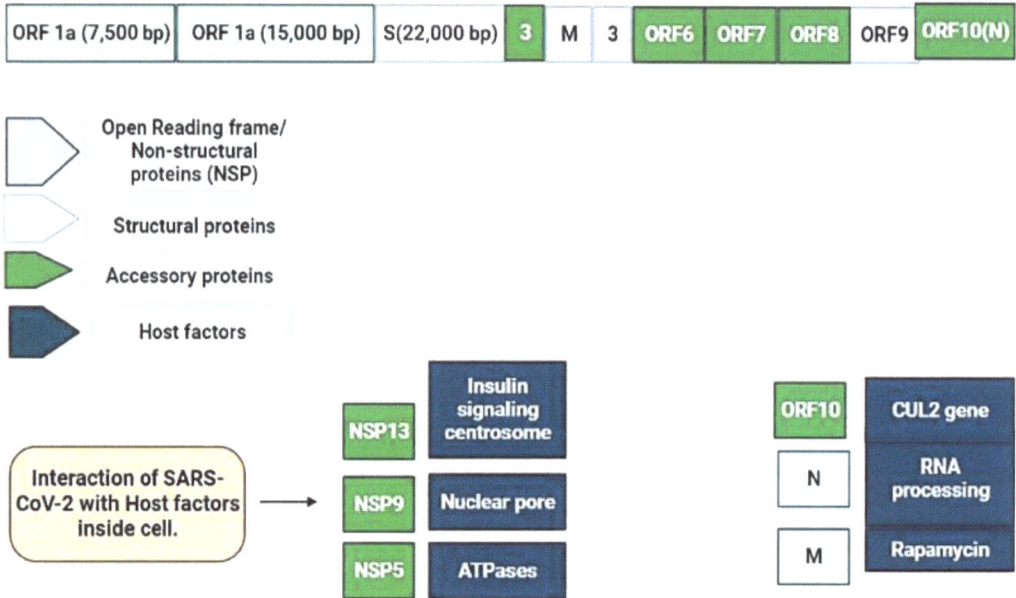

Fig. (**2**). The SARS-CoV-2 genes' interaction with host factors.

CONCLUSION

NSP13 is associated with centrosomes and insulin signals in humans, NSP5 is associated with ATPases of the host cell, and NSP9 is associated with the host proteins of the nuclear pore. The ORF8ab and ORF8b avoid the host immune responses and inhibit the signaling cascade of INF-β. Cytokine storm is associated with TLR2, FOXO1, and MYC genes of SARS-CoV-2 that further cause host cell death during infection. STAT1, IFIH1, IRF9, OAS1-3, and PML are associated with the immune response to SARS-CoV-2 infection, particularly the production of type I interferon. The SARS-CoV-2 entry is affected by the TMEM106B gene, and this gene can prevent virus-induced cell death. Moreover, replication of SARS-CoV-2 was reduced due to deletions in TMEM106B and VAC14 genes. Genetic variants also influence the host susceptibility in the major HLA. The susceptibility of COVID-19 is considerably associated with the genetic variation in HLA and plays a significant role in identifying populations at higher risk. Conclusively, host-directed therapies are beneficial as they allow pre-existing drugs to be repurposed and deliver broad-spectrum inhibition against various viral infections. In comparison with anti-viral treatment, host-directed therapies are preferable for rapidly mutating viruses, particularly for SARS-CoV-2.

ACKNOWLEDGEMENTS

The authors wish to thank and acknowledge their respective universities and institutes.

REFERENCES

[1]   2020.https://www.who.int/docs/default-source/coronaviruse/situation-reports/20200121-sitrep-1-2019-ncov.pdf

[2]   Zhu N, Zhang D, Wang W, *et al.* China Novel Coronavirus, I., and Research, T.(2020) A Novel Coronavirus from Patients with Pneumonia in China. N Engl J Med 2020; 382: 727-33.
[http://dx.doi.org/10.1056/NEJMoa2001017] [PMID: 31978945]

[3]   2020.https://www.who.int/internal-publications-detail/clinical-management-of-severe-acute-respiratory-infection-when-novel-coronavirus-(ncov)-infection-is-suspected

[4]   Hasan A, Paray BA, Hussain A, *et al.* A review on the cleavage priming of the spike protein on coronavirus by angiotensin-converting enzyme-2 and furin. J Biomol Struct Dyn 2020; 9: 1-9.
[PMID: 32274964]

[5]   Novel Coronavirus 2019.https://www.who.int/docs/defaultsource/

[6]   Cowley JA, Dimmock CM, Spann KM, Walker PJ. Gill-associated virus of Penaeus monodon prawns: an invertebrate virus with ORF1a and ORF1b genes related to arteri- and coronaviruses. J Gen Virol 2000; 81(6): 1473-84.
[http://dx.doi.org/10.1099/0022-1317-81-6-1473] [PMID: 10811931]

[7]   Schoeman D, Fielding BC. Coronavirus envelope protein: current knowledge. Virol J 2019; 16(1): 69.
[http://dx.doi.org/10.1186/s12985-019-1182-0] [PMID: 31133031]

[8]   Chan JFW, To KKW, Tse H, Jin DY, Yuen KY. Interspecies transmission and emergence of novel viruses: lessons from bats and birds. Trends Microbiol 2013; 21(10): 544-55.
[http://dx.doi.org/10.1016/j.tim.2013.05.005] [PMID: 23770275]

[9]   Woo PCY, Huang Y, Lau SKP, Yuen KY. Coronavirus genomics and bioinformatics analysis. Viruses 2010; 2(8): 1804-20.
[http://dx.doi.org/10.3390/v2081803] [PMID: 21994708]

[10]   Woo PCY, Wang M, Lau SKP, *et al.* Comparative analysis of twelve genomes of three novel group 2c and group 2d coronaviruses reveals unique group and subgroup features. J Virol 2007; 81(4): 1574-85.
[http://dx.doi.org/10.1128/JVI.02182-06] [PMID: 17121802]

[11]   Lau SKP, Woo PCY, Yip CCY, *et al.* Isolation and characterization of a novel Betacoronavirus subgroup A coronavirus, rabbit coronavirus HKU14, from domestic rabbits. J Virol 2012; 86(10): 5481-96.
[http://dx.doi.org/10.1128/JVI.06927-11] [PMID: 22398294]

[12]   Lau SKP, Poon RWS, Wong BHL, *et al.* Coexistence of different genotypes in the same bat and serological characterization of Rousettus bat coronavirus HKU9 belonging to a novel Betacoronavirus subgroup. J Virol 2010; 84(21): 11385-94.
[http://dx.doi.org/10.1128/JVI.01121-10] [PMID: 20702646]

[13]   Zhang W, Zheng XS, Agwanda B, *et al.* Serological evidence of MERS-CoV and HKU8-related CoV co-infection in Kenyan camels. Emerg Microbes Infect 2019; 8(1): 1528-34.
[http://dx.doi.org/10.1080/22221751.2019.1679610] [PMID: 31645223]

[14]   Liu DX, Fung TS, Chong KKL, Shukla A, Hilgenfeld R. Accessory proteins of SARS-CoV and other coronaviruses. Antiviral Res 2014; 109: 97-109.
[http://dx.doi.org/10.1016/j.antiviral.2014.06.013] [PMID: 24995382]

[15]   Narayanan K, Huang C, Makino S. SARS coronavirus accessory proteins. Virus Res 2008; 133(1): 113-21.
[http://dx.doi.org/10.1016/j.virusres.2007.10.009] [PMID: 18045721]

[16]   Lai MMC, Cavanagh D. The molecular biology of coronaviruses. Adv Virus Res 1997; 48: 1-100.
[http://dx.doi.org/10.1016/S0065-3527(08)60286-9] [PMID: 9233431]

[17]   Neuman BW, Kiss G, Kunding AH, *et al.* A structural analysis of M protein in coronavirus assembly and morphology. J Struct Biol 2011; 174(1): 11-22.
[http://dx.doi.org/10.1016/j.jsb.2010.11.021] [PMID: 21130884]

[18]   Richman DD, Whitley RJ, Hayden FG. Clinic virol. John Wiley & Sons 2016.
[http://dx.doi.org/10.1128/9781555819439]

[19]   Fehr AR, Perlman S. Coronaviruses: an overview of their replication and pathogenesis. Methods Mol Biol 2015; 1282: 1-23.
[http://dx.doi.org/10.1007/978-1-4939-2438-7_1] [PMID: 25720466]

[20]   Wu A, Peng Y, Huang B, *et al.* Genome composition and divergence of the novel coronavirus (2019-nCoV) originating in China. Cell Host Microbe 2020; 27(3): 325-8.
[http://dx.doi.org/10.1016/j.chom.2020.02.001] [PMID: 32035028]

[21]   Chan JFW, Kok KH, Zhu Z, *et al.* Genomic characterization of the 2019 novel human-pathogenic coronavirus isolated from a patient with atypical pneumonia after visiting Wuhan. Emerg Microbes Infect 2020; 9(1): 221-36.
[http://dx.doi.org/10.1080/22221751.2020.1719902] [PMID: 31987001]

[22]   Uddin M, Mustafa F, Rizvi TA, *et al.* SARS-CoV-2/COVID-19: viral genomics, epidemiology, vaccines, and therapeutic interventions. Viruses 2020; 12(5): 526.
[http://dx.doi.org/10.3390/v12050526] [PMID: 32397688]

[23]   Belouzard S, Millet JK, Licitra BN, Whittaker GR. Mechanisms of coronavirus cell entry mediated by the viral spike protein. Viruses 2012; 4(6): 1011-33.
[http://dx.doi.org/10.3390/v4061011] [PMID: 22816037]

[24]   Bolles M, Donaldson E, Baric R. SARS-CoV and emergent coronaviruses: viral determinants of interspecies transmission. Curr Opin Virol 2011; 1(6): 624-34.
[http://dx.doi.org/10.1016/j.coviro.2011.10.012] [PMID: 22180768]

[25]   Li F. Structure, function, and evolution of coronavirus spike proteins. Annu Rev Virol 2016; 3(1): 237-61.
[http://dx.doi.org/10.1146/annurev-virology-110615-042301] [PMID: 27578435]

[26]   Ashour HM, Elkhatib WF, Rahman MM, Elshabrawy HA. Insights into the recent 2019 novel coronavirus (SARS-CoV-2) in light of past human coronavirus outbreaks. Pathogens 2020; 9(3): 186.
[http://dx.doi.org/10.3390/pathogens9030186] [PMID: 32143502]

[27]   Duffy S. Why are RNA virus mutation rates so damn high? PLoS Biol 2018; 16(8): e3000003.
[http://dx.doi.org/10.1371/journal.pbio.3000003] [PMID: 30102691]

[28]   Kautz TF, Forrester NL. RNA virus fidelity mutants: a useful tool for evolutionary biology or a complex challenge? Viruses 2018; 10(11): 600.
[http://dx.doi.org/10.3390/v10110600] [PMID: 30388745]

[29]   Smith EC. The not-so-infinite malleability of RNA viruses: Viral and cellular determinants of RNA virus mutation rates. PLoS Pathog 2017; 13(4): e1006254.
[http://dx.doi.org/10.1371/journal.ppat.1006254] [PMID: 28448634]

[30]   Xiao Y, Rouzine IM, Bianco S, *et al.* RNA recombination enhances adaptability and is required for virus spread and virulence. Cell Host Microbe 2016; 19(4): 493-503.
[http://dx.doi.org/10.1016/j.chom.2016.03.009] [PMID: 27078068]

[31]   Tang X, Wu C, Li X, *et al.* On the origin and continuing evolution of SARS-CoV-2. Natl Sci Rev

2020; 7(6): 1012-23.
[http://dx.doi.org/10.1093/nsr/nwaa036] [PMID: 34676127]

[32]   Kim JS, Jang JH, Kim JM, Chung YS, Yoo CK, Han MG. Genome-wide identification and characterization of point mutations in the SARS-CoV-2 genome. Osong Public Health Res Perspect 2020; 11(3): 101-11.
[http://dx.doi.org/10.24171/j.phrp.2020.11.3.05] [PMID: 32528815]

[33]   https://www.who.int/internal-publications-detail/clinical-management-of-severe-acute-resp-ratory-infection-when-novel-coronavirus-(ncov)-infection-is-suspected2020.

[34]   Zhou Y, Hou Y, Shen J, Huang Y, Martin W, Cheng F. Network-based drug repurposing for novel coronavirus 2019-nCoV/SARS-CoV-2. Cell Discov 2020; 6(1): 14.
[http://dx.doi.org/10.1038/s41421-020-0153-3] [PMID: 32194980]

[35]   Andersen KG, Rambaut A, Lipkin WI, Holmes EC, Garry RF. The proximal origin of SARS-CoV-2. Nat Med 2020; 26(4): 450-2.
[http://dx.doi.org/10.1038/s41591-020-0820-9] [PMID: 32284615]

[36]   Zhu N, Zhang D, Wang W, *et al.* A novel coronavirus from patients with pneumonia in China, 2019. N Engl J Med 2020; 382(8): 727-33.
[http://dx.doi.org/10.1056/NEJMoa2001017] [PMID: 31978945]

[37]   Liu DX, Fung TS, Chong KKL, Shukla A, Hilgenfeld R. Accessory proteins of SARS-CoV and other coronaviruses. Antiviral Res 2014; 109: 97-109.
[http://dx.doi.org/10.1016/j.antiviral.2014.06.013] [PMID: 24995382]

[38]   Cowley JA, Dimmock CM, Spann KM, Walker PJ. Gill-associated virus of Penaeus monodon prawns: an invertebrate virus with ORF1a and ORF1b genes related to arteri- and coronaviruses. J Gen Virol 2000; 81(6): 1473-84.
[http://dx.doi.org/10.1099/0022-1317-81-6-1473] [PMID: 10811931]

[39]   Lai MMC, Cavanagh D. The molecular biology of coronaviruses. Adv Virus Res 1997; 48: 1-100.
[http://dx.doi.org/10.1016/S0065-3527(08)60286-9] [PMID: 9233431]

[40]   Neuman BW, Kiss G, Kunding AH, *et al.* A structural analysis of M protein in coronavirus assembly and morphology. J Struct Biol 2011; 174(1): 11-22.
[http://dx.doi.org/10.1016/j.jsb.2010.11.021] [PMID: 21130884]

[41]   Richman DD, Whitley RJ, Hayden FG. Clinic virol. John Wiley & Sons 2016.
[http://dx.doi.org/10.1128/9781555819439]

[42]   Kim D, Lee JY, Yang JS, Kim JW, Kim VN, Chang H. The architecture of SARS-CoV-2 transcriptome. Cell 2020; 181(4): 914-921.e10.
[http://dx.doi.org/10.1016/j.cell.2020.04.011] [PMID: 32330414]

[43]   Gordon DE, Jang GM, Bouhaddou M, *et al.* A SARS-CoV-2 protein interaction map reveals targets for drug repurposing. Nature 2020; 583(7816): 459-68.
[http://dx.doi.org/10.1038/s41586-020-2286-9] [PMID: 32353859]

[44]   Kim JS, Jang JH, Kim JM, Chung YS, Yoo CK, Han MG. Genome-wide identification and characterization of point mutations in the SARS-CoV-2 genome. Osong Public Health Res Perspect 2020; 11(3): 101-11.
[http://dx.doi.org/10.24171/j.phrp.2020.11.3.05] [PMID: 32528815]

[45]   Wu F, Zhao S, Yu B, *et al.* A new coronavirus associated with human respiratory disease in China. Nature 2020; 579(7798): 265-9.
[http://dx.doi.org/10.1038/s41586-020-2008-3] [PMID: 32015508]

[46]   Zhang Y, Zhang J, Chen Y, *et al.* The ORF8 protein of SARS-CoV-2 mediates immune evasion through potently downregulating MHC-I. biorxiv 2020.
[http://dx.doi.org/10.1101/2020.05.24.111823]

[47]   Li JY, Liao CH, Wang Q, *et al.* The ORF6, ORF8 and nucleocapsid proteins of SARS-CoV-2 inhibit type I interferon signaling pathway. Virus Res 2020; 286: 198074.
[http://dx.doi.org/10.1016/j.virusres.2020.198074] [PMID: 32589897]

[48]   Wong HH, Fung TS, Fang S, Huang M, Le MT, Liu DX. Accessory proteins 8b and 8ab of severe acute respiratory syndrome coronavirus suppress the interferon signaling pathway by mediating ubiquitin-dependent rapid degradation of interferon regulatory factor 3. Virology 2018; 515: 165-75.
[http://dx.doi.org/10.1016/j.virol.2017.12.028] [PMID: 29294448]

[49]   Li JY, Liao CH, Wang Q, *et al.* The ORF6, ORF8 and nucleocapsid proteins of SARS-CoV-2 inhibit type I interferon signaling pathway. Virus Res 2020; 286: 198074.
[http://dx.doi.org/10.1016/j.virusres.2020.198074] [PMID: 32589897]

[50]   Koyama T, Platt D, Parida L. Variant analysis of SARS-CoV-2 genomes. Bull World Health Organ 2020; 98(7): 495-504.
[http://dx.doi.org/10.2471/BLT.20.253591] [PMID: 32742035]

[51]   Wan Y, Shang J, Graham R, Baric RS, Li F. Receptor recognition by the novel coronavirus from Wuhan: an analysis based on decade-long structural studies of SARS coronavirus. J Virol 2020; 94(7): e00127-20.
[http://dx.doi.org/10.1128/JVI.00127-20] [PMID: 31996437]

[52]   Niemeyer D, Mösbauer K, Klein EM, *et al.* The papain-like protease determines a virulence trait that varies among members of the SARS-coronavirus species. PLoS Pathog 2018; 14(9): e1007296.
[http://dx.doi.org/10.1371/journal.ppat.1007296] [PMID: 30248143]

[53]   Vuille-dit-Bille RN, Camargo SM, Emmenegger L, *et al.* Human intestine luminal ACE2 and amino acid transporter expression increased by ACE-inhibitors. Amino Acids 2015; 47(4): 693-705.
[http://dx.doi.org/10.1007/s00726-014-1889-6] [PMID: 25534429]

[54]   Kuba K, Imai Y, Ohto-Nakanishi T, Penninger JM. Trilogy of ACE2: A peptidase in the renin–angiotensin system, a SARS receptor, and a partner for amino acid transporters. Pharmacol Ther 2010; 128(1): 119-28.
[http://dx.doi.org/10.1016/j.pharmthera.2010.06.003] [PMID: 20599443]

[55]   Ellinghaus D, Degenhardt F, Bujanda L, *et al.* The ABO blood group locus and a chromosome 3 gene cluster associate with SARS-CoV-2 respiratory failure in an Italian-Spanish genome-wide association analysis. MedRxiv 2020: 2020-05.
[http://dx.doi.org/10.1101/2020.05.31.20114991]

[56]   Blanco-Melo D, Nilsson-Payant BE, Liu WC, *et al.* Imbalanced host response to SARS-CoV-2 drives development of COVID-19. Cell 2020; 181(5): 1036-1045.e9.
[http://dx.doi.org/10.1016/j.cell.2020.04.026] [PMID: 32416070]

[57]   Sun J, Zhuang Z, Zheng J, *et al.* Generation of a broadly useful model for COVID-19 pathogenesis, vaccination, and treatment. Cell 2020; 182(3): 734-743.e5.
[http://dx.doi.org/10.1016/j.cell.2020.06.010] [PMID: 32643603]

[58]   Wilk AJ, Rustagi A, Zhao NQ, *et al.* A single-cell atlas of the peripheral immune response in patients with severe COVID-19. Nat Med 2020; 26(7): 1070-6.
[http://dx.doi.org/10.1038/s41591-020-0944-y] [PMID: 32514174]

[59]   Liao M, Liu Y, Yuan J, *et al.* Single-cell landscape of bronchoalveolar immune cells in patients with COVID-19. Nat Med 2020; 26(6): 842-4.
[http://dx.doi.org/10.1038/s41591-020-0901-9] [PMID: 32398875]

[60]   Butler DJ, Mozsary C, Meydan C, *et al.* Shotgun transcriptome and isothermal profiling of SARS-CoV-2 infection reveals unique host responses, viral diversification, and drug interactions. BioRxiv 2020.
[http://dx.doi.org/10.1101/2020.04.20.048066]

[61]   Di Giorgio S, Martignano F, Torcia MG, Mattiuz G, Conticello SG. Evidence for host-dependent RNA

editing in the transcriptome of SARS-CoV-2. Sci Adv 2020; 6(25): eabb5813.
[http://dx.doi.org/10.1126/sciadv.abb5813] [PMID: 32596474]

[62]   O'Connell MA, Mannion NM, Keegan LP. The epitranscriptome and innate immunity. PLoS Genet 2015; 11(12): e1005687.
[http://dx.doi.org/10.1371/journal.pgen.1005687] [PMID: 26658668]

[63]   Eisenberg E, Levanon EY. A-to-I RNA editing — immune protector and transcriptome diversifier. Nat Rev Genet 2018; 19(8): 473-90.
[http://dx.doi.org/10.1038/s41576-018-0006-1] [PMID: 29692414]

[64]   Harris RS, Dudley JP. APOBECs and virus restriction. Virology 2015; 479-480: 131-45.
[http://dx.doi.org/10.1016/j.virol.2015.03.012] [PMID: 25818029]

[65]   Salter JD, Smith HC. Modeling the embrace of a mutator: APOBEC selection of nucleic acid ligands. Trends Biochem Sci 2018; 43(8): 606-22.
[http://dx.doi.org/10.1016/j.tibs.2018.04.013] [PMID: 29803538]

[66]   Rosani U, Bai CM, Maso L, *et al.* A-to-I editing of Malacoherpesviridae RNAs supports the antiviral role of ADAR1 in mollusks. BMC Evol Biol 2019; 19(1): 149.
[http://dx.doi.org/10.1186/s12862-019-1472-6] [PMID: 31337330]

[67]   Peretti A, Geoghegan EM, Pastrana DV, *et al.* Characterization of BK polyomaviruses from kidney transplant recipients suggests a role for APOBEC3 in driving in-host virus evolution. Cell Host Microbe 2018; 23(5): 628-635.e7.
[http://dx.doi.org/10.1016/j.chom.2018.04.005] [PMID: 29746834]

[68]   Newman ENC, Holmes RK, Craig HM, *et al.* Antiviral function of APOBEC3G can be dissociated from cytidine deaminase activity. Curr Biol 2005; 15(2): 166-70.
[http://dx.doi.org/10.1016/j.cub.2004.12.068] [PMID: 15668174]

[69]   Pollpeter D, Parsons M, Sobala AE, *et al.* Deep sequencing of HIV-1 reverse transcripts reveals the multifaceted antiviral functions of APOBEC3G. Nat Microbiol 2017; 3(2): 220-33.
[http://dx.doi.org/10.1038/s41564-017-0063-9] [PMID: 29158605]

[70]   Milewska A, Kindler E, Vkovski P, *et al.* APOBEC3-mediated restriction of RNA virus replication. Sci Rep 2018; 8(1): 5960.
[http://dx.doi.org/10.1038/s41598-018-24448-2] [PMID: 29654310]

[71]   Albin JS, Haché G, Hultquist JF, Brown WL, Harris RS. Long-term restriction by APOBEC3F selects human immunodeficiency virus type 1 variants with restored Vif function. J Virol 2010; 84(19): 10209-19.
[http://dx.doi.org/10.1128/JVI.00632-10] [PMID: 20686027]

[72]   Sadler HA, Stenglein MD, Harris RS, Mansky LM. APOBEC3G contributes to HIV-1 variation through sublethal mutagenesis. J Virol 2010; 84(14): 7396-404.
[http://dx.doi.org/10.1128/JVI.00056-10] [PMID: 20463080]

[73]   Perelygina L, Chen M, Suppiah S, *et al.* Infectious vaccine-derived rubella viruses emerge, persist, and evolve in cutaneous granulomas of children with primary immunodeficiencies. PLoS Pathog 2019; 15(10): e1008080.
[http://dx.doi.org/10.1371/journal.ppat.1008080] [PMID: 31658304]

[74]   Josset L, Menachery VD, Gralinski LE, *et al.* Cell host response to infection with novel human coronavirus EMC predicts potential antivirals and important differences with SARS coronavirus. MBio 2013; 4(3): e00165-13.
[http://dx.doi.org/10.1128/mBio.00165-13] [PMID: 23631916]

[75]   Lely AT, Hamming I, van Goor H, Navis GJ. Renal ACE2 expression in human kidney disease. The Journal of Pathology: A Journal of the Pathological Society of Great Britain and Ireland. 2004; 204(5): 587-93.
[http://dx.doi.org/10.1002/path.1670]

[76] Zou X, Chen K, Zou J, Han P, Hao J, Han Z. Single-cell RNA-seq data analysis on the receptor ACE2 expression reveals the potential risk of different human organs vulnerable to 2019-nCoV infection. Front Med 2020; 14(2): 185-92.
[http://dx.doi.org/10.1007/s11684-020-0754-0] [PMID: 32170560]

[77] Alsamman AM, Zayed H. The transcriptomic profiling of SARS-CoV-2 compared to SARS, MERS, EBOV, and H1N1. PLoS One 2020; 15(12): e0243270.
[http://dx.doi.org/10.1371/journal.pone.0243270] [PMID: 33301474]

[78] Pinto BGG, Oliveira AER, Singh Y, *et al.* ACE2 expression is increased in the lungs of patients with comorbidities associated with severe COVID-19. J Infect Dis 2020; 222(4): 556-63.
[http://dx.doi.org/10.1093/infdis/jiaa332] [PMID: 32526012]

[79] Carter-Timofte ME, Jørgensen SE, Freytag MR, *et al.* Deciphering the role of host genetics in susceptibility to severe COVID-19. Front Immunol 2020; 11: 1606.
[http://dx.doi.org/10.3389/fimmu.2020.01606] [PMID: 32695122]

[80] Li MY, Li L, Zhang Y, Wang XS. Expression of the SARS-CoV-2 cell receptor gene ACE2 in a wide variety of human tissues. Infect Dis Poverty 2020; 9(1): 45.
[http://dx.doi.org/10.1186/s40249-020-00662-x] [PMID: 32345362]

[81] Li W, Moore MJ, Vasilieva N, *et al.* Angiotensin-converting enzyme 2 is a functional receptor for the SARS coronavirus. Nature 2003; 426(6965): 450-4.
[http://dx.doi.org/10.1038/nature02145] [PMID: 14647384]

[82] Huang C, Wang Y, Li X, *et al.* Clinical features of patients infected with 2019 novel coronavirus in Wuhan, China. Lancet 2020; 395(10223): 497-506.
[http://dx.doi.org/10.1016/S0140-6736(20)30183-5] [PMID: 31986264]

[83] Qin C, Ziwei MP, Tao SY, Ke PC, Shang MM. Shang MM. Dysregulation of immune response in patients with COVID-19 in Wuhan, China. Clin Infect Dis 2020; 71(15): 762-8.
[http://dx.doi.org/10.1093/cid/ciaa248]

[84] Pedersen SF, Ho YC. SARS-CoV-2: a storm is raging. J Clin Invest 2020; 130(5): 2202-5.
[http://dx.doi.org/10.1172/JCI137647] [PMID: 32217834]

[85] Diao B, Wang C, Tan Y, *et al.* Reduction and functional exhaustion of T cells in patients with coronavirus disease 2019 (COVID-19). Front Immunol 2020; 11: 827.
[http://dx.doi.org/10.3389/fimmu.2020.00827] [PMID: 32425950]

[86] Huang C, Wang Y, Li X, *et al.* Clinical features of patients infected with 2019 novel coronavirus in Wuhan, China. Lancet 2020; 395(10223): 497-506.
[http://dx.doi.org/10.1016/S0140-6736(20)30183-5] [PMID: 31986264]

[87] Chen G, Wu D, Guo W, *et al.* Clinical and immunological features of severe and moderate coronavirus disease 2019. J Clin Invest 2020; 130(5): 2620-9.
[http://dx.doi.org/10.1172/JCI137244] [PMID: 32217835]

[88] Zheng HY, Zhang M, Yang CX, *et al.* Elevated exhaustion levels and reduced functional diversity of T cells in peripheral blood may predict severe progression in COVID-19 patients. Cell Mol Immunol 2020; 17(5): 541-3.
[http://dx.doi.org/10.1038/s41423-020-0401-3] [PMID: 32203186]

[89] Wang D, Hu B, Hu C, *et al.* Clinical characteristics of 138 hospitalized patients with 2019 novel coronavirus–infected pneumonia in Wuhan, China. JAMA 2020; 323(11): 1061-9.
[http://dx.doi.org/10.1001/jama.2020.1585] [PMID: 32031570]

[90] Liao M, Liu Y, Yuan J, *et al.* Single-cell landscape of bronchoalveolar immune cells in patients with COVID-19. Nat Med 2020; 26(6): 842-4.
[http://dx.doi.org/10.1038/s41591-020-0901-9] [PMID: 32398875]

[91] Hamano E, Hijikata M, Itoyama S, *et al.* Polymorphisms of interferon-inducible genes OAS-1 and

MxA associated with SARS in the Vietnamese population. Biochem Biophys Res Commun 2005; 329(4): 1234-9.
[http://dx.doi.org/10.1016/j.bbrc.2005.02.101] [PMID: 15766558]

[92]   He J, Feng D, de Vlas SJ, *et al.* Association of SARS susceptibility with single nucleic acid polymorphisms of OAS1 and MxA genes: a case-control study. BMC Infect Dis 2006; 6(1): 106.
[http://dx.doi.org/10.1186/1471-2334-6-106] [PMID: 16824203]

[93]   Kumaki Y, Ennis J, Rahbar R, *et al.* Single-dose intranasal administration with mDEF201 (adenovirus vectored mouse interferon-alpha) confers protection from mortality in a lethal SARS-CoV BALB/c mouse model. Antiviral Res 2011; 89(1): 75-82.
[http://dx.doi.org/10.1016/j.antiviral.2010.11.007] [PMID: 21093489]

[94]   Moriguchi H, Sato C. Treatment of SARS with human interferons. Lancet 2003; 362(9390): 1159.
[http://dx.doi.org/10.1016/S0140-6736(03)14484-4] [PMID: 14550718]

[95]   Song WC, FitzGerald GA. COVID-19, microangiopathy, hemostatic activation, and complement. J Clin Invest 2020; 130(8): 3950-3.
[PMID: 32459663]

[96]   Bosmann M. Complement activation during critical illness: current findings and an outlook in the era of COVID-19. Am J Respir Crit Care Med 2020; 202(2): 163-5.
[http://dx.doi.org/10.1164/rccm.202005-1926ED]

[97]   Kulasekararaj AG, Lazana I, Large J, *et al.* Terminal complement inhibition dampens the inflammation during COVID-19. Br J Haematol 2020; 190(3): e141-3.
[http://dx.doi.org/10.1111/bjh.16916] [PMID: 32495372]

[98]   Quinti I, Lougaris V, Milito C, *et al.* A possible role for B cells in COVID-19? Lesson from patients with agammaglobulinemia. J Allergy Clin Immunol 2020; 146(1): 211-213.e4.
[http://dx.doi.org/10.1016/j.jaci.2020.04.013] [PMID: 32333914]

[99]   Lagunas-Rangel FA, Chávez-Valencia V. High IL-6/IFN-γ ratio could be associated with severe disease in COVID-19 patients. J Med Virol 2020; 92(10): 1789-90.
[http://dx.doi.org/10.1002/jmv.25900] [PMID: 32297995]

[100] Henderson LA, Canna SW, Schulert GS, *et al.* On the alert for cytokine storm: immunopathology in COVID-19. Arthritis Rheumatol 2020; 72(7): 1059-63.
[http://dx.doi.org/10.1002/art.41285] [PMID: 32293098]

[101] Cao X. COVID-19: immunopathology and its implications for therapy. Nat Rev Immunol 2020; 20(5): 269-70.
[http://dx.doi.org/10.1038/s41577-020-0308-3] [PMID: 32273594]

[102] Matzaraki V, Kumar V, Wijmenga C, Zhernakova A. The MHC locus and genetic susceptibility to autoimmune and infectious diseases. Genome Biol 2017; 18(1): 76.
[http://dx.doi.org/10.1186/s13059-017-1207-1] [PMID: 28449694]

[103] Dimarco AD. COVID-19 and ethnicity: it's too early to point to healthcare provider attitudes as a cause of poorer outcomes. BMJ 2020; 369: m2181.
[http://dx.doi.org/10.1136/bmj.m2181] [PMID: 32487546]

[104] Lassale C, Gaye B, Hamer M, Gale CR, Batty GD. Ethnic disparities in hospitalisation for COVID-19 in England: The role of socioeconomic factors, mental health, and inflammatory and pro-inflammatory factors in a community-based cohort study. Brain Behav Immun 2020; 88: 44-9.
[http://dx.doi.org/10.1016/j.bbi.2020.05.074] [PMID: 32497776]

[105] Galloway JB, Norton S, Barker RD, *et al.* A clinical risk score to identify patients with COVID-19 at high risk of critical care admission or death: An observational cohort study. J Infect 2020; 81(2): 282-8.
[http://dx.doi.org/10.1016/j.jinf.2020.05.064] [PMID: 32479771]

[106] Zachariah P, Johnson CL, Halabi KC, *et al.* Epidemiology, clinical features, and disease severity in

patients with coronavirus disease 2019 (COVID-19) in a children's hospital in New York City, New York. JAMA Pediatr 2020; 174(10): e202430.
[http://dx.doi.org/10.1001/jamapediatrics.2020.2430] [PMID: 32492092]

[107] Price-Haywood EG, Burton J, Fort D, Seoane L. Hospitalization and mortality among black patients and white patients with Covid-19. N Engl J Med 2020; 382(26): 2534-43.
[http://dx.doi.org/10.1056/NEJMsa2011686] [PMID: 32459916]

[108] Manthiram K, Zhou Q, Aksentijevich I, Kastner DL. The monogenic autoinflammatory diseases define new pathways in human innate immunity and inflammation. Nat Immunol 2017; 18(8): 832-42.
[http://dx.doi.org/10.1038/ni.3777] [PMID: 28722725]

[109] Stawiski EW, Diwanji D, Suryamohan K, *et al.* Human ACE2 receptor polymorphisms predict SARS-CoV-2 susceptibility. BioRxiv 2020.
[http://dx.doi.org/10.1101/2020.04.07.024752]

[110] Asselta R, Paraboschi EM, Mantovani A, Duga S. ACE2 and TMPRSS2 variants and expression as candidates to sex and country differences in COVID-19 severity in Italy. Aging (Albany NY) 2020; 12(11): 10087-98.
[http://dx.doi.org/10.18632/aging.103415]

[111] Ozato K, Tsujimura H, Tamura T. Toll-like receptor signaling and regulation of cytokine gene expression in the immune system. Biotechniques 2002; 33(sup4) (Suppl.): 66-68, 70, 72 passim.
[http://dx.doi.org/10.2144/Oct0208] [PMID: 12395929]

[112] Debnath M, Banerjee M, Berk M. Genetic gateways to COVID-19 infection: Implications for risk, severity, and outcomes. FASEB J 2020; 34(7): 8787-95.
[http://dx.doi.org/10.1096/fj.202001115R] [PMID: 32525600]

[113] Gralinski LE, Menachery VD, Morgan AP, *et al.* Allelic variation in the toll-like receptor adaptor protein ticam2 contributes to SARS-coronavirus pathogenesis in mice. G3: Genes, Genomes. G3 (Bethesda) 2017; 7(6): 1653-63.
[http://dx.doi.org/10.1534/g3.117.041434] [PMID: 28592648]

[114] Barreiro LB, Ben-Ali M, Quach H, *et al.* Evolutionary dynamics of human Toll-like receptors and their different contributions to host defense. PLoS Genet 2009; 5(7): e1000562.
[http://dx.doi.org/10.1371/journal.pgen.1000562] [PMID: 19609346]

[115] Cao Y, Li L, Feng Z, *et al.* Comparative genetic analysis of the novel coronavirus (2019-nCoV/SAR-CoV-2) receptor ACE2 in different populations. Cell Discov 2020; 6(1): 11.
[http://dx.doi.org/10.1038/s41421-020-0147-1] [PMID: 32133153]

[116] Hussain M, Jabeen N, Raza F, *et al.* Structural variations in human ACE2 may influence its binding with SARS-CoV-2 spike protein. J Med Virol 2020; 92(9): 1580-6.
[http://dx.doi.org/10.1002/jmv.25832] [PMID: 32249956]

[117] Reddy Gaddam R, Chambers S, Bhatia M. ACE and ACE2 in inflammation: a tale of two enzymes. Inflamm Allergy Drug Targets 2014; 13(4): 224-34.
[http://dx.doi.org/10.2174/1871528113666140713164506.]

[118] Thomas MC, Pickering RJ, Tsorotes D, *et al.* Genetic Ace2 deficiency accentuates vascular inflammation and atherosclerosis in the ApoE knockout mouse. Circ Res 2010; 107(7): 888-97.
[http://dx.doi.org/10.1161/CIRCRESAHA.110.219279] [PMID: 20671240]

[119] Hoffmann HH, Sánchez-Rivera FJ, Schneider WM, *et al.* Functional interrogation of a SARS-CoV-2 host protein interactome identifies unique and shared coronavirus host factors. Cell Host Microbe 2021; 29(2): 267-280.e5.
[http://dx.doi.org/10.1016/j.chom.2020.12.009] [PMID: 33357464]

[120] Ng K, Attig J, Bolland W, *et al.* Tissue-specific and interferon-inducible expression of non-functional ACE2 through endogenous retrovirus co-option. BioRxiv 2020.
[http://dx.doi.org/10.1101/2020.07.24.219139]

[121] Baggen J, Persoons L, Jansen S, *et al.* Identification of TMEM106B as proviral host factor for SARS-CoV-2. BioRxiv 2020.
[http://dx.doi.org/10.1101/2020.09.28.316281]

[122] Jiang Q, Du G, Wang J, *et al.* The accessible promoter–mediated supplementary effect of ACE2 provides new insight into the tissue tropism of SARS-CoV-2. Mol Ther Nucleic Acids 2022; 28(249): 258.
[http://dx.doi.org/10.1016/j.omtn.2022.03.010]

[123] Cuadrado A, Rojo AI, Wells G, *et al.* Therapeutic targeting of the NRF2 and KEAP1 partnership in chronic diseases. Nat Rev Drug Discov 2019; 18(4): 295-317.
[http://dx.doi.org/10.1038/s41573-018-0008-x] [PMID: 30610225]

[124] Wang R, Simoneau CR, Kulsuptrakul J, Bouhaddou M, Travisano K, Hayashi JM, Carlson-Stevermer J, Oki J, Holden K, Krogan NJ, Ott M. Functional genomic screens identify human host factors for SARS-CoV-2 and common cold coronaviruses. BioRxiv. 2020 Sep 24.
[http://dx.doi.org/10.1101/2020.09.24.312298] [PMID: 32995787]

[125] Olagnier D, Farahani E, Thyrsted J, *et al.* SARS-CoV2-mediated suppression of NRF2-signaling reveals potent antiviral and anti-inflammatory activity of 4-octyl-itaconate and dimethyl fumarate. Nat Commun 2020; 11(1): 4938.
[http://dx.doi.org/10.1038/s41467-020-18764-3] [PMID: 31911652]

[126] Klein ZA, Takahashi H, Ma M, *et al.* Loss of TMEM106B ameliorates lysosomal and frontotemporal dementia-related phenotypes in progranulin-deficient mice. Neuron 2017; 95(2): 281-296.e6.
[http://dx.doi.org/10.1016/j.neuron.2017.06.026] [PMID: 28728022]

[127] Daniels LB, Sitapati AM, Zhang J, *et al.* Relation of statin use prior to admission to severity and recovery among COVID-19 inpatients. Am J Cardiol 2020; 136: 149-55.
[http://dx.doi.org/10.1016/j.amjcard.2020.09.012] [PMID: 32946859]

[128] Zhang XJ, Qin JJ, Cheng X, *et al.* In-hospital use of statins is associated with a reduced risk of mortality among individuals with COVID-19. Cell Metab 2020; 32(2): 176-187.e4.
[http://dx.doi.org/10.1016/j.cmet.2020.06.015] [PMID: 32592657]

[129] Wu F, Zhao S, Yu B, *et al.* A new coronavirus associated with human respiratory disease in China. Nature 2020; 579(7798): 265-9.
[http://dx.doi.org/10.1038/s41586-020-2008-3] [PMID: 32015508]

[130] Chong WP, Ip WKE, Tso GHW, *et al.* The interferon gamma gene polymorphism +874 A/T is associated with severe acute respiratory syndrome. BMC Infect Dis 2006; 6(1): 82.
[http://dx.doi.org/10.1186/1471-2334-6-82] [PMID: 16672072]

[131] He J, Feng D, de Vlas SJ, *et al.* Association of SARS susceptibility with single nucleic acid polymorphisms of OAS1 and MxA genes: a case-control study. BMC Infect Dis 2006; 6(1): 106.
[http://dx.doi.org/10.1186/1471-2334-6-106] [PMID: 16824203]

[132] Ng MW, Zhou G, Chong WP, *et al.* The association of RANTES polymorphism with severe acute respiratory syndrome in Hong Kong and Beijing Chinese. BMC Infect Dis 2007; 7(1): 50.
[http://dx.doi.org/10.1186/1471-2334-7-50] [PMID: 17540042]

[133] Yuan FF, Boehm I, Chan PKS, *et al.* High prevalence of the CD14-159CC genotype in patients infected with severe acute respiratory syndrome-associated coronavirus. Clin Vaccine Immunol 2007; 14(12): 1644-5.
[http://dx.doi.org/10.1128/CVI.00100-07] [PMID: 17913858]

[134] Chan KY, Xu MS, Ching JC, *et al.* Association of a single nucleotide polymorphism in the CD209 (DC-SIGN) promoter with SARS severity. Hong Kong Med J 2010; 16(5 Suppl 4): 37-42.
[PMID: 20864747]

[135] Tu X, Chong WP, Zhai Y, *et al.* Functional polymorphisms of the CCL2 and MBL genes cumulatively increase susceptibility to severe acute respiratory syndrome coronavirus infection. J Infect 2015;

71(1): 101-9.
[http://dx.doi.org/10.1016/j.jinf.2015.03.006] [PMID: 25818534]

[136] Zhu X, Wang Y, Zhang H, *et al.* Genetic variation of the human α-2-Heremans-Schmid glycoprotein (AHSG) gene associated with the risk of SARS-CoV infection. PLoS One 2011; 6(8): e23730.
[http://dx.doi.org/10.1371/journal.pone.0023730] [PMID: 21904596]

[137] Klaassen K, Stankovic B, Zukic B, *et al.* Functional prediction and comparative population analysis of variants in genes for proteases and innate immunity related to SARS-CoV-2 infection. Infect Genet Evol 2020; 84: 104498.
[http://dx.doi.org/10.1016/j.meegid.2020.104498] [PMID: 32771700]

[138] Kenney AD, Dowdle JA, Bozzacco L, *et al.* Human genetic determinants of viral diseases. Annu Rev Genet 2017; 51: 241-63.
[http://dx.doi.org/10.1146/annurev-genet-120116-023425] [PMID: 28853921]

[139] Williams FM, Freydin M, Mangino M, *et al.* Self-reported symptoms of COVID-19 including symptoms most predictive of SARS-CoV-2 infection, are heritable. MedRxiv 2020.
[http://dx.doi.org/10.1101/2020.04.22.20072124]

[140] Lu G, Wang Q, Gao GF. Bat-to-human: spike features determining 'host jump' of coronaviruses SARS-CoV, MERS-CoV, and beyond. Trends Microbiol 2015; 23(8): 468-78.
[http://dx.doi.org/10.1016/j.tim.2015.06.003] [PMID: 26206723]

[141] Wrapp D, Wang N, Corbett KS, *et al.* Cryo-EM structure of the 2019-nCoV spike in the prefusion conformation. Science 2020; 367(6483): 1260-3.
[http://dx.doi.org/10.1126/science.abb2507] [PMID: 32075877]

[142] Hoffmann M, Kleine-Weber H, Schroeder S, *et al.* SARS-CoV-2 cell entry depends on ACE2 and TMPRSS2 and is blocked by a clinically proven protease inhibitor. Cell 2020; 181(2): 271-80.
[http://dx.doi.org/10.1016/j.cell.2020.02.052]

[143] Wang R, Simoneau CR, Kulsuptrakul J, *et al.* Genetic screens identify host factors for SARS-CoV-2 and common cold coronaviruses. Cell 2021; 184(1): 106-119.e14.
[http://dx.doi.org/10.1016/j.cell.2020.12.004] [PMID: 33333024]

[144] Sungnak W, Huang N, Bécavin C, *et al.* SARS-CoV-2 entry factors are highly expressed in nasal epithelial cells together with innate immune genes. Nat Med 2020; 26(5): 681-7.
[http://dx.doi.org/10.1038/s41591-020-0868-6] [PMID: 32327758]

[145] Daniloski Z, Jordan TX, Wessels HH, *et al.* Identification of required host factors for SARS-CoV-2 infection in human cells. Cell 2021; 184(1): 92-105.e16.
[http://dx.doi.org/10.1016/j.cell.2020.10.030] [PMID: 33147445]

[146] Coutard B, Valle C, de Lamballerie X, Canard B, Seidah NG, Decroly E. The spike glycoprotein of the new coronavirus 2019-nCoV contains a furin-like cleavage site absent in CoV of the same clade. Antiviral Res 2020; 176: 104742.
[http://dx.doi.org/10.1016/j.antiviral.2020.104742] [PMID: 32057769]

[147] Zhao R, Ali G, Nie HG, *et al.* Plasmin improves blood–gas barrier function in oedematous lungs by cleaving epithelial sodium channels. Br J Pharmacol 2020; 177(13): 3091-106.
[http://dx.doi.org/10.1111/bph.15038] [PMID: 32133621]

[148] Ji HL, Zhao R, Matalon S, Matthay MA. Elevated plasmin (ogen) as a common risk factor for COVID-19 susceptibility. Physiol Rev 2020; 100(3): 1065-75.
[http://dx.doi.org/10.1152/physrev.00013.2020] [PMID: 32216698]

[149] Lin M, Tseng HK, Trejaut JA, *et al.* Association of HLA class I with severe acute respiratory syndrome coronavirus infection. BMC Med Genet 2003; 4(1): 9.
[http://dx.doi.org/10.1186/1471-2350-4-9] [PMID: 12969506]

[150] Surveillances V. The epidemiological characteristics of an outbreak of 2019 novel coronavirus diseases (COVID-19)—China, 2020. China CDC weekly. 2020; 2(8): 113-22.

[PMID: 34594836] [PMCID: 8392929]

[151] Kim IC, Kim JY, Kim HA, Han S. COVID-19-related myocarditis in a 21-year-old female patient. Eur Heart J 2020; 41(19): 1859.
[http://dx.doi.org/10.1093/eurheartj/ehaa288] [PMID: 32282027]

[152] Li YC, Bai WZ, Hashikawa T. The neuroinvasive potential of SARS-CoV2 may play a role in the respiratory failure of COVID-19 patients. J Med Virol 2020; 92(6): 552-5.
[http://dx.doi.org/10.1002/jmv.25728] [PMID: 32104915]

[153] Conde Cardona G, Quintana Pájaro LD, Quintero Marzola ID, Ramos Villegas Y, Moscote Salazar LR. Neurotropism of SARS-CoV 2: Mechanisms and manifestations. J Neurol Sci 2020; 412: 116824.
[http://dx.doi.org/10.1016/j.jns.2020.116824] [PMID: 32299010]

[154] Ottaviano G, Carecchio M, Scarpa B, Marchese-Ragona R. Olfactory and rhinological evaluations in SARS-CoV-2 patients complaining of olfactory loss. Rhinology 2020; 58(4): 400-1.
[http://dx.doi.org/10.4193/Rhin20.136] [PMID: 32338254]

[155] Baig AM. Neurological manifestations in COVID-19 caused by SARS-CoV-2. CNS Neurosci Ther 2020; 26(5): 499-501.
[http://dx.doi.org/10.1111/cns.13372] [PMID: 32266761]

[156] Ellegren H, Parsch J. The evolution of sex-biased genes and sex-biased gene expression. Nat Rev Genet 2007; 8(9): 689-98.
[http://dx.doi.org/10.1038/nrg2167] [PMID: 17680007]

[157] von Brunn A, Ciesek S, von Brunn B, Carbajo-Lozoya J. Genetic deficiency and polymorphisms of cyclophilin A reveal its essential role for Human Coronavirus 229E replication. Curr Opin Virol 2015; 14: 56-61.
[http://dx.doi.org/10.1016/j.coviro.2015.08.004] [PMID: 26318518]

[158] https://www.nihr. ac.uk/covid-studies/study-detail.htm?entryId=1896762020.

[159] Neuman BW, Joseph JS, Saikatendu KS, et al. Proteomics analysis unravels the functional repertoire of coronavirus nonstructural protein 3. J Virol 2008; 82(11): 5279-94.
[http://dx.doi.org/10.1128/JVI.02631-07] [PMID: 18367524]

[160] Shang J, Wan Y, Luo C, et al. Cell entry mechanisms of SARS-CoV-2. Proc Natl Acad Sci USA 2020; 117(21): 11727-34.
[http://dx.doi.org/10.1073/pnas.2003138117] [PMID: 32376634]

[161] Hoffmann M, Kleine-Weber H, Schroeder S, et al. SARS-CoV-2 cell entry depends on ACE2 and TMPRSS2 and is blocked by a clinically proven protease inhibitor. Cell 2020; 181(2): 271-80.
[http://dx.doi.org/10.1016/j.cell.2020.02.052]

[162] Ou X, Liu Y, Lei X, et al. Characterization of spike glycoprotein of SARS-CoV-2 on virus entry and its immune cross-reactivity with SARS-CoV. Nat Commun 2020; 11(1): 1620.
[http://dx.doi.org/10.1038/s41467-020-15562-9] [PMID: 32221306]

[163] Wei J, Alfajaro M, Hanna R, et al. Genome-wide CRISPR screen reveals host genes that regulate SARS-CoV-2 infection. Biorxiv 2020.
[http://dx.doi.org/10.1101/2020.06.16.155101]

[164] Menachery VD, Eisfeld AJ, Schäfer A, et al. Pathogenic influenza viruses and coronaviruses utilize similar and contrasting approaches to control interferon-stimulated gene responses. MBio 2014; 5(3): e01174-14.
[http://dx.doi.org/10.1128/mBio.01174-14] [PMID: 24846384]

[165] Simpson J, Loh Z, Ullah MA, et al. Respiratory syncytial virus infection promotes necroptosis and HMGB1 release by airway epithelial cells. Am J Respir Crit Care Med 2020; 201(11): 1358-71.
[http://dx.doi.org/10.1164/rccm.201906-1149OC] [PMID: 32105156]

[166] Andersson U, Ottestad W, Tracey KJ. Extracellular HMGB1: a therapeutic target in severe pulmonary

inflammation including COVID-19? Mol Med 2020; 26(1): 42.
[http://dx.doi.org/10.1186/s10020-020-00172-4] [PMID: 32380958]

[167] Manti S, Harford TJ, Salpietro C, Rezaee F, Piedimonte G. Induction of high-mobility group Box-1 *in vitro* and *in vivo* by respiratory syncytial virus. Pediatr Res 2018; 83(5): 1049-56.
[http://dx.doi.org/10.1038/pr.2018.6] [PMID: 29329282]

[168] Hatayama K, Nosaka N, Yamada M, *et al.* Combined effect of anti-high-mobility group box-1 monoclonal antibody and peramivir against influenza A virus-induced pneumonia in mice. J Med Virol 2019; 91(3): 361-9.
[http://dx.doi.org/10.1002/jmv.25330] [PMID: 30281823]

[169] Avgousti DC, Herrmann C, Kulej K, *et al.* A core viral protein binds host nucleosomes to sequester immune danger signals. Nature 2016; 535(7610): 173-7.
[http://dx.doi.org/10.1038/nature18317] [PMID: 27362237]

[170] Zhao X, Nicholls JM, Chen YG. Severe acute respiratory syndrome-associated coronavirus nucleocapsid protein interacts with Smad3 and modulates transforming growth factor-β signaling. J Biol Chem 2008; 283(6): 3272-80.
[http://dx.doi.org/10.1074/jbc.M708033200] [PMID: 18055455]

[171] Zhu N, Zhang D, Wang W, *et al.* A Novel Coronavirus from Patients with Pneumonia in China, 2019. N Engl J Med 2020; 382(8): 727-33.
[http://dx.doi.org/10.1056/NEJMoa2001017] [PMID: 31978945]

[172] Wang D, Hu B, Hu C, *et al.* Clinical characteristics of 138 hospitalized patients with 2019 novel coronavirus–infected pneumonia in Wuhan, China. JAMA 2020; 323(11): 1061-9.
[http://dx.doi.org/10.1001/jama.2020.1585] [PMID: 32031570]

[173] Smith JC, Sausville EL, Girish V, *et al.* Cigarette smoke exposure and inflammatory signaling increase the expression of the SARS-CoV-2 receptor ACE2 in the respiratory tract. Dev Cell 2020; 53(5): 514-529.e3.
[http://dx.doi.org/10.1016/j.devcel.2020.05.012] [PMID: 32425701]

[174] Yang J, Feng X, Zhou Q, *et al.* Pathological Ace2-to-Ace enzyme switch in the stressed heart is transcriptionally controlled by the endothelial Brg1–FoxM1 complex. Proc Natl Acad Sci USA 2016; 113(38): E5628-35.
[http://dx.doi.org/10.1073/pnas.1525078113] [PMID: 27601681]

[175] Peng D, Si D, Zhang R, *et al.* Deletion of SMARCA4 impairs alveolar epithelial type II cells proliferation and aggravates pulmonary fibrosis in mice. Genes Dis 2017; 4(4): 204-14.
[http://dx.doi.org/10.1016/j.gendis.2017.10.001] [PMID: 30258924]

[176] Spagnolo P, Balestro E, Aliberti S, *et al.* Pulmonary fibrosis secondary to COVID-19: a call to arms? Lancet Respir Med 2020; 8(8): 750-2.
[http://dx.doi.org/10.1016/S2213-2600(20)30222-8] [PMID: 32422177]

[177] Shiina T, Hosomichi K, Inoko H, Kulski JK. The HLA genomic loci map: expression, interaction, diversity and disease. J Hum Genet 2009; 54(1): 15-39.
[http://dx.doi.org/10.1038/jhg.2008.5] [PMID: 19158813]

[178] Kachuri L, Francis SS, Morrison ML, *et al.* The landscape of host genetic factors involved in immune response to common viral infections. Genome Med 2020; 12(1): 93.
[http://dx.doi.org/10.1186/s13073-020-00790-x] [PMID: 33109261]

[179] Lin M, Tseng HK, Trejaut JA, *et al.* Association of HLA class I with severe acute respiratory syndrome coronavirus infection. BMC Med Genet 2003; 4(1): 9.
[http://dx.doi.org/10.1186/1471-2350-4-9] [PMID: 12969506]

[180] Hajeer A, Balkhy H, Johani S, Yousef M, Arabi Y. Association of human leukocyte antigen class II alleles with severe Middle East respiratory syndrome-coronavirus infection. Ann Thorac Med 2016; 11(3): 211-3.

[http://dx.doi.org/10.4103/1817-1737.185756] [PMID: 27512511]

[181] Luckey D, Weaver EA, Osborne DG, Billadeau DD, Taneja V. Immunity to Influenza is dependent on MHC II polymorphism: study with 2 HLA transgenic strains. Sci Rep 2019; 9(1): 19061.
[http://dx.doi.org/10.1038/s41598-019-55503-1] [PMID: 31836763]

[182] Lan NTP, Kikuchi M, Huong VTQ, *et al.* Protective and enhancing HLA alleles, HLA-DRB1*0901 and HLA-A*24, for severe forms of dengue virus infection, dengue hemorrhagic fever and dengue shock syndrome. PLoS Negl Trop Dis 2008; 2(10): e304.
[http://dx.doi.org/10.1371/journal.pntd.0000304] [PMID: 18827882]

[183] Nishida N, Ohashi J, Khor SS, *et al.* Understanding of HLA-conferred susceptibility to chronic hepatitis B infection requires HLA genotyping-based association analysis. Sci Rep 2016; 6(1): 24767.
[http://dx.doi.org/10.1038/srep24767] [PMID: 27091392]

[184] Johnson A, Leke R, Harun L, *et al.* Interaction of HLA and age on levels of antibody to Plasmodium falciparum rhoptry-associated proteins 1 and 2. Infect Immun 2000; 68(4): 2231-6.
[http://dx.doi.org/10.1128/IAI.68.4.2231-2236.2000] [PMID: 10722624]

[185] Dragin N, Nancy P, Villegas J, Roussin R, Le Panse R, Berrih-Aknin S. Balance between estrogens and proinflammatory cytokines regulates chemokine production involved in thymic germinal center formation. Sci Rep 2017; 7(1): 7970.
[http://dx.doi.org/10.1038/s41598-017-08631-5] [PMID: 28801669]

[186] Minchenko DO. Insulin resistance in obese adolescents affects the expression of genes associated with immune response. Endocr Regul 2019; 53(2): 71-82.
[http://dx.doi.org/10.2478/enr-2019-0009] [PMID: 31517622]

[187] Langton DJ, Bourke SC, Lie BA, *et al.* The influence of hla genotype on susceptibility to, and severity of, COVID-19 infection. medRxiv 2021.
[http://dx.doi.org/10.1101/2020.12.31.20249081]

[188] Blackwell JM, Jamieson SE, Burgner D. HLA and infectious diseases. Clin Microbiol Rev 2009; 22(2): 370-85.
[http://dx.doi.org/10.1128/CMR.00048-08] [PMID: 19366919]

[189] Crux NB, Elahi S. Human leukocyte antigen (HLA) and immune regulation: how do classical and non-classical HLA alleles modulate immune response to human immunodeficiency virus and hepatitis C virus infections? Front Immunol 2017; 8: 832.
[http://dx.doi.org/10.3389/fimmu.2017.00832] [PMID: 28769934]

[190] Pisanti S, Deelen J, Gallina AM, *et al.* Correlation of the two most frequent HLA haplotypes in the Italian population to the differential regional incidence of Covid-19. J Transl Med 2020; 18(1): 352.
[http://dx.doi.org/10.1186/s12967-020-02515-5] [PMID: 32933522]

[191] Brierley AS, Fernandes PG, Brandon MA, *et al.* Antarctic krill under sea ice: elevated abundance in a narrow band just south of ice edge. Science 2002; 295(5561): 1890-2.
[http://dx.doi.org/10.1126/science.1068574] [PMID: 11884754]

[192] Nishida N, Sugiyama M, Ohashi J, *et al.* Importance of HBsAg recognition by HLA molecules as revealed by responsiveness to different hepatitis B vaccines. Sci Rep 2021; 11(1): 3703.
[http://dx.doi.org/10.1038/s41598-021-82986-8] [PMID: 33654122]

[193] Zhu M, Dai J, Wang C, *et al.* Fine mapping the MHC region identified four independent variants modifying susceptibility to chronic hepatitis B in Han Chinese. Hum Mol Genet 2016; 25(6): 1225-32.
[http://dx.doi.org/10.1093/hmg/ddw003] [PMID: 26769676]

[194] Duggal P, Thio CL, Wojcik GL, *et al.* Genome-wide association study of spontaneous resolution of hepatitis C virus infection: data from multiple cohorts. Ann Intern Med 2013; 158(4): 235-45.
[http://dx.doi.org/10.7326/0003-4819-158-4-201302190-00003] [PMID: 23420232]

[195] Grasselli G, Zangrillo A, Zanella A, *et al.* Baseline characteristics and outcomes of 1591 patients infected with SARS-CoV-2 admitted to ICUs of the Lombardy Region, Italy. JAMA 2020; 323(16):

1574-81.
[http://dx.doi.org/10.1001/jama.2020.5394] [PMID: 32250385]

[196]   Lin M, Tseng HK, Trejaut JA, *et al.* Association of HLA class I with severe acute respiratory syndrome coronavirus infection. BMC Med Genet 2003; 4(1): 9.
[http://dx.doi.org/10.1186/1471-2350-4-9] [PMID: 12969506]

[197]   Chen YMA, Liang SY, Shih YP, *et al.* Epidemiological and genetic correlates of severe acute respiratory syndrome coronavirus infection in the hospital with the highest nosocomial infection rate in Taiwan in 2003. J Clin Microbiol 2006; 44(2): 359-65.
[http://dx.doi.org/10.1128/JCM.44.2.359-365.2006] [PMID: 16455884]

[198]   Keicho N, Itoyama S, Kashiwase K, *et al.* Association of human leukocyte antigen class II alleles with severe acute respiratory syndrome in the Vietnamese population. Hum Immunol 2009; 70(7): 527-31.
[http://dx.doi.org/10.1016/j.humimm.2009.05.006] [PMID: 19445991]

[199]   Wang SF, Chen KH, Chen M, *et al.* Human-leukocyte antigen class I Cw 1502 and class II DR 0301 genotypes are associated with resistance to severe acute respiratory syndrome (SARS) infection. Viral Immunol 2011; 24(5): 421-6.
[http://dx.doi.org/10.1089/vim.2011.0024] [PMID: 21958371]

[200]   Falk K, Rötzschke O, Stevanovié S, Jung G, Rammensee HG. Allele-specific motifs revealed by sequencing of self-peptides eluted from MHC molecules. Nature 1991; 351(6324): 290-6.
[http://dx.doi.org/10.1038/351290a0] [PMID: 1709722]

[201]   Gross G, Margalit A. Targeting tumor-associated antigens to the MHC class I presentation pathway. Endocrine, Metabolic & Immune Disorders - Drug Targets 2007; 7: (2).
[http://dx.doi.org/10.2174/187153007780832064]

[202]   Nguyen A, David JK, Maden SK, *et al.* Human leukocyte antigen susceptibility map for severe acute respiratory syndrome coronavirus 2. J Virol 2020; 94(13): e00510-20.
[http://dx.doi.org/10.1128/JVI.00510-20] [PMID: 32303592]

[203]   Ahmed SF, Quadeer AA, McKay MR. Preliminary identification of potential vaccine targets for the COVID-19 coronavirus (SARS-CoV-2) based on SARS-CoV immunological studies. Viruses 2020; 12(3): 254.
[http://dx.doi.org/10.3390/v12030254] [PMID: 32106567]

[204]   Barquera R, Collen E, Di D, *et al.* Binding affinities of 438 HLA proteins to complete proteomes of seven pandemic viruses and distributions of strongest and weakest HLA peptide binders in populations worldwide. HLA 2020; 96(3): 277-98.
[http://dx.doi.org/10.1111/tan.13956]

[205]   Baruah V, Bose S. Immunoinformatics-aided identification of T cell and B cell epitopes in the surface glycoprotein of 2019-nCoV. J Med Virol 2020; 92(5): 495-500.
[http://dx.doi.org/10.1002/jmv.25698] [PMID: 32022276]

[206]   Bhattacharya M, Sharma AR, Patra P, *et al.* Development of epitope-based peptide vaccine against novel coronavirus 2019 (SARS-COV-2): Immunoinformatics approach. J Med Virol 2020; 92(6): 618-31.
[http://dx.doi.org/10.1002/jmv.25736] [PMID: 32108359]

[207]   Grifoni A, Sidney J, Zhang Y, Scheuermann RH, Peters B, Sette A. A sequence homology and bioinformatic approach can predict candidate targets for immune responses to SARS-CoV-2. Cell Host Microbe 2020; 27(4): 671-680.e2.
[http://dx.doi.org/10.1016/j.chom.2020.03.002] [PMID: 32183941]

[208]   Sacchi N, Castagnetta M, Miotti V, Garbarino L, Gallina A. High-resolution analysis of the HLA-A, -B, -C and -DRB1 alleles and national and regional haplotype frequencies based on 120 926 volunteers from the Italian Bone Marrow Donor Registry. HLA 2019; 94(3): 285-95.
[http://dx.doi.org/10.1111/tan.13613] [PMID: 31207125]

[209] Nguyen A, David JK, Maden SK, *et al.* Human leukocyte antigen susceptibility map for severe acute respiratory syndrome coronavirus 2. J Virol 2020; 94(13): e00510-20.
[http://dx.doi.org/10.1128/JVI.00510-20] [PMID: 32303592]

[210] Li X, Geng M, Peng Y, Meng L, Lu S. Molecular immune pathogenesis and diagnosis of COVID-19. J Pharm Anal 2020; 10(2): 102-8.
[http://dx.doi.org/10.1016/j.jpha.2020.03.001] [PMID: 32282863]

[211] Wang W, Zhang W, Zhang J, He J, Zhu F. Distribution of HLA allele frequencies in 82 Chinese individuals with coronavirus disease-2019 (COVID-19). HLA 2020; 96(2): 194-6.
[http://dx.doi.org/10.1111/tan.13941] [PMID: 32424945]

[212] Simmonds MJ, Gough SCL. Genetic insights into disease mechanisms of autoimmunity. Br Med Bull 2005; 71(1): 93-113.
[http://dx.doi.org/10.1093/bmb/ldh032] [PMID: 15701924]

[213] Li S, Jiao H, Yu X, *et al.* Human leukocyte antigen class I and class II allele frequencies and HIV-1 infection associations in a Chinese cohort. J Acquir Immune Defic Syndr 2007; 44(2): 121-31.
[http://dx.doi.org/10.1097/01.qai.0000248355.40877.2a] [PMID: 17106278]

[214] Vejbaesya S, Thongpradit R, Kalayanarooj S, *et al.* HLA class I supertype associations with clinical outcome of secondary dengue virus infections in ethnic Thais. J Infect Dis 2015; 212(6): 939-47.
[http://dx.doi.org/10.1093/infdis/jiv127] [PMID: 25740956]

[215] Hudson LE, Allen RL. Leukocyte Ig-like receptors–a model for MHC class I disease associations. Front Immunol 2016; 7: 281.
[http://dx.doi.org/10.3389/fimmu.2016.00281] [PMID: 27504110]

[216] Rallón N, Restrepo C, Vicario JL, *et al.* Human leucocyte antigen (HLA)- DQB 1*03:02 and HLA -A*02:01 have opposite patterns in their effects on susceptibility to HIV infection. HIV Med 2017; 18(8): 587-94.
[http://dx.doi.org/10.1111/hiv.12494] [PMID: 28218480]

[217] Rallón N, Restrepo C, Vicario JL, *et al.* Human leucocyte antigen (HLA)- DQB 1*03:02 and HLA -A*02:01 have opposite patterns in their effects on susceptibility to HIV infection. HIV Med 2017; 18(8): 587-94.
[http://dx.doi.org/10.1111/hiv.12494] [PMID: 28218480]

[218] Falfán-Valencia R, Narayanankutty A, Reséndiz-Hernández JM, *et al.* An increased frequency in HLA Class I alleles and haplotypes suggests genetic susceptibility to influenza A (H1N1) 2009 pandemic: a case-control study. J Immunol Res 2018; 2018: 1-12.
[http://dx.doi.org/10.1155/2018/3174868] [PMID: 29682588]

[219] Correale P, Saladino RE, Nardone V, *et al.* Could PD-1/PDL1 immune checkpoints be linked to HLA signature? Immunotherapy 2019; 11(18): 1523-6.
[http://dx.doi.org/10.2217/imt-2019-0160]

[220] Jung ES, Cheon JH, Lee JH, *et al.* HLA-C* 01 is a risk factor for Crohn's disease. Inflamm Bowel Dis 2016; 22(4): 796-806.
[http://dx.doi.org/10.1097/MIB.0000000000000693] [PMID: 26891255]

[221] Johnston DT, Mehaffey G, Thomas J, *et al.* Increased frequency of HLA-B44 in recurrent sinopulmonary infections (RESPI). Clin Immunol 2006; 119(3): 346-50.
[http://dx.doi.org/10.1016/j.clim.2006.02.001] [PMID: 16542878]

[222] Fadda L, Körner C, Kumar S, *et al.* HLA-Cw*0102-restricted HIV-1 p24 epitope variants can modulate the binding of the inhibitory KIR2DL2 receptor and primary NK cell function. PLoS Pathog 2012; 8(7): e1002805.
[http://dx.doi.org/10.1371/journal.ppat.1002805] [PMID: 22807681]

[223] Mori M, Wichukchinda N, Miyahara R, *et al.* Impact of HLA allele-KIR pairs on disease outcome in HIV-infected Thai population. J Acquir Immune Defic Syndr 2018; 78(3): 356-61.

[http://dx.doi.org/10.1097/QAI.0000000000001676] [PMID: 29528943]

[224] Pende D, Falco M, Vitale M, *et al.* Killer Ig-like receptors (KIRs): their role in NK cell modulation and developments leading to their clinical exploitation. Front Immunol 2019; 10: 1179.
[http://dx.doi.org/10.3389/fimmu.2019.01179] [PMID: 31231370]

[225] Correale P, Mutti L, Pentimalli F, *et al.* HLA-B* 44 and C* 01 prevalence correlates with Covid19 spreading across Italy. Int J Mol Sci 2020; 21(15): 5205.
[http://dx.doi.org/10.3390/ijms21155205] [PMID: 32717807]

[226] Bloom DE, Cadarette D. Infectious disease threats in the twenty-first century: strengthening the global response. Front Immunol 2019; 10: 549.
[http://dx.doi.org/10.3389/fimmu.2019.00549] [PMID: 30984169]

[227] Li C, Zhao C, Bao J, Tang B, Wang Y, Gu B. Laboratory diagnosis of coronavirus disease-2019 (COVID-19). Int J Clinic Chem 2020; 510: 35-46.
[PMID: 32621814]

[228] Sardar R, Satish D, Gupta D. Identification of novel SARS-CoV-2 drug targets by host microRNAs and transcription factors co-regulatory interaction network analysis. Front Genet 2020; 11: 571274.
[http://dx.doi.org/10.3389/fgene.2020.571274] [PMID: 33173539]

[229] Kaufmann SH, Dorhoi A, Hotchkiss RS, Bartenschlager R. Host-directed therapies for bacterial and viral infections. Nature reviews Drug discovery. 2018 Jan; 17(1): 35-56.
[http://dx.doi.org/10.1038/nrd.2017.162]

[230] Gassen NC, Niemeyer D, Muth D, *et al.* SKP2 attenuates autophagy through Beclin1-ubiquitination and its inhibition reduces MERS-Coronavirus infection. Nat Commun 2019; 10(1): 5770.
[http://dx.doi.org/10.1038/s41467-019-13659-4] [PMID: 31852899]

[231] Wang X, Dhindsa R, Povysil G, *et al.* Transcriptional inhibition of host viral entry proteins as a therapeutic strategy for SARS-CoV-2. Preprints 2020; 2020030360.
[http://dx.doi.org/10.20944/preprints202003.0360.v1]

[232] Saçar Demirci MD, Adan A. Computational analysis of microRNA-mediated interactions in SARS-CoV-2 infection. PeerJ 2020; 8: e9369.
[http://dx.doi.org/10.7717/peerj.9369] [PMID: 32547891]

[233] Chen L, Zhong L. Lung adenocarcinoma patients own higher risk of SARS-CoV-2 infection. Preprints 2020.

[234] Lai-Jiang C, Xu R, Hui-Min Y, Chang Q, Zhong JC. The ACE2/Apelin Signaling, MicroRNAs, and Hypertension. Int J Hypertens 2015; 2015: 896861.
[http://dx.doi.org/10.1155/2015/896861]

CHAPTER 8

Epigenetic Mutations and Coronaviruses

Amjad Islam Aqib[1,*], Yasir Razzaq Khan[1], Tean Zaheer[2], Rabia Liaqat[3], Muhammad Luqman Sohail[1], Ahmad Ali[1], Hina Afzal Sajid[4], Firasat Hussain[5] and Saadia Muneer[6]

[1] *Department of Medicine, Faculty of Veterinary Science, Cholistan University of Veterinary and Animal Sciences (CUVAS), Bahawalpur 63100, Pakistan*

[2] *Department of Parasitology, University of Agriculture, Faisalabad, Pakistan*

[3] *Department of Pathology, University of Agriculture, Faisalabad, Pakistan*

[4] *Centre of Excellence in Molecular Biology, University of the Punjab, Lahore, Pakistan*

[5] *Department of Microbiology, Cholistan University of Veterinary and Animal Sciences (CUVAS), Bahawalpur 63100, Pakistan*

[6] *Institute of Microbiology, University of Agriculture, Faisalabad, Pakistan*

Abstract: All genetic variations are the outcome of mutations in the genetic material. The greater the mutation ratio, the greater will be the genomic diversity. Currently, epigenomics enables us to locate, read, and translate the epigenetic mechanism that monitors and reins the whole genome of coronaviruses at different stages. Many researchers reported the role of epigenetic mutations in the development and progression of several common viral infections, especially age-related diseases. Many families of viruses can counter the immune response by utilizing a cascade of epigenetic events and taking over the regulatory capacity for their benefit. Coronaviruses possess the same mechanism to affect epigenetic machinery, *i.e.*, by improving mutations in the epigenetic code, DNA methylation, post-translational alterations of histone proteins and other proteins linked with epigenome, or direct dysregulation of enzymes.

Keywords: Epigenetic mutations, Enzyme dysregulation, DNA methylation, Post-translational alterations.

INTRODUCTION

Coronaviruses are enveloped viruses; they have a crown-like appearance under an electron microscope with an RNA genome that is single-stranded and a positive sense strand. Their genome size ranges from 26-32 kilobases (kb) in length. It is

* **Corresponding author Amjad Islam Aqib:** Department of Medicine, Faculty of Veterinary Science, Cholistan University of Veterinary and Animal Sciences (CUVAS), Bahawalpur 63100, Pakistan; Tel: +92 343 7474583; E-mail: amjadwaseer@cuvas.edu.pk

Kamal Niaz, Muhammad Sajjad Khan & Muhammad Farrukh Nisar (Eds.)

known that coronaviruses have giant RNA genomes. These have been structured into three classes, namely γ- coronaviruses, β- coronaviruses, and α-coronaviruses, based on their genetic portfolio and antigenicity. Coronaviruses primarily infect birds and mammals by crossing species barriers and causing various infections ranging from general cold to further serious illnesses, such as the Middle East respiratory syndrome (MERS) and SAR, which particularly impact the farming industry. Recently, in 2019, they destroyed the world, causing severe respiratory diseases that eventually led to global lockdowns that stalled life on Earth with millions of deaths. The disease symptoms range from upper respiratory tract infection (URTI), like the common cold and flu, to infection of the lower respiratory tract (LRTI), for instance, bronchitis, pneumonia, and even severe acute respiratory syndrome (SARS). Transmission of coronaviruses results from close contact and *via* respiratory droplets generated by sneezing and coughing [1, 2]. Coronaviruses have been known to circulate among other animals and have been identified to infect human beings, as in SARS and MERS. Four other coronaviruses cause respiratory indications resembling the cold [3, 4].

A novel coronavirus, designated coronavirus disease-2019 (COVID-19), was identified when a number of pneumonia cases were discovered in Wuhan, China, and its province Hubei by the end of 2019 [5]. In late January 2020, thousands of coronavirus cases were confirmed by laboratories in China, with a constant rise in cases in adjacent areas eventually spreading throughout China first and then the rest of the world. Epidemiologic investigation in Wuhan associated the coronavirus with a seafood bazaar where the most patients had visited or worked [6, 7]. This market was eventually closed for sterilization. The seafood marketplace also sold living bats, snakes, rabbits, and different kinds of animals [8]. However, as the virus spread, many laboratories claimed that it had no contact with this market. There was a surge in cases recognized among healthcare labors and other interactions of coronavirus-infected patients.

In China, transmission through human-to-human contact was confirmed, including in the United States [9, 10]. A report of a trivial cluster using five cases recommended that there has been a spread from an asymptomatic patient that occurred all through the incubation period; eventually, all sufferers that fall in this group are known to have mild infection [11].

There is a small E protein in the coronavirus, and 76 to 109 amino acids are present in its integral membrane protein. Further studies on prime and secondary configuration suggested that E has an amino terminus that is hydrophilic, containing 7 to 12 amino acids. It is small and tracked by a bulky transmembrane domain (TMD) that is hydrophobic, consisting of 25 amino acids, as it finishes with a hydrophilic carboxyl terminus that is long and consists of the bulk of the protein. A pore in membranes is ion-conductive, formed by the amphipathic α-helix TMD [12].

Why are Viral Mutations Important?

All genetic variations are the outcome of mutations in the genetic material. Mutations result from hereditary material or nucleic acid damage and are not restricted to replication only [13]. The mutation is the first step of evolution as it yields new strands of DNA/RNA for a particular gene, ending up creating a new allele. New DNA/RNA strand sequences (a new allele) can also be produced by recombination technology that creates a specific gene. The mutation rate is a variation in genetic material when passed to the subsequent generation of an organism, and it is described as a probability. Usually, in the case of viruses, a generation is determined by a cell infection phase; this comprises adherence to the cell exterior, fusion of the cell membrane, uncoating, replication, gene expression, encapsulation, and finally, discharge of the infective particles. The frequency at which mutations occur in the virus should not be confused with the virus's mutation rate, as both go different ways. The former is a measure of genomic disparity, which is the combination of several factors, such as recombination, random genetic drift, and natural selection. The greater the mutation ratio, the larger will be the genomic diversity. Even though genetic diversity is always dependent on several factors, the mutation level is of prime concern as it is the crucial basis of genomic variation [14]. Likewise, alteration rates must not be tangled through molecular evolutionary ratios. According to the neutral theory of molecular evolution, these two have a linear association. However, the mutation is an inherited/biochemical procedure. Molecular evolution is linked to the infatuation of novel alleles in populations. Understanding pharmacogenomics and viral modification rates is crucial for better consideration and managing the pathogenesis, medication resistance, vaccination, immune avoidance, and the emergence of new strains causing new illnesses [15].

The Baltimore taxonomy of viruses is built conforming to the genomic material of the virion: positive-strand RNA viruses such as tobacco mosaic virus, rhinoviruses, noroviruses, and hepatitis C virus, and negative-strand RNA viruses such as rabies virus, influenza virus, and Ebola virus; likewise there are RNA viruses that are double-stranded for instance rotaviruses and bursal disease virus; also there are retroviruses, for example, human T cell leukemia virus, HIV, *etc.*, and para-retroviruses, *i.e.*, hepatitis B viruses [13]. After the classification of RNA viruses, there are single-stranded DNA viruses (including bacteriophage and parvoviruses) and double-stranded (including herpes viruses, papillomaviruses, adenoviruses, and poxviruses). Viruses are non-living infectious particles that entirely rely on human cell machinery to replicate, and in biological systems, they have extensive disparity in mutation rates. There is often a massive difference between DNA and RNA viruses [16]. Table **1** presents rates of mutation of different viruses. In terms of mutation rate variations and despite the fact of some doubts, it could be yielded that alteration rates limit unevenly between 10^{-8} to 10^{-4} switches per nucleotide per cell septicity. It ranges from 10^{-8}–10^{-6} for DNA viruses, and between 10^{-6}–10^{-4} is reserved for RNA viruses [17]. Such alterations have multiple mechanical bases. Firstly, the polymerase activity of the bulk of RNA viruses is lacking with 3′ exonuclease proofreading action; thus, these are more susceptible to errors and mutation than DNA viruses [18]. However, the exception lies with this rule in the case of coronaviruses, RNA virus family that are positive strands. These encode a composite of RNA-dependent RNA polymerase containing 3′ exonuclease proofreading domain [19, 20]. The 3′ exonuclease activity is also absent in Reverse Transcriptase viruses and, therefore, retroviruses (virions containing RNA and cellular DNA phase) and para-retroviruses (cellular RNA) DNA) when mutated develop at rates comparable to non-reverse transcribing RNA viruses.

The latter is also known as rhinoviruses [21]. Certain DNA viruses develop at rates near to that of RNA viruses. This includes human parvovirus, emerging canine parvovirus strains, tomato yellow leaf curl geminivirus, African swine fever virus, beak-and-feather disease circovirus, and others [22 - 26]. This highlights the evidence that numerous factors contribute to evolution other than mutation rate. It must be noted that the modification levels are unfamiliar for several DNA viruses and can be higher in some instances than what is presently believed. Current studies suggest that hominoid cytomegalovirus (CMV) has a genome-wide average of 2×10^{-7}s/n/c, the rate that is to some extent higher than what was formerly supposed for DNA virus double-stranded, though this was devious [27]. Since various DNA and RNA viruses have many similarities, the query may explain why alteration rates evolve so adversely in both DNA and RNA virus groups. Fast mutators are found to be single-strand DNA viruses compared to double-strand DNA viruses. However, this difference is found in work carried out with bacteriophages. So far, there have been no mutation level approximations found for eukaryotic single-strand DNA viruses. Similarly, there were no obvious dissimilarities in mutation rate within RNA viruses in Baltimore classes [28]. Again, the mechanism underlying these differences in mutation rates among different virion groups is still not well understood.

Table 1. Mutation rate of viruses.

Class	Virus	Genome Size (kb)	Average Mutation Rate (s/n/c)
Ss (+) RNA	Bacteriophage Qβ^{c}	4.22	1.4×10^{-4}
-	Tobacco mosaic virus	6.40	8.7×10^{-6}
-	Human rhinovirus 14	7.13	6.9×10^{-5}
-	Poliovirus 1	7.44	9.0×10^{-5}
-	Human norovirus G1	7.65	1.5×10^{-4}
-	Tobacco *etc* hes virus	9.49	1.2×10^{-5}
-	Hepatitis C virus	9.65	3.8×10^{-5}
-	Murine hepatitis virus	31.4	3.5×10^{-6}
Ss (-) RNA	Vesicular stomatitis virus	11.2	3.7×10^{-5}
-	Influenza A virus	13.6	2.5×10^{-5}
-	Measles virus	15.9	3.5×10^{-5}
dsRNA	Bacteriophage Φ6	13.4	1.6×10^{-6}
Reverse transcribing	Duck hepatitis B virus	3.03	2.0×10^{-5}
-	Spleen necrosis virus	7.80	3.7×10^{-5}
-	Murine leukemia virus	8.33	3.0×10^{-5}
-	Bovine leukemia virus	8.42	1.7×10^{-5}
-	Human T-cell leukemia virus	8.50	1.6×10^{-5}
-	HIV-1 (free virions)	9.18	6.3×10^{-5}
-	HIV-1 (cellular DNA)	9.18	4.4×10^{-3}
-	Foamy virus	13.2	2.1×10^{-5}
-	Rous sarcoma virus	9.40	1.4×10^{-4}
ssDNA	Bacteriophage ΦX174	5.39	1.1×10^{-6}
-	Bacteriophage m13	6.41	7.9×10^{-7}
dsDNA	Bacteriophage λ	48.5	5.4×10^{-7}
-	Herpes simplex virus	152	5.9×10^{-8}
-	Bacteriophage T2	169	9.8×10^{-8}
-	Human cytomegalovirus	235	2.0×10^{-7}

Epigenetic Mutations in Human Coronaviruses

Epigenetics has been witnessing a continuous surge over the past decades as a new field of science since its emergence in 1940. It involves the study of firmly heritable phenotype because of alterations in the activation of chromatin or structural status without changing the primary DNA sequences. This property makes epigenetic mutations flexible, reversible, and quickly responsive to other exposures and environmental factors. Currently, epigenomics enables us to locate, read and translate the epigenetic mechanism that monitors and reins the whole genome at different stages [29]. Many researchers reported the role of epigenetic mutations in the development and progression of several common virus infections, especially age-related diseases. Human cells become epigenetically affected after prolonged exposure to changed metabolic conditions. Tracing the epigenetic mutations at the pathophysiological level might provide essential information to design innovative treatment regimes, leading to a better understanding of the host immune response [30]. Some viruses, especially influenza and corona families, might change the host epigenome, but they usually do not have the potential to hack the host genetic sequence. Currently, researchers have focused on how viruses use epigenetic machinery for spreading and persistence of infection. It has been reported that many families of viruses can counter the immune response by utilizing a cascade of epigenetic events and taking over the regulatory capacity for their benefit. Coronaviruses possess the same mechanism to affect epigenetic machinery, *i.e.*, by improving mutations in the epigenetic code, DNA methylation, post-translational alterations of histone proteins and other proteins linked with epigenome, or direct dysregulation of enzymes [31].

SARS-CoV

Human coronaviruses have been described as a significant pathogen that causes respiratory diseases. The first lethal outbreak of coronavirus, namely "severe acute respiratory syndrome coronavirus" (SARS-CoV), was reported in 2003 in China, having zoonotic origin from bats and causing case fatality rates (CFR) of 10% [32]. Reports indicate that some viruses use the host cellular mechanism, including epigenetic machinery, for division and propagation as they cannot incorporate into the host DNA [33]. SARS and MERS-CoVs have evolved mechanisms that delay or antagonize viral recognition and interferon-stimulated gene functions. Many proteins encoded by SARS-CoV oppose interferon induction, evading the host immune response. Several non-structural proteins, including non-structural proteins (Nsp1, 3, 14, and 16), antagonize NF-kB, different sensing and signaling pathways, and play a crucial part in capping viral messenger RNAs. Epigenetic mutations in SARS-CoV induce alterations in the basal state of host chromatin that cause enrichment of H3K4me3 incorporation and diminution of H3K27. In open transcription, active chromatin inhibited interferon-stimulated gene expression. SARS-CoVs have the potential to turn the identification off by the immune system by encoding various exclusive proteins [34]. RNA and N6-methyadenosine have also been associated with SARS-CoVs and play essential roles in replicating viruses [35]. Spike (S) proteins of SARS-CoV are cleaved by trypsin, factor Xa, and cathepsin L, resulting in cleavage of S protein into S1 and S2, allowing viral entry into the cytoplasm of fibroblast and epithelial cells showing angiotensin-converting enzyme 2 (ACE2) receptor induces IL-8 production in response to spike protein through the AP-1 pathway. Furthermore, RNA methylation of viruses can be directed at sequences only. Overall, epigenetic mutations either encourage or discourage the replication or propagation of viruses [36], as shown in Table **2**.

The Case of MERS-CoV

MERS-CoV was first reported in 2013 in the Arabian Peninsula from dromedary camels, with case fatality rates of 20% and can change immune response [37]. World Health Organization (WHO) included both SARS and MERS-CoVs in the priority list of pathogens in 2017. Epigenetic mutations in MERS-CoV enrich H3K27me3 levels at promoter regions and depletion of H3K4me3 for a gene subset that favors a closed chromatin conformation and inhibition of gene expression stimulated by interferon, such that viruses can aim at innate immunity triggered by interferon [38]. MERS-CoV interferes with the host's epigenetic mechanism and influences immune functions by infection-mediated histone alterations with lower gene expression despite the activation of many transcription factors leading to stimulation by interferon. Reports indicate that MERS-CoV interferes with the immune system *via* various epigenetic mechanisms (Table **2**). These viruses have the potential to antagonize the NF-kB signaling to evade the host defense system by specific accessory proteins. Notably, DNA methylation plays a vital role in antigen presentation and host immune response [38].

Table 2. Epigenetic mutations in coronavirus infections.

Epigenetic Mutations	Virus Infection	Target	Functions	References
DNA methylation	SARS-CoV	-	Delayed pathogen identification and ISG expression pattern modulation.	[34]
	MERS-CoV	-	Loss of antigen-presenting molecules	[35]
RNA methylation	SARS-CoV	5mC	Mutation in virus structure and replication	[36]
Histone methylation	SARS-CoV	H3K4me	Promotes ISG expression and active transcription	[37]
	MERS-CoV	H3K27me3	Down-regulation of ISGs	[36, 37]

The Case of SARS-CoV-2

COVID-19 is a significant public health issue and a prominent cause of morbidities and mortalities throughout the world as viruses have possessed several critical mechanisms to efficiently multiply inside the host cells by fine-tuning the host epigenetic process, leading to evasion from both innate and adaptive immune responses. The epigenetic mechanism of SARS-CoV-2 involves its entry into lung epithelial cells by methylation of the ACE2 gene across three CpG sites (*i.e.*, cg03536816, cg04013915, and cg08559914) [39]. SARS-CoV-2 also has the potential to regulate the expression of the ACE2 gene by controlling the KDM5B and SIRT1 activity. Epigenetic modifications lead to significantly delayed antigen presentation and interferon-stimulated gene expression as well as regulation of type I and III interferon response by modulating H3K4me3 and H3K27me3 histone marks. Acetylation and deacetylation of histone induce monocytes and macrophage-mediated inflammatory response. Histone imitation of SARS-CoV-2 exhibits as a basis for gene expression modulation and evasion from the host immune mechanism. SARS-CoV-2 also modulates innate epigenetic signaling mechanism by regulating the NF-kB signaling by recruitment of p65 chromatin and mimicry of the host's cap1 structure by 2'-O-MTases that play an influential role in immune response evasion (Table **3**). Coronaviruses also use the Hsp90-mediated epigenetic mechanism to hijack the infected host cells [40].

Table 3. Epigenetic mutations associated with SARS-CoV-2 infections.

Viral Components	Host Machinery	Epigenetic Mutations	Response	References
Spike protein	ACE2R	CpG site methylation	Viral entry, pathogenesis	[38]
Protein 3b	RUNX1b	Recruitment	T cell activities cytokine response	[41]
Nsp5	TRMT1 HDAC2	TRMT1 HDAC2	It prevents HDAC2 movements to the nucleus and induces localization of HDAC2 to mitochondria	[42]
Nsp16 Nsp13 Nsp14	2'-O-MT activity Helicase and 5'-triphosphatase activity N7MT activity	Methylation of Cap1 structure	Immune evasion mechanism from interferon response	[43]
COVID-19	NF-$_k$P MCP-1 TNF-α	HDAC2, HDAC5	Inflammation	[44]
NL63/IDP	Host SLiM protein	Mimics histone (H$_3$)	Immune evasion	[45]

(Table 3) cont.....

Viral Components	Host Machinery	Epigenetic Mutations	Response	References
MERS-CoV	TNF-α interferon	H3K27me3	Antagonizes antigen presentation immune evasion	[46]
CoV infection	BRD2	Mimics histone (H2A)	Host immune evasion	[41, 42, 46]

Epigenetic Mutations in Other Human Coronaviruses

The four strains of human coronaviruses (HCoV-229E, HKU1, NL63, and OC43) primarily infect the upper respiratory tract, while other strains of zoonotic origin, namely MERS, SARS-CoV, and SARS-CoV-2 cause severe LRTI. Epigenetic mutations in the case of HCoV-229E lead to histone modifications (H3K36ac, H3K4me1, H3K27ac, H3k9ac, and H4K5ac), Ser5-phosphorylated RNA polymerase II recruitment, and genome-wide expression changes. Thus, the human coronavirus can fine-tune the host-chromatin landscape and signal NF-kB at multiple steps. Activation of NF-kB allows the production of the A20 protein necessary for the efficient replication of viruses [47].

Epigenetic Mutations and Control of Coronaviruses

The quick transmission and the variety of hosts of SARS-CoV-2 feature the requirement of to-bottom comprehension of its structure and natural ability. Changes that manage the structure of chromatin significantly affect the genome adjustment and maintain cellular homeostasis and are involved in the pathophysiology of the disease. The epigenetic guideline of quality articulation depends on post-translational alterations in the chromatin level at DNA and RNA, along with essential methylation, acetylation, and phosphorylation. Such guideline spans genotypes without changing the primary DNA grouping sequence. The transcriptomic and epi-transcriptomic examination has demonstrated essential significance in investigating infections by deciding their design and work, consequently giving important data. Ongoing information by the Center for RNA Research, the Korean National Organization of Health, has portrayed a guide to SARS-CoV-2 [48]. Nanopore RNA sequencing was done to recognize 41 RNA alteration locations on viral records. AAGAA was noticed most frequently in the genome of the virus. The poly (A) tail assumes a significant part in RNA turnover, and it was proposed that such inside adjustment can add to RNA security and interpretation productivity to be invulnerable [48, 49].

Genetics of Host and SARS-CoV-2 Infection

SARS-CoV-2 is a β-variety Covid. It is a single-stranded, enveloped, 29Kb long RNA genome with a positive sense. It displays partial similarity with SARS-CoV and MERS-CoV (80%). Initially, it was considered an enzootic infection in warm-blooded animals; transmission across the species is conceivable, bringing about human outbreaks. The entry point of infection is the ACE2 type I-layer receptor in the blood vessel and the endothelial cells of veins, enterocytes in the small intestine, lung type II alveolar cells, and smooth muscle cells in blood vessels of various organs, including brainstem and cerebral cortex [48]. ACE2 is a metalloenzyme having zinc (Zn) with a peptidase M2 and renal amino acid, which counterbalance by converting angiotensin I into vasoconstricting angiotensin II. Thus, the phenylalanine is separated from the carboxyl-terminal of angiotensin II by ACE2 and produces angiotensin, which vasodilates [50, 51]. After entering the host, infection imitates a genomic RNA comprising 9 open reading frames. There is a total of 9 sub-genomic RNAs translated from the genomic RNA, encoding and conserving structural proteins, in particular, an envelope protein (E), spike protein (S), nucleocapsid protein (N), and membrane protein (M) [49, 50]. Information has revealed that protease enzymes cut SARS-CoV proteins; for example, Cathepsin L (CTSL), Furin, and transmembrane serine protease 2 (TMPRSS2) coupled with primary amino acid breaks the enzyme (FURIN) into S1 and S2, individually.

SARS-CoV-2 utilizes the receptor-binding domain of the S1 protein, having the main structure and a receptor-binding motif for binding the external receptor surface to enter host tissues/cells [50]. Human ACE2 has two hot spot areas to bind and mutate the virus, whereas mutation at the RBM typically occurs close to these areas, which decides the scope of the infection in hosts [52]. As indicated by the underlying investigation, SARS-CoV-2 contains high human ACE2 [52]. A solitary N501T mutation at point 501 was identified, elevating the SARS-CoV-2 receptor binding domain capability. Similar mutation has already been identified in humans, and it is imperative to judiciously monitor 501 of ACE2 for novel mutation later [52]. A new cross-tissue examination showed that cells having ACE2 co-express the protease CTSL or TMPRSS2, such as pancreas cardiomyocytes and oligodendrocytes, are associated with extreme illness [51].

In this way, ACE2 makes the virus entry point, and almost certainly, these comorbidities impact ACE2 levels that influence viral transmission [53, 54]. Besides, ACE2 was also up-regulated in airways, multi-ciliated, and epithelial cells in individuals who smoke. Curiously, single-cell RNA-sequence reports have uncovered lesser ACE2 expression in pediatrics, showing the absence of accessibility of chromatin in the ACE2 locus [55]. Moreover, hyper-methylation of ACE2 may occur in a child's lungs, reducing its performance [56]. Noteworthy, ACE2 expression was altogether raised in renal papillary cell carcinoma tissues and endometrial carcinoma, related to immune cell penetration and expectation; in this way, recommending a potential vulnerability to SARS-CoV-2 necessitates deeper investigations [57]. In any case, it ought to be evident that the expression of ACE2 in various tissues is mind-boggling and possibly influenced by disease just as by regular treatments.

SARS-CoV-2 and Host Epigenetics Association of X Inactivation with COVID-19

The SARS-CoV-2 receptor, the ACE2 gene, is situated at the X chromosome and focuses on a more critical look at the developmental cycle of XCI, regulated by epigenetics. One X chromosome in females goes through an XCI measure when differentiating to attain compensation in dose in females and males. The female-explicit non-coding RNA Xist is transcribed from the XCI focus and disseminated on the whole X chromosome, making a dormant scene by recruiting polycomb (PRC1) and PRC2, the histone-modifying proteins. Histone H2A is catalyzed by PRC1 on the lysine 119 (H2AK119ub), whereas PRC2 tri-methylates histone H3 on the lysine 27 (H3K27me3) and essentially keeps up the silencing of genes during interaction with XCI, giving a guideline stage and prompting the silent state triggered through the Xist RNA [58].

Notwithstanding, XCI is inadequate in humans, with $1/3^{rd}$ of X-chromosome genes expressed from both inactive (Xi) and active (Xa) X chromosomes in females have genes that get away from XCI being called escapers [58, 59]. A new report plotted the XCI over a few human tissues. The researchers efficiently analyzed over 5000 transcriptomes found in 29 tissues of the genotype tissue expression project. By exploring the variations in long non-coding RNA and X-chromosomal protein-coding expression in both genders, uniformity was found across human tissues in XCI, but some variations can occur in cells, tissues, and people. The information revealed that inadequate XCI controlled at least 7 escaper genes and 23% of X-chromosomal. Escape from XCI appeared to bring about gender predispositions in gene expression and phenotype variation. ACE2 was noted in those genes that got away from XCI in the lung tissue of females, depicting a more heterogeneous gender predisposition. Additionally, ACE2 expression was somewhat higher in males than female tissues, and open chromatin marks were observed related to its demeanor portfolio, perhaps proving more respiratory tract infections in males than females [60].

Histone Modifications and DNA Methylation at ACE2 Gene Locus

The reports involving DNA methylation to regulate the ACE2 demonstrate that the host's epigenome might pose a threat to COVID-19. When DNA methylation profiles were examined from 4 distinct public information bases for lung tissue, they had the option to evaluate for contrasts among both genders on 2 CpGs sites on the ACE2. Researchers have utilized Illumina DNA methylation, which exhibits information from tests of various ages, and recognized that CpG (cg085599149), which was close to the ACE2 transcription site, revealed diminished methylation levels. Also, DNA methylation, reliant on age, was found closer to the transcription start in ACE2 of epithelial cells of the airways [61]. Whole-genome bisulfite sequencing is used to draw more differential methylated CpG islands controlling ACE2 in an age-dependent fashion [62]. Previous investigations have proclaimed that worldwide DNA methylation levels are diminished with aging, prompting variable methylation patterns to be identified with inflammation, aging, and immune response. It was uncovered that DNA methylation is highjacked by MERS-CoV, the principal mechanism to counter antigen-presenting genes and modulate the immune response. This information might clarify the higher morbidity rate of the disease in aged patients with hidden ailments [62, 63].

Moreover, the ACE2 promoter was found hypo-methylated in renal papillary cells and endometrial carcinoma, which caused expanded ACE2 expression, proposing its ratification itself and provoking its levels [58]. When SARS-CoV-2 influenced such individuals, the ACE2 level was diminished, and immunity weakened, influencing the disease condition. Focusing on SARS-CoV-2 disease aside from ACE2, the TMPRSS2 controls the infective capability of SARS-CoV-2. During disease, SARS-CoV-2 binds with ACE2 through Spike protein (S). The S proteins are prepared by the membranous serine protease TMPRSS2, allowing its breakage at S1/S2, while S2 permits cellular union with the viral membrane [48 - 50, 52]. Along with the antibodies against the S protein, a progression of substance compounds is being tried to impede the action and joining potential of TMPRSS2 and ACE2. A protease inhibitor (serine) was uncovered to hamper TMPRSS2 and block the SARS-2-S controlled entrance, proposing its ability as an effective remedy [64].

Not many investigations have explained the significance of medications focusing on the ACE2 gene expression. Researchers screened the two data sets of genome-wide transcriptional expression information, JeaMoon Map (JMap) and connectivity Map (CMap), and distinguished various competitor agents (Fulvestrant, Pirinixic Acid, AG - 013608, Staurosporine, and Azathioprine), which decline ACE2 expression in respiratory tract epithelium along with the azathioprine [65]. Besides, a significant job for epi-transcriptomic and epigenetic components was anticipated in controlling the ACE2 X-related expression ability regarding COVID-19. H3K4 methylation and DNA methylation on the gene promoter impacted its demeanor portfolio [66]. Additionally, an investigation of the roadmap epigenomics project information uncovered that the H3K27ac and p300 acetyltransferase were discovered on the promoter location of the ACE2. The highly homologous cyclic AMP (cAMP), HATs, response element-binding protein, and p300 are grounded indicators of dynamic enhancers. The restraint of the p300 HAT activity lessens the H3K27Ac levels [67, 68].

Prevention of SARS-CoV-2

The study on disease transmission of SARS-CoV-2 is yet muddled, and information accessibility is restricted. In this way, it is essential to follow preventive measures and security insurance given by well-being specialists to restrict contact with the infection and decrease further transmission. General hygienic measures ought to be carried out, for example:

• Wash hands regularly with a cleanser or a liquor-based hand sanitizer
• Hack or sniffle behavior, suggesting covering of the mouth
• Trying not to contact eyes, nose, and mouth without cleaning hands
• Prevent close contact with debilitated people
• Abstaining from sharing utensils and other things with infected/suspected individuals
• Cleaning and sterilization of top surfaces that are frequently contacted
• Remaining at home from work, school, and public zones when feeling exhausted

The transmission course of SARS-CoV-2 is likely not just through the hack, respiratory droplets, or potentially debased surfaces [69, 70] but also *via* fecal-oral transmission [71]. Subsequently, severe clean measures should be followed, particularly in crowded urban communities or rural spaces [72]. Since the SARS-CoV-2 spread is determined by movement and screening of travellers exposed to pandemic zones for conceivable SARS-CoV-2 disease, passage screening systems are important at airports. Likewise, general hygienic precautions during movement are vigorously suggested. Travelers who experience intense respiratory infections should be tried and checked by general well-being specialists [73]. Furthermore, individuals ought to be urged to tell and report about movement history and close contacts if there should be an occurrence of SARS-CoV-2.

Asymptomatic carriers and patients after convalescence from the intense disease are likewise viewed as possible sources of infection [74, 75]. Thorough sterile measures ought to be carried out to hamper the infection transmission to medical personnel, laborers, and different contacts, *i.e.*, the position of SARS-CoV-2 suspected or confirmed patients in single-individual rooms and wearing personal protective equipment (PPE) like veils, goggles, and defensive outfits. Since early determination and discovery of asymptomatic carriers of SARS-CoV-2 are fruitful variables for the treatment and avoidance of transmission, welfare specialists should dispense examination facilities to execute tests for fast and precise findings [76]. The control of COVID-19 depends on biosecurity viewing creatures just as on shifts in food propensities, including debilitating the utilization of bushmeat and items without suitable cooking [77]. Boycotts of wet commercial centers where dead creatures are present should be carried out. Observation of individuals who have contact with untamed life and improvement of biosecurity regarding natural life exchange are critically expected to anticipate the pandemic outbreak [78].

Challenges and Future Perspectives of SARS-CoV-2

The study of disease transmission of SARS-CoV-2 is yet muddled. Numerous uncertain inquiries identified with SARS-CoV-2 in studying disease transmission and pathogenicity present incredible difficulties for analysts. These uncertain inquiries include:

- What is the source of SARS-CoV-2?
- What is the intermediate host that transfers the infection from bats?
- For what reason does the infection cause severe sickness and mortality in the older population or those with comorbidities, while it is milder in kids?
- Are airborne, salivation, dung, pee, and food the lone transmission courses? What are the other obscure courses of transmission?

Control of the SARS-CoV-2 outbreak and future scourges requires worldwide activities among clinical and veterinary clinicians, diagnosticians, disease transmission specialists, general health specialists, vaccinologists, drug businesses, financial experts, and governments to execute a One-Health approach [78]. These actions should include:

- Composing strategies and supporting initiatives needed for the execution of One Health, counteraction, and control measures
- Recruiting prepared and expert staff
- Finding quick and precise solutions and treatments for affected people
- Production of vaccination to control infection in people
- Directing observation among wildlife for the identification and description of potential sources and investigation among individuals who are in contact with natural life to distinguish risk factors in human practices and living climate
- Improving sterile measures
- Evaluating the social and monetary effects of COVID-19 on the public

- Using veterinary involvement for the sterilization of premises under the management of health specialists to lessen incidents in people
- Giving antiviral medications to treat the illnesses of people
- Expanding general health mindfulness about the infection and its transmission.

CONCLUSION

In conclusion, the chapter summarizes all the aspects of viruses' epigenetic mutation rates, especially focusing on coronaviruses. Coronaviruses have spread among other animals and human beings, as in SARS and MERS. A novel coronavirus, designated as COVID-2019, was identified when groups of pneumonia cases were discovered in Wuhan, China, and its province Hubei in 2019. Mutation in the viruses is crucial because it is the first step of evolution as it yields new strands of DNA/RNA for a particular gene, ending up creating a new allele. The greater the mutation ratio, the greater will be the genomic diversity. Even though genetic diversity is always dependent on several factors, the mutation level is of prime concern as it is the crucial basis of genomic variation. Higher mutation rate is found in single-stranded DNA viruses compared to double-stranded DNA viruses. However, this difference is found in work carried out on bacteriophages. So far, there have been no mutation level approximations found for eukaryotic single-stranded DNA viruses.

Similarly, there were no apparent dissimilarities in the mutation rate of RNA viruses in Baltimore classes. Epigenetics has been witnessing a continuous surge over the past decades as a new field of science. Epigenomics enables us to locate, study and explain the epigenetic machinery that monitors the whole genome at different stages. It has been reported that many families of viruses can counter the immune response by utilizing a cascade of epigenetic events and taking over the regulatory capacity for their benefit. Coronaviruses possess the same mechanism to affect epigenetic machinery, *i.e.*, either by improving mutations in the epigenetic code, DNA methylation, post-translational alterations of histone proteins and other proteins linked with epigenome, or directly dysregulating enzymes. Epigenomic search can open novel ways to develop antiviral agents through the targeted evaluation of particular epigenetic modulators and probing novel chromatin-based treatment regimens for various viruses, which can uncover new dimensions of virus and host interaction and the role they play in developing the severity of the disease. This chapter describes the comprehensive understanding of epigenetic aspects linked with coronavirus infections and explains the potential of different epigenetic therapies. This study tells the importance of understanding the epigenetic regulation of immune response, which can surely assist in designing specific strategies for the prevention and treatment of infection. The study of disease transmission of SARS-CoV-2 is yet muddled, and information accessibility is restricted. In this way, it is basic to follow preventive measures and security insurance given by well-being specialists to restrict contact with the infection and decrease further spread. Control of the SARS-CoV-2 outbreak and future scourges requires worldwide activities.

ACKNOWLEDGEMENTS

The authors wish to thank and acknowledge their respective universities and institutes.

REFERENCES

[1]   Novel coronavirus situation report-2 2020. Available from: https://www.who.int/docs/defaultsource/coronaviruse/situation-reports/20200122-sitrep-2-2019-ncov.pdf

[2]   Sajid HA, Ali A, Khan YR, *et al.* COVID-19: Third Wave Feared as Cases Soar and Precautionary Measures. Am J Life Sci 2021; 9: 19-24.
[http://dx.doi.org/10.11648/j.ajls.20210902.11]

[3]   Chan JFW, Kok KH, Zhu Z, *et al.* Genomic characterization of the 2019 novel human-pathogenic coronavirus isolated from a patient with atypical pneumonia after visiting Wuhan. Emerg Microbes Infect 2020; 9(1): 221-36.
[http://dx.doi.org/10.1080/22221751.2020.1719902] [PMID: 31987001]

[4]   Mankar SD, Jadhav RS, Gaikwad K. Corona Viruses -Current Knowledge -A Review. Res J Sci Tech 2020; 12(2): 163-6.
[http://dx.doi.org/10.5958/2349-2988.2020.00021.2]

[5]   Sajid HA, Ali A, Afzal A. COVID-19: Recent Trends in the World and Precautionary Measures. Am J Life Sci 2020; 8: 41-4.
[http://dx.doi.org/10.11648/j.ajls.20200803.12]

[6]   McIntosh K, Dees JH, Becker WB, Kapikian AZ, Chanock RM. Recovery in tracheal organ cultures of novel viruses from patients with respiratory disease. Proc Natl Acad Sci USA 1967; 57(4): 933-40.
[http://dx.doi.org/10.1073/pnas.57.4.933] [PMID: 5231356]

[7]   Manandhar S, Nakarmi P, Baniya N. A novel coronavirus emerging in the world—key questions for developing countries and underdeveloped countries. Nor Am Acad Res 2020; 3: 473-97.
[http://dx.doi.org/10.5281/zenodo.3690311]

[8]   Oyeagu CE, Ezeuko AS, Lewu FB, *et al.* The impact of COVID-19 on the livestock industry and the way forward: A review. Adv Anim Vet Sci 2021; 9: 941-55.
[http://dx.doi.org/10.17582/journal.aavs/2021/9.6.941.955]

[9]   Rabaan AA, Al-Ahmed SH, Haque S, *et al.* SARS-CoV-2, SARS-CoV, and MERS-COV: a comparative overview. Infez Med 2020; 28(2): 174-84.
[PMID: 32275259]

[10]   Enjuanes L, Smerdou C, Castilla J, *et al.* Development of protection against coronavirus-induced diseases Adv Exp Med Biol 1995; 380: 197-211.
[http://dx.doi.org/10.1007/978-1-4615-1899-0_34]

[11]   Ujike M, Taguchi F. Incorporation of spike and membrane glycoproteins into coronavirus virions. Viruses 2015; 7(4): 1700-25.
[http://dx.doi.org/10.3390/v7041700] [PMID: 25855243]

[12]   Kuo L, Masters PS. Genetic evidence for a structural interaction between the carboxy termini of the membrane and nucleocapsid proteins of mouse hepatitis virus. J Virol 2002; 76(10): 4987-99.
[http://dx.doi.org/10.1128/JVI.76.10.4987-4999.2002] [PMID: 11967315]

[13]   Sanjuán R, Nebot MR, Chirico N, Mansky LM, Belshaw R. Viral mutation rates. J Virol 2010; 84(19): 9733-48.
[http://dx.doi.org/10.1128/JVI.00694-10] [PMID: 20660197]

[14]   Duffy S, Shackelton LA, Holmes EC. Rates of evolutionary change in viruses: patterns and determinants. Nat Rev Genet 2008; 9(4): 267-76.
[http://dx.doi.org/10.1038/nrg2323] [PMID: 18319742]

[15]   Sanjuán R. From molecular genetics to phylodynamics: evolutionary relevance of mutation rates across viruses. PLoS Pathog 2012; 8(5): e1002685.
[http://dx.doi.org/10.1371/journal.ppat.1002685] [PMID: 22570614]

[16]   Roberts JD, Bebenek K, Kunkel TA. The accuracy of reverse transcriptase from HIV-1. Science 1988; 242(4882): 1171-3.
[http://dx.doi.org/10.1126/science.2460925] [PMID: 2460925]

[17]   Steinhauer DA, Domingo E, Holland JJ. Lack of evidence for proofreading mechanisms associated with an RNA virus polymerase. Gene 1992; 122(2): 281-8.
[http://dx.doi.org/10.1016/0378-1119(92)90216-C] [PMID: 1336756]

[18]   Muzyczka N, Poland RL, Bessman MJ. Studies on the biochemical basis of spontaneous mutation. I. A comparison of the deoxyribonucleic acid polymerases of mutator, antimutator, and wild type strains of bacteriophage T4. J Biol Chem 1972; 247(22): 7116-22.
[http://dx.doi.org/10.1016/S0021-9258(19)44602-4] [PMID: 4565077]

[19]   Hong YB, Choi Y, Jung G. Increased DNA polymerase fidelity of the Lamivudine resistant variants of human hepatitis B virus DNA polymerase. J Biochem Mol Biol 2004; 37(2): 167-76.
[PMID: 15469692]

[20]   Menéndez-Arias L. Mutation rates and intrinsic fidelity of retroviral reverse transcriptases. Viruses 2009; 1(3): 1137-65.
[http://dx.doi.org/10.3390/v1031137] [PMID: 21994586]

[21]   Biek R, Pybus OG, Lloyd-Smith JO, Didelot X. Measurably evolving pathogens in the genomic era. Trends Ecol Evol 2015; 30(6): 306-13.
[http://dx.doi.org/10.1016/j.tree.2015.03.009] [PMID: 25887947]

[22]   Shackelton LA, Parrish CR, Truyen U, Holmes EC. High rate of viral evolution associated with the emergence of carnivore parvovirus. Proc Natl Acad Sci USA 2005; 102(2): 379-84.
[http://dx.doi.org/10.1073/pnas.0406765102] [PMID: 15626758]

[23]   Shackelton LA, Holmes EC. Phylogenetic evidence for the rapid evolution of human B19 erythrovirus. J Virol 2006; 80(7): 3666-9.
[http://dx.doi.org/10.1128/JVI.80.7.3666-3669.2006] [PMID: 16537636]

[24]   Duffy S, Holmes EC. Phylogenetic evidence for rapid rates of molecular evolution in the single-stranded DNA begomovirus tomato yellow leaf curl virus. J Virol 2008; 82(2): 957-65.
[http://dx.doi.org/10.1128/JVI.01929-07] [PMID: 17977971]

[25]   Sarker S, Patterson EI, Peters A, *et al.* Mutability dynamics of an emergent single stranded DNA virus in a naïve host. PLoS One 2014; 9(1): e85370.
[http://dx.doi.org/10.1371/journal.pone.0085370] [PMID: 24416396]

[26]   Michaud V, Randriamparany T, Albina E. Comprehensive phylogenetic reconstructions of African swine fever virus: proposal for a new classification and molecular dating of the virus. PLoS One 2013; 8(7): e69662.
[http://dx.doi.org/10.1371/journal.pone.0069662] [PMID: 23936068]

[27]   Renzette N, Pokalyuk C, Gibson L, *et al.* Limits and patterns of cytomegalovirus genomic diversity in humans. Proc Natl Acad Sci USA 2015; 112(30): E4120-8.
[http://dx.doi.org/10.1073/pnas.1501880112] [PMID: 26150505]

[28] Sanjuán R, Domingo-Calap P. Mechanisms of viral mutation. Cell Mol Life Sci 2016; 73(23): 4433-48.
[http://dx.doi.org/10.1007/s00018-016-2299-6] [PMID: 27392606]

[29] Shirato K, Kawase M, Watanabe O, *et al.* Differences in neutralizing antigenicity between laboratory and clinical isolates of HCoV-229E isolated in Japan in 2004–2008 depend on the S1 region sequence of the spike protein. J Gen Virol 2012; 93(9): 1908-17.
[http://dx.doi.org/10.1099/vir.0.043117-0] [PMID: 22673931]

[30] Smale ST, Tarakhovsky A, Natoli G. Chromatin contributions to the regulation of innate immunity. Annu Rev Immunol 2014; 32(1): 489-511.
[http://dx.doi.org/10.1146/annurev-immunol-031210-101303] [PMID: 24555473]

[31] Vavougios GD. A data-driven hypothesis on the epigenetic dysregulation of host metabolism by SARS coronaviral infection: potential implications for the SARS-CoV-2. Medical Hypotheses 2020; 140: 109759.
[http://dx.doi.org/10.1016/j.mehy.2020.109759]

[32] Guarner J. Three emerging coronaviruses in two decades: the story of SARS, MERS, and now COVID-19. Am J Clin Pathol 2020; 153(4): 420-1.
[http://dx.doi.org/10.1093/ajcp/aqaa029] [PMID: 32053148]

[33] Kennedy PGE, Rovnak J, Badani H, Cohrs RJ. A comparison of herpes simplex virus type 1 and varicella-zoster virus latency and reactivation. J Gen Virol 2015; 96(7): 1581-602.
[http://dx.doi.org/10.1099/vir.0.000128] [PMID: 25794504]

[34] Liang Y, Vogel JL, Narayanan A, Peng H, Kristie TM. Inhibition of the histone demethylase LSD1 blocks α-herpesvirus lytic replication and reactivation from latency. Nat Med 2009; 15(11): 1312-7.
[http://dx.doi.org/10.1038/nm.2051] [PMID: 19855399]

[35] Schäfer A, Baric R. Epigenetic landscape during coronavirus infection. Pathogens 2017; 6(1): 8.
[http://dx.doi.org/10.3390/pathogens6010008] [PMID: 28212305]

[36] Kaikkonen MU, Lam MTY, Glass CK. Non-coding RNAs as regulators of gene expression and epigenetics. Cardiovasc Res 2011; 90(3): 430-40.
[http://dx.doi.org/10.1093/cvr/cvr097] [PMID: 21558279]

[37] Li Q, Guan X, Wu P, *et al.* Early transmission dynamics in Wuhan, China, of novel coronavirus–infected pneumonia. N Engl J Med 2020; 382(13): 1199-207.
[http://dx.doi.org/10.1056/NEJMoa2001316] [PMID: 31995857]

[38] Seo YL, Heo S, Jang KL. Hepatitis C virus core protein overcomes H2O2-induced apoptosis by downregulating p14 expression *via* DNA methylation. J Gen Virol 2015; 96(4): 822-32.
[http://dx.doi.org/10.1099/vir.0.000032] [PMID: 25535325]

[39] Mudersbach T, Siuda D, Kohlstedt K, Fleming I. Epigenetic control of the angiotensin-converting enzyme in endothelial cells during inflammation. PLoS One 2019; 14(5): e0216218.
[http://dx.doi.org/10.1371/journal.pone.0216218] [PMID: 31042763]

[40] Hummel B, Hansen EC, Yoveva A, Aprile-Garcia F, Hussong R, Sawarkar R. The evolutionary capacitor HSP90 buffers the regulatory effects of mammalian endogenous retroviruses. Nat Struct Mol Biol 2017; 24(3): 234-42.
[http://dx.doi.org/10.1038/nsmb.3368] [PMID: 28134929]

[41] Liu G, Zhong M, Guo C, *et al.* Autophagy is involved in regulating influenza A virus RNA and protein synthesis associated with both modulation of Hsp90 induction and mTOR/p70S6K signaling pathway. Int J Biochem Cell Biol 2016; 72: 100-8.
[http://dx.doi.org/10.1016/j.biocel.2016.01.012] [PMID: 26794463]

[42] Obermann WMJ. A motif in HSP90 and P23 that links molecular chaperones to efficient estrogen receptor α methylation by the lysine methyltransferase SMYD2. J Biol Chem 2018; 293(42): 16479-87.

[http://dx.doi.org/10.1074/jbc.RA118.003578] [PMID: 30190324]

[43] Kox M, Waalders NJB, Kooistra EJ, Gerretsen J, Pickkers P. Cytokine levels in critically ill patients with COVID-19 and other conditions. JAMA 2020; 324(15): 1565-7.
[http://dx.doi.org/10.1001/jama.2020.17052] [PMID: 32880615]

[44] Gordon D, Jang GM, Bouhaddou M, *et al.* A SARS-CoV-2-Human Protein-Protein Interaction Map Reveals Drug Targets and Potential Drug Repurposing. Nature 2020; 583: 459-68.
[http://dx.doi.org/10.1038/s41586-020-2286-9] [PMID: 32353859]

[45] Pyrc K, Berkhout B, van der Hoek L. The novel human coronaviruses NL63 and HKU1. J Virol 2007; 81(7): 3051-7.
[http://dx.doi.org/10.1128/JVI.01466-06] [PMID: 17079323]

[46] Law HKW, Cheung CY, Ng HY, *et al.* Chemokine up-regulation in SARS-coronavirus–infected, monocyte-derived human dendritic cells. Blood 2005; 106(7): 2366-74.
[http://dx.doi.org/10.1182/blood-2004-10-4166] [PMID: 15860669]

[47] Becares M, Pascual-Iglesias A, Nogales A, Sola I, Enjuanes L, Zuñiga S. Mutagenesis of coronavirus nsp14 reveals its potential role in the modulation of the innate immune response. J Virol 2016; 90(11): 5399-414.
[http://dx.doi.org/10.1128/JVI.03259-15] [PMID: 27009949]

[48] Kim D, Lee JY, Yang JS, Kim JW, Kim VN, Chang H. The architecture of SARS-CoV-2 transcriptome. Cell 2020; 181(4): 914-921.e10.
[http://dx.doi.org/10.1016/j.cell.2020.04.011] [PMID: 32330414]

[49] Kim JM, Chung YS, Jo HJ, *et al.* Identification of coronavirus isolated from a patient in Korea with COVID-19. Osong Public Health Res Perspect 2020; 11(1): 3-7.
[http://dx.doi.org/10.24171/j.phrp.2020.11.1.02] [PMID: 32149036]

[50] Verdecchia P, Cavallini C, Spanevello A, Angeli F. The pivotal link between ACE2 deficiency and SARS-CoV-2 infection. Eur J Intern Med 2020; 76: 14-20.
[http://dx.doi.org/10.1016/j.ejim.2020.04.037] [PMID: 32336612]

[51] Jia HP, Look DC, Shi L, *et al.* ACE2 receptor expression and severe acute respiratory syndrome coronavirus infection depend on differentiation of human airway epithelia. J Virol 2005; 79(23): 14614-21.
[http://dx.doi.org/10.1128/JVI.79.23.14614-14621.2005] [PMID: 16282461]

[52] Wan Y, Shang J, Graham R, Baric RS, Li F. Receptor recognition by the novel coronavirus from Wuhan: an analysis based on decade-long structural studies of SARS coronavirus. J Virol 2020; 94(7): e00127-20.
[http://dx.doi.org/10.1128/JVI.00127-20] [PMID: 31996437]

[53] Pinto BGG, Oliveira AER, Singh Y, *et al.* ACE2 expression is increased in the lungs of patients with comorbidities associated with severe COVID-19. J Infect Dis 2020; 222(4): 556-63.
[http://dx.doi.org/10.1093/infdis/jiaa332] [PMID: 32526012]

[54] Sawalha AH, Zhao M, Coit P, Lu Q. Epigenetic dysregulation of ACE2 and interferon-regulated genes might suggest increased COVID-19 susceptibility and severity in lupus patients. Clin Immunol 2020; 215: 108410.
[http://dx.doi.org/10.1016/j.clim.2020.108410] [PMID: 32276140]

[55] Barbry P, Muus C, Luecken M, *et al.* Integrated analyses of single-cell atlases reveal age, gender, and smoking status associations with cell type-specific expression of mediators of SARS-CoV-2 viral entry and highlight inflammatory programs in putative target cells. bioRxiv 2020.
[http://dx.doi.org/10.1101/2020.04.19.049254]

[56] Holmes L Jr, Lim A, Comeaux CR, Dabney KW, Okundaye O. DNA methylation of candidate genes (ACE II, IFN-Γ, AGTR 1, CKG, ADD1, SCNN1B and TLR2) in essential hypertension: A systematic review and quantitative evidence synthesis. Int J Environ Res Public Health 2019; 16(23): 4829.

[http://dx.doi.org/10.3390/ijerph16234829] [PMID: 31805646]

[57] Yang J, Li H, Hu S, Zhou Y. ACE2 correlated with immune infiltration serves as a prognostic biomarker in endometrial carcinoma and renal papillary cell carcinoma: implication for COVID-19. Aging (Albany NY) 2020; 12(8): 6518-35.
[http://dx.doi.org/10.18632/aging.103100] [PMID: 32339157]

[58] Galupa R, Heard E. X-chromosome inactivation: a crossroads between chromosome architecture and gene regulation. Annu Rev Genet 2018; 52(1): 535-66.
[http://dx.doi.org/10.1146/annurev-genet-120116-024611] [PMID: 30256677]

[59] Żylicz JJ, Bousard A, Žumer K, *et al.* The implication of early chromatin changes in X chromosome inactivation. Cell 2019; 176(1-2): 182-197.e23.
[http://dx.doi.org/10.1016/j.cell.2018.11.041] [PMID: 30595450]

[60] Tukiainen T, Villani AC, Yen A, *et al.* Landscape of X chromosome inactivation across human tissues. Nature 2017; 550(7675): 244-8.
[http://dx.doi.org/10.1038/nature24265] [PMID: 29022598]

[61] Li F. Structure, function, and evolution of coronavirus spike proteins. Annu Rev Virol 2016; 3(1): 237-61.
[http://dx.doi.org/10.1146/annurev-virology-110615-042301] [PMID: 27578435]

[62] Corley MJ, Ndhlovu LC. DNA methylation analysis of the COVID-19 host cell receptor, angiotensin I converting enzyme 2 gene (ACE2) in the respiratory system reveals age and gender differences. Preprints 2020; 2020030295.
[http://dx.doi.org/10.20944/preprints202003.0295.v1]

[63] Menachery VD, Schäfer A, Burnum-Johnson KE, *et al.* MERS-CoV and H5N1 influenza virus antagonize antigen presentation by altering the epigenetic landscape. Proc Natl Acad Sci USA 2018; 115(5): E1012-21.
[http://dx.doi.org/10.1073/pnas.1706928115] [PMID: 29339515]

[64] Hoffmann M, Kleine-Weber H, Schroeder S, *et al.* SARS-CoV-2 cell entry depends on ACE2 and TMPRSS2 and is blocked by a clinically proven protease inhibitor. Cell 2020; 181(2): 271-280.e8.
[http://dx.doi.org/10.1016/j.cell.2020.02.052] [PMID: 32142651]

[65] Cui Q, Huang C, Ji X, *et al.* Possible inhibitors of ACE2, the receptor of 2019-nCoV. Preprints 2020; 2020020047.
[http://dx.doi.org/10.20944/preprints202002.0047.v1]

[66] Raisner R, Kharbanda S, Jin L, *et al.* Enhancer activity requires CBP/P300 bromodomain-dependent histone H3K27 acetylation. Cell Rep 2018; 24(7): 1722-9.
[http://dx.doi.org/10.1016/j.celrep.2018.07.041] [PMID: 30110629]

[67] Lasko LM, Jakob CG, Edalji RP, *et al.* Discovery of a selective catalytic p300/CBP inhibitor that targets lineage-specific tumours. Nature 2017; 550(7674): 128-32.
[http://dx.doi.org/10.1038/nature24028] [PMID: 28953875]

[68] Karamouzis MV, Konstantinopoulos PA, Papavassiliou AG. Roles of CREB-binding protein (CBP)/p300 in respiratory epithelium tumorigenesis. Cell Res 2007; 17(4): 324-32.
[http://dx.doi.org/10.1038/cr.2007.10] [PMID: 17372613]

[69] Chan JFW, Lau SKP, To KKW, Cheng VCC, Woo PCY, Yuen KY. Middle East respiratory syndrome coronavirus: another zoonotic betacoronavirus causing SARS-like disease. Clin Microbiol Rev 2015; 28(2): 465-522.
[http://dx.doi.org/10.1128/CMR.00102-14] [PMID: 25810418]

[70] Phan LT, Nguyen TV, Luong QC, *et al.* Importation and human-to-human transmission of a novel coronavirus in Vietnam. N Engl J Med 2020; 382(9): 872-4.
[http://dx.doi.org/10.1056/NEJMc2001272] [PMID: 31991079]

[71] Holshue ML, DeBolt C, Lindquist S, *et al.* First case of 2019 novel coronavirus in the United States. N

Engl J Med 2020; 382(10): 929-36.
[http://dx.doi.org/10.1056/NEJMoa2001191] [PMID: 32004427]

[72]   Neiderud CJ. How urbanization affects the epidemiology of emerging infectious diseases. Infect Ecol Epidemiol 2015; 5(1): 27060.
[http://dx.doi.org/10.3402/iee.v5.27060] [PMID: 26112265]

[73]   Available from: https://www.ecdc.europa.eu/sites/default/files/documents/SARS-CoV-2-risk-assessment-14-feb-2020.pdf

[74]   Rothe C, Schunk M, Sothmann P, *et al.* Transmission of 2019-nCoV infection from an asymptomatic contact in Germany. N Engl J Med 2020; 382(10): 970-1.
[http://dx.doi.org/10.1056/NEJMc2001468] [PMID: 32003551]

[75]   Available from: https://www.who.int/publications-detail/infection-prevention-and-control-during-health-care-when-novel-coronavirus-(ncov)-infection-is-suspected-20200125

[76]   Kock RA, Karesh WB, Veas F, *et al.* 2019-nCoV in context: lessons learned? Lancet Planet Health 2020; 4(3): e87-8.
[http://dx.doi.org/10.1016/S2542-5196(20)30035-8] [PMID: 32035507]

[77]   Daszak P, Olival KJ, Li H. A strategy to prevent future epidemics similar to the 2019-nCoV outbreak. Biosafety and Health 2020; 2(1): 6-8.
[http://dx.doi.org/10.1016/j.bsheal.2020.01.003] [PMID: 32562482]

[78]   Fawzy M, Helmy YA. The One Health approach is necessary for the control of Rift Valley fever infections in Egypt: a comprehensive review. Viruses 2019; 11(2): 139.
[http://dx.doi.org/10.3390/v11020139] [PMID: 30736362]

CHAPTER 9

Neurological Complications of SARS-CoV, MERS-CoV, and SARS-CoV-2

Amjad Islam Aqib[1,*], Tean Zaheer[2], Rabia Liaqat Khan[3], Yasir Razzaq Khan[1], Ahmad Ali[1], Hina Afzal Sajid[4], Vishal Kiran[5], C-Neen Fatima Zaheer[6], Firasat Hussain[7] and Muhammad Ashir Nabeel[8]

[1] *Department of Medicine, Faculty of Veterinary Science, Cholistan University of Veterinary and Animal Sciences (CUVAS), Bahawalpur 63100, Pakistan*

[2] *Department of Parasitology, University of Agriculture, Faisalabad, Pakistan*

[3] *Department of Pathology, University of Agriculture, Faisalabad, Pakistan*

[4] *Center of Excellence Molecular Biology, University of the Punjab, Lahore, Pakistan*

[5] *Government College University Lahore, Lahore, Pakistan*

[6] *Faculty of Veterinary Science, University of Agriculture, Faisalabad, Pakistan*

[7] *Department of Microbiology, Cholistan University of Veterinary and Animal Sciences (CUVAS), Bahawalpur 63100, Pakistan*

[8] *Department of Theriogenology, University of Agriculture, Faisalabad, Pakistan*

Abstract: This chapter comprises the neurological pathogenesis of Coronaviridae in the central nervous system (CNS). These viruses manifest their virulence factors involving multiple organs of the body, initiating from febrile conditions, respiratory distress, and hypoproteinemia leading to edematous fluid accumulation. They pave their path to CNS by directly affecting the cranial plus vagus nerve fibers and synapses or through systematic circulation. The viruses can have an affinity with various receptor sites present on organs that help in hematogenous and retrograde mobility towards CNS. Comorbidities occur excessively due to these viruses in the living system involving vital organs such as the liver, heart, and lungs. Neurological dissemination of these viruses is characterized by a permanent loss of nerves or part of the CNS, either entirely or partially. Prevention is suggested, accompanied by adequate treatment and care management to avoid extensive spreading of the virus throughout CNS.

Keywords: Comorbidities, MERS-COV, Neurological complications, SARS COV-2, SARS-COV.

* **Corresponding author Amjad Islam Aqib:** Department of Medicine, Faculty of Veterinary Science, Cholistan University of Veterinary and Animal Sciences (CUVAS), Bahawalpur 63100, Pakistan; E-mail: amjadislamaqib@cuvas.edu.pk

Kamal Niaz, Muhammad Sajjad Khan & Muhammad Farrukh Nisar (Eds.)

INTRODUCTION

Coronaviruses are classified as enveloped viruses and belong to the Nedovirals and Coronaviridae families. There are four genera: *Alpha*, *Beta*, *Gamma*, and *Delta*. Their genome is positive-sense, single-stranded RNA [1]. Among them, all the genera except gamma coronaviruses are responsible for the infection in a variety of mammals. Despite the ability of all four genera to transmit between species, they all harm humans by causing severe respiratory syndromes like the Middle East respiratory syndrome, which is brought on by MERS-CoV. Additionally, SARS-CoV is involved in respiratory syndrome with severe acuteness (SARS), and SARS-CoV-2 has recently been linked to the COVID-19 virus [2]. Scientists first described the CoV disease in 1931, and in 1965, they isolated the first humanoid virus (HCoV-229E). Only two types were available in late 2002. Among coronaviruses, HCoV-OC43 and HCoV-229E were known to exist when the prevalence of SARS was first observed. Since then, six more coronaviruses have been discovered that affect humans. Wuhan, China, saw the first SARS-CoV-2 detection in December 2019, which quickly became a global pandemic within months [3]. The pandemic has had an important impact on the world economy, social interactions, and public health, resulting in a rise in mortality rates worldwide [4]. COVID-19, a disease caused by SARS-CoV-2, is a recognized medical condition. Symptoms of COVID-19 are similar to those of the common flu, including fever (90%) and cough (70%), as well as myalgia and lethargy (50%). Headache (8%), diarrhea (5%), ageusia, and anosmia can also occur as the first signs [4]. In contrast, the lesser fraction of severe cases showed some severe lower respiratory tract infections that frequently needed respiratory aid. 5% of asymptomatic cases of this virus have also been detected [5].

The worst condition of the pandemic has led the health systems to prevent and combat COVID-19. Evidence shows that patients and clinical settings face more problems in gaining access to health benefactors despite a considerable upsurge in telemedicine. For example, it has been reported that deaths due to cardiac arrest at home increased by about 800% due to the COVID-19 pandemic in New York. On the other hand, it was predicted that individuals with neurological disorders faced problems in receiving help from their neurologists. The neurological community is offering the utmost caution to their patients with all the suffering faced due to the COVID-19 virus.

Transmission to CNS

Coronaviruses' Potential Mechanism of Nervous System Infection

Aside from the respiratory system, coronaviruses can evade immune responses and infect other organs, like the central nervous system. Since coronaviruses can be detected in brain tissue using *in situ* hybridization, which demonstrates there are viral remnants in the brain of infection, this neuroinvasive nature of coronaviruses has been demonstrated. Autopsy studies have provided proof of the opportunistic capacity of these pathogens to infect the brain [6]. Additionally, research has shown that coronaviruses can enter the nasal cavity and infect the brain. The infection can enter the central nervous system to peripheral nerve terminals and then travel through synapses in the CNS either retrogradely or trans-synaptically from infected tissues. Coronaviruses can result in cognitive and behavioral impairments as a result of this invasion [7]. The SARS-CoV's capacity to spread throughout the body *via* systemic circulation enables the virus to enter infected individuals' cerebral circulation. This slow flow increases the chance for the virus spike protein to interact with the ACE2 receptor and can explain why the virus is more successful in infecting the endothelial cells of the microcirculation. This interaction is the first step in the virus' ability to spread throughout the body. The cribriform plate is connected to the nasal cavity and has a porous structure, allowing for easy passage of the virus. The olfactory bulb is responsible for sensing odors, providing another potential entry point for the virus. The virus might be able to enter the brain as a result of this movement [8]. Another possible mechanism for the invasion of the brain by coronaviruses is through the lymphatic or hematogenous route. These mechanisms allow coronaviruses to possess neurotropic and neuroinvasive characteristics. The virus may initially infect neurons, glial cells, white blood cells, or even the blood-brain barrier's endothelial cells (BBB), which can result in cell death and neurodegeneration [9]. According to the scant research on COVID-19's neurological effects, it appears that SARS-CoV-2 can harm the nervous system in two different ways:

¬ Direct invasion of neural tissue
¬ Maladaptive inflammatory responses

The central nervous system (CNS) can become infected by SARS-CoV-2 directly through hematogenous and neuronal regurgitation pathways. The virus can attack by infecting CNS endothelial cells, which are prevalent in ACE2. The virus then uses the infected cells to enter the CSF and gain access to the nervous system. From there, it can spread to other areas of the brain and spinal cord, leading to inflammation and tissue damage [10]. The investigation produced data that supported this hypothesis. SARS-CoV-2 is believed to be capable of attaching to the arterial endothelium, breaking the blood-brain barrier and entering nerve tissues through hemogenous pathways. Transmission electron microscopy (TEM) studies have shown that viral particles are captured by cytoplasmic vacuoles at the endothelial-neural cell interface. In addition to the hematogenous route, there is evidence that neuronal regressive transmission may also be a means by which the virus can enter the CNS.

When a virus enters the CNS, it typically first targets nerve terminals. Studies conducted on animals infected with OC43-CoV and SARS-CoV indicate that the virus can disrupt the nasal epithelium, infiltrate the brain, and spread through the nervous system through inhalation. Given the similarities between SARS-CoV-2, SARS-CoV, and OC43-CoV, COVID-19 may use the same route. Although upper respiratory symptoms are not always present, recent research suggests that COVID-19 patients are more likely to experience loss of smell (anosmia) and taste (dysgesia). The overexpression of ACE2 and other SARS-CoV-2 genes by sustentacular and nonneuronal cells in the olfactory neuroepithelium of humans may be the cause of these symptoms in COVID-19 patients [11]. While the regrowth of neurons may be a possible transmission route for SARS-CoV-2 to the CNS, further research is necessary to confirm this. Neurological symptoms of COVID-19 have also been linked to poor inflammatory responses, particularly in patients in whom viral RNA was not found in cerebrospinal fluid (CSF). Inflammatory cytokines such as IL-1, IFN, TNF, IL-4, and IL-10 are secreted in large amounts during the early stages of COVID-19. This cytokine storm is a distinguishing feature of the disease caused by rapid viral replication and secondary cellular damage. High levels of these cytokines have been observed in the plasma of ICU patients, indicating cytokine storms in severe cases. This cytokine storm, which can also disrupt the blood-brain barrier and cause neuroinflammation in sepsis, can lead to various neurological symptoms [12].

This can lead to worse outcomes and even death in some cases. Therefore, it is important to understand the consequences of such treatments before they are used in clinical settings. Close monitoring of patients is essential to minimize the potential risks. This can lead to some serious health complications, including acute respiratory distress syndrome and acute lung injury. In some cases, these complications can be fatal. In the current case series of neurological symptoms in severe SARS-CoV-2 infection, elevated levels of IgG and oligoclonal bands were found in the cerebrospinal fluid, indicating that there may be a "double-edged sword" in the immune system's functioning [12]. Furthermore, the coronavirus can cause an overactive immune system, which can trigger the onset or worsening of neurological symptoms. MERS-CoV infection can be more severe due to rapid infection and replication in human macrophages, dendritic cells, and primary T cells, resulting in the production of proinflammatory chemokines and cytokines that impair immune responses and cause significant amounts of reactive apoptosis [6].

Comorbidities and Coronaviruses

Comorbidities

Comorbidity depicts the influence of all further conditions that an individual may have other than the prime condition of importance, while it can be psychological or physiological. In medicine, comorbidity is a term used to manifest one or other surplus conditions that are frequently co-occurring (associated or concurrent) using a principal condition. In the case of mental wellbeing, comorbidity is known as a series of ailments that are frequently concurrent with each other, like anxiety disorders and depression. The term "comorbid" can be defined in three different ways:

- It indicates a medical condition that exists simultaneously but independently with an alternative condition in a patient.
- Indicating a health condition in an affected individual triggered by or linked to an extra disorder in a similar patient [13].
- Indicating binary or other medical settings that are prevailing simultaneously irrespective of their connection with each other [14].

Coronaviruses

SARS-CoV

Reports suggest that the virus infects adults aged 25 to 70. In comparison, limited cases have also been reported in adolescents (aged 15 years). The duration of infection is between 2 and 7 days and sometimes between 10 days. During this period, infected people may have a low-grade fever with some cold and flu-like signs such as high and severe fever, headaches, muscle pain, and sore throat. Respiratory problems also start with thirst and cough 3 to 7 days after infection. They result in trouble breathing, and depletion of blood oxygen takes place in 10-20% of cases [15]. SARS can be characterized by mainly two experimental stages. In the former stage, the indications are relatively mild and linked to the higher portion of the respiratory organization (signs of cold, exertion in-breath, and cough). Whereas in the later phase, the lower respiratory system, due to occupation of the virus, might cause shortness of breath, cough, and eventually the depletion of blood oxygen level [16]. However, the severity of symptoms may fluctuate, but all of the described symptoms happen in adults as well as in children.

MERS-CoV

MERS-CoV may cause a large variety of indications, from trivial fever, respirational indications (higher respiratory region infection), weakness, diarrhea, and lethargy to advanced renal failure, respiratory letdown, or several organ failures in Spartan cases. Respiratory symptoms and fever are the most common indications of this disease, and all affected patients experience respirational symptoms all through their infection [17]. Patients affected with MERS-CoV have also been observed to have symptoms of intravascular coagulation, coagulopathy, and anemia. Reports also illustrate more potassium levels, troponin, serum transaminases, C-reactive (CRP) protein, creatine kinase, procalcitonin, and lactate dehydrogenase, and reduced albumin and serum sodium levels [18]. The two viruses, MERS-CoV and SARS, display similar symptoms, but the former has an altered clinical sequence and significant 35-50% mortality proportions. The death rate from MERS is greater in men, plus fatalities from primary infections.

SARS-CoV-2

As reported in a preliminary study on people infected with the latest coronavirus (SARS-CoV-2), the duration of the virus's rearing is about five days, ranging from 4 to 7 days. As confirmed by the current pandemic, the incubation period of COVID-19 is different from 1-14 days, which fluctuates from 3-7 days. The virus SARS-CoV-2 can reproduce in cells in the lower respiratory tract [19]. At the beginning phase of septicity through SARS-CoV-2, patients display common nonspecific indications such as dry cough, body aches, fatigue, fever, nausea, and diarrhea. Infected individuals may also develop neurological signs such as anosmia and headache [20]. The data available is limited for SARS-CoV-2 due to comparatively novel and understudied illness. Rapidly emerging cases demonstrate that comorbidities can increase the rate of infection. According to recent evidence and medical expertise, aged individuals, those in durable precaution facilities, and people with severe underlying health settings are at a greater risk of receiving SARS-CoV-2. The aged are becoming a more susceptible population, having prolonged health situations such as cardiovascular or lung disease and diabetes. They are not merely at a greater risk of having serious infection but are also at a larger risk of disease after getting infected with the virus. Individuals who have underlying uncontrolled health conditions, for example, hypertension, diabetes, liver, lung, and kidney disease, smokers, people with cancer on chemotherapy, patients taking steroids frequently, and transplant receivers are at larger risk of SARS-CoV-2 septicity [1]. These comorbidities described in Tables **1** and **2** are linked with severe COVID-19 infection in grown people of all ages. The record of the comorbidities having recognized risk features is more reliable and broader compared to the comorbidities scheduled as potential risk dynamics. The probability of severe infection also surges gradually with age. Underlying health conditions are also related to severe illness in children, but associated evidence is restricted. Children with the following situations can be at more significant risk for severe illnesses like medical complexity, obesity, severe neurologic disarrays, severe genomic disorders, genetic metabolic ailments, congenital heart disease, sickle cell disease, chronic kidney infection, asthma, and other chronic lung illness, diabetes, and immunosuppression because of immune-weakening medicines or malignancy [21].

Table 1. Mortality rate of COVID-19 (SARS-CoV-2) patients with comorbidities [1].

Disease	Countries		
	USA	China	Italy
Obesity	55.0	13.0	8.5
Hypertension	Not Reported	9.5	73.8
Diabetes	58	7.4	35.5
Cardiovascular Diseases (CVD)	9.0	7.3	42.5
Chronic Obstructive Pulmonary Disease (COPD)	4.0	7.0	13.7
Liver Diseases	0.6	2.4	3.7
Renal Diseases	21	0.7	20.2
Malignancy	9.5	2.0	5.0

Table 2. Comorbidities are categorized by the Centres for Disease Control and Prevention as known and potential risk factors for severe SARS-CoV-2 infection [22].

Established Risk Factors	Possible Risk Factors
Cancer	Asthma
Chronic Renal Diseases	Liver Diseases
Chronic Obstructive Pulmonary Disease	Pulmonary Fibrosis
Pregnancy	Cerebrovascular Disease
Obesity	Hypertension
Down Syndrome	Neurological Conditions
Immunocompromised from Solid Organ Transplant	Immunocompromised from Hematopoietic Cell Transplant
Cardiovascular Diseases (CVD)	Overweight
Heart failure/ coronary artery disease	Thalassemia
Sickle Cell Disease	Cystic Fibrosis
Type 2 Diabetes Mellitus	Type 1 Diabetes Mellitus

Multi-Organ Involvement in Coronaviruses

The emergence and spread of COVID-19 is believed to be linked to a zoonotic event that likely occurred in wild animal markets in China. Since the emergence of the disease, there have been reports of multiorgan involvement during the diagnostic process [23]. The widespread transmission of the disease is thought to be influenced by the presence of comorbidities and injury to the lungs. COVID-19 was initially identified as an uncommon pneumonia but has since transformed into a severe acute respiratory syndrome with multiple clinical presentations and the development of a dynamic and versatile disease. The fact that it is transmitted through droplets has made it a difficult task to control its spread, especially when human angiotensin-converting enzyme-2 (HACE2) receptors, which facilitate its transmission, are widely distributed throughout the body. As a result, COVID-19 can cause multi-organ dysfunction, with SARS-CoV-2 exhibiting organ-specific pathophysiology that can result in a range of manifestations, including myocardial dysfunction, neurological illness, dermatological complications, gastrointestinal symptoms, and hepatic and renal injury. Different comorbidities due to SARS-CoV, MERS CoV, and SARS-CoV-2 are the following:

In SARS-CoV

Heart

SARS-CoV-2 is associated with various cardiovascular complications such as transient cardiomegaly, paroxysmal atrial fibrillation, myocardial infarction, hypotension, tachycardia, and acute coronary syndrome.

Lungs

Acute lung strengthening, focal hemorrhage, alveolar and septal fibrosis, edema, alveolar hemorrhage, hyalin membrane formation, fibrin excretion in alveolar spaces, and respiratory injury are just a few manifestations of the lung that can appear during the acute phase of SARS-CoV infection.

Kidney

SARS-CoV causes severe kidney failure.

Liver

Liver injury is characterized by high AST and ALT levels and hepatitis.

Central Nervous System

Vision problems are linked to the presence of a chemokine called Mug in the patient's brain, as well as the chemotactic attraction of immune cells by infected brain cells [24].

In MERS-CoV

Heart

A long-lasting acute 3 arterial disease characterized by coronary angiography is caused by MERS-CoV.

Lungs

Rapidly developing pneumonitis and respiratory failure can result in septic shock, acute respiratory distress syndrome (ARDS), and even mild upper respiratory disease.

Liver

Liver damage caused by SARS-CoV-2 can result in hepatocytes dying in hepatic sinuses, invading activated Kupffer cells and macrophages, and increasing pro-inflammatory cytokines. These changes can result in lymphocyte infiltration into the liver, leading to increased AST and ALT levels. Furthermore, hepatic parenchyma can have minor portal tract involvement as well as mild cellular hydropic degeneration.

Central Nervous System

Vomiting, fever, confusion, and ataxia are just a few of the symptoms that the MERS-CoV infection can produce. Moreover, the virus has been found to affect the bilateral basal ganglia, leading to the presence of multiple patchy areas of decreased density in the periventricular region, as well as a significant region of decreased density in the anterior half of the corpus callosum that extends towards the middle of the body. Severe infections in the central nervous system caused by the virus may also spread bilaterally in the deep watershed and parasital region, with diffuse areas of focus in the cortical and subcortical regions of the parietal and temporal lobes [24].

In SARS-CoV-2

Heart

Increased troponin levels and decreased ACE2 receptor levels cause cardiac arrest and injury.

Lungs

SARS-CoV-2 in the lungs can cause edema, protein growth, formation of hyaline membranes, focal reactive hyperplasia of pneumocytes with inflammatory cellular infiltration into the lungs, multinucleated giant cells, and ARDS and SARS.

Acute kidney injury (AKI) and hematuria are symptoms of SARS-CoV-2 in the kidney.

Liver

Liver damage due to SARS-CoV-2 is characterized by increased levels of GGT, AST and ALT and decreased levels of bilirubin.

The Digestive System

SARS-CoV-2 viral load is detected in the rectum and duodenum epithelial cytoplasm in diarrhea and nausea.

Nervous System, Central

SARS-CoV-2 causes nausea, vomiting, and headaches [24].

Potential Mechanisms of Neurological Manifestation of Coronaviruses

The coronavirus family, named for its crown-like appearance, includes viruses that affect the respiratory and gastrointestinal systems. While four other coronaviruses are responsible for mild respiratory infections, SARS-CoV-2 is the seventh coronavirus to infect humans and can cause life-threatening disease. The symptoms of COVID-19 are varied, and our knowledge of the disease is still evolving. Further studies are likely to follow as more cases are reported [25, 26].

The prevalence of neurological symptoms in COVID-19 patients varies depending on the population studied, disease severity, and diagnostic methods. It has also been linked to mental health issues such as anxiety and depression, as well as cognitive problems such as confusion and difficulty concentrating. Additionally, recent research suggests that long-term neurological effects may occur in some patients. Further research is needed to better comprehend the neurological effects of COVID-19 and develop appropriate therapies for affected patients [27].

The mechanism of neural contribution in COVID-19 has been previously determined. All these factors can lead to psychiatric symptoms, cognitive dysfunctions, and neurological changes. These can be long-term and can have a lasting impact on an individual's mental and physical health. The exact mechanisms remain to be understood [28]. The data collected from Wuhan predicts that utmost problems have an initial beginning that suggests the persistent nervous system through the virus is directly involved in it. This is not similar to SARS-CoV, whose neural conclusions show a late start, suggesting a fundamental autoimmune mechanism.

Deficiency of some factors such as myoclonus, chorea, ataxia, and opsoclonus, and the inadequacy of cases of severe demyelinating polyradiculopathy expected in COVID-19 immune facilitated phenomena that are not frequently general. However, caution is indicated in depicting such statistics, as most autoimmune indicators have an extended delay. Individuals with COVID-19 infection have been found to exhibit ataxia, stroke linked to antiphospholipid antibodies, and Guillain-Barré syndrome (GBS) [29]. The question of whether pre-existing neurological conditions increase the risk of severe complications, such as respiratory failure in COVID-19, is raised by the interaction between SARS-Co-2 and the nervous system. It is evident that conditions associated with respiratory issues (*e.g.*, neuropathies, severe myopathies, and neuromuscular junction syndrome), as well as progressive Parkinson's disease (PD), increase susceptibility to a new severe course of COVID-19 infection. In addition, despite the lack of data, it is also possible that the COVID-19 virus may exacerbate neurological conditions. The authors' unpublished observations suggest that this may be the case for PD, which is not surprising given that patients with primary degenerative diseases, including dementing conditions, are significantly and often irreversibly affected by experimental instability. The absence of exercise due to social quarantine and home and public isolation poses significant challenges for individuals with neurological diseases [30].

CNS-Based Neurological Complications in Coronaviruses

Cerebrovascular Events

Initial reports propose a massive danger of thrombotic occasions, including stroke, in patients hospitalized with COVID-19. Nonetheless, there is minimal information on stroke rates and events, especially among culturally mixed residents [31]. A higher-than-average thrombotic incident rate, including severe cerebrovascular episodes in young patients, has been linked to the coronavirus

[32]. A few sources, however, have documented a decline in severe cardiovascular and cerebrovascular cases and low rates of such incidents among hospitalized COVID-19 patients during the pandemic [33]. An increased frequency of thrombotic cases, including stroke, has been linked to COVID-19. However, it is unclear what COVID-19 stroke patients' characteristics and prognoses are [34]. Of the 277 stroke victims, 105 (38.0%) had COVID-19 positive results. COVID-19-positive patients had higher rates of cryptogenic causes of stroke (51.8 *versus* 22.3%, P0.0001) and ischemic stroke in the temporal, parietal, occipital, and cerebellar regions (P=0.02, 0.002, and 0.028, respectively) compared to COVID-19-negative patients [35].

Stroke

The results of these studies suggest that stroke is present in a small but significant proportion of hospitalized COVID-19 patients. The rate of stroke appears to be higher in patients with severe COVID-19 symptoms compared to those with milder symptoms. Further research is needed to better understand the link between stroke and SARS-CoV-2 infection. Another report noted that the proportion of patients with a history of stroke infected with severe COVID-19 was 2.5. In the first observational study, which reviewed 221 patients, 11 (5%) had an acute ischemic stroke, 1 (0%) had cerebral venous sinus thrombosis (CVST), and 1 (0%) had a cerebral hemorrhage. The second prospective investigation of 288 patients revealed that 9 (2.5%) had an ischemic stroke. Among the nine case reports and case series, 21 patients were discussed, of whom 16 were men and 5 were women. The average age was 59.8 years (63.1 years for men and 49.8 years for women), although a case series of young strokes may have inadvertently skewed the data [35, 36]. Most of the strokes [19] were ischemic, although three changed to a hemorrhagic type and two began as hemorrhagic. Eight of the 19 ischemic cases had multiple infarcts. Imaging revealed blood clot formation in 13 patients: 6 in the central cerebral hemisphere, 2 in the posterior cerebral hemisphere, 3 in the spinal cord/basilar region, and 1 in the inner carotid. In another case, there were multiple sites of blood clotting. The remaining two were lacunar infected. All six patients had thrombus formation, but they were not visible because four of them were stable with major artery obstructions. There have been reports of additional thrombotic events. Pneumonic emboli were found in four patients (three bilaterally), myocardial infarction was observed in one, and there were also ischemic organs and kidney infections described in some reports. Of the 19 patients with ischemic stroke, four died, six needed to stay in the intensive care unit (ICU), one needed to stay in the stroke unit, two needed to go to a stroke rehabilitation center, and five recovered. In one instance, the result was not stated [37].

COVID-19 patients with D-dimer levels (1,000 g/l) and anti-cardiolipin antibodies were detected in nine cases. Lupus anticoagulant was detected in four cases, with varying results. A medium titer of IgM anti-cardiolipin antibodies was detected in one patient with five out of six positive lupus anticoagulant cases. The antibodies to anti-cardiolipin IgA and anti-2-glycoprotein IIGA and IgG were positive in two patients from Beijing, though none of them had lupus anticoagulant activity [7].

Guillain-Barré Syndrome and Variants

As of May 1, 2020, eight reports were published [38]. Describing a total of 13 cases of para-COVID-19 or post-coronavirus Glenberry syndrome (GBS), including six single case reports and two case series with 2-5 patients [39]. There were 10 men and 3 women in this group, with an average age of 58.9 (males were 55.8 and females were 69.7). Two patients, however, tested negative for SARS-CoV-2 RT-QPCR. One patient was identified 24 days after the onset of COVID-19 respiratory symptoms despite having a CT chest deformity [1] in the majority of cases. Another instance saw the onset of GBS 8 days prior to respiratory side effects.

Eight reports on para-COVID-19 or post-coronavirus GBS cases were released as of May 1, 2020. Of the 13 cases, 11 had flexic flaccid tetraparesis, five had bilateral facial weakness, and seven needed intubation and ventilation [39]. A Miller-Fisher mutation was present in two instances [1]. Between 3 and 28 days, or an average of 11, passed between the onset of respiratory symptoms and the onset of neurological symptoms. IVIG was administered to 12 out of 13 cases, with 2 patients requiring continuous mechanical ventilation in the ICU, 3 undergoing rehabilitation, 4 discharged, and 1 deceased within a month. The outcomes of the remaining 3 patients are unknown. Between the first and fifth day of neurological symptoms, lumbar punctures were done on 11 patients, with white cell counts typically normal or slightly elevated (1-9/L in 5 cases). In 3 cases, protein levels were within the normal range; in the remaining 8 cases, they were above the normal range (range: 48–193 mg/dL; normal: 104.6 mg/dL). All 8 cases tested for SARS-COV2 PCR in CSF tested negative. Ten patients underwent neurophysiological evaluations between days 3 and 12 of neurological symptoms, and six of them displayed changes that were consistent with demyelination and four with axonal GBS. Only 4 cases of anti-ganglioside antibody testing were reported, 3 of which were negative. One Miller Fisher patient tested positive for the GD1b antibody but negative for the GQ1b antibody.

Encephalitis, Meningoencephalitis, and Encephalopathy

As of May 1, 2020, eight reports were published, of which seven were single case reports [40], and one was a case series (n = 2) [41]. Five of the nine cases that were reported involved females, three involved males, and one did not include a gender designation. The gender split was 42.0 for men and 60.8 for women, making the average age 55.5. Fever and confusion were frequent clinical signs. Three patients had meningitis, four had headaches, three had seizures, and three had symptoms of frontal release [40]. Three cases—two with encephalopathy and one with seizures—were examined using EEG, and all displayed general slowing [43]. Seven of the nine cases that were published underwent CSF testing for SARS-CoV-2, while the other two noted that CSF testing was unavailable at their institutions [40]. While five cases tested negative for SARS-CoV-2 by CSF PCR, two cases tested positive [41].

Broad-spectrum antibiotics and antiviral drugs were the mainstays of the majority of patients' initial treatments. In two cases, supportive care and symptomatic treatment helped patients recover quickly within four days. One patient received high doses of steroids in addition to hydroxychloroquine and recovered dramatically after responding poorly to antiviral therapy. He was released after two weeks. Mannitol infusion [44] and hydroxychloroquine [45] were used to treat two additional patients who did not respond well to the initial course of treatment. In the intensive care unit (ITU), two patients required ongoing mechanical ventilation [42] and the prognosis for two additional cases was unknown [40].

Demyelinating Disease

The majority of patients' initial treatments were primarily comprised of broad-spectrum antibiotics and antiviral medications. In two instances, patients recovered fully within four days with the aid of supportive care and symptomatic treatment. After failing to respond to antiviral therapy, one patient received high doses of steroids in addition to hydroxychloroquine and made a remarkable recovery. After two weeks, he was discharged. Two additional patients who did not respond well to the initial course of treatment were treated with mannitol infusion [44] and hydroxychloroquine [45]. The prognosis for two additional cases in the intensive care unit (ITU) was unknown [40], and two patients in the ITU required ongoing mechanical ventilation [42].

The discovery of SARS-CoV-2 in a patient's cerebrospinal fluid (CSF) in a recent report, which was supported by deep sequencing, raises the possibility that COVID-19 and demyelinating diseases, even without respiratory symptoms, are related to each other [46]. For the first time in this report, deep sequencing was used to confirm the presence of SARS-CoV-2 in CSF. Research is still underway to determine how the virus enters the CNS. The ghalan nerve [47], or hematogenous route, which has been observed in other coronaviruses, is thought to be a possible entry route of SARS-CoV-2 into the central nervous system. A patient had respiratory symptoms for three weeks before taking an oropharyngeal swab, which led to a negative result of SARS-CoV-2 in a PCR test. Since the CNS is an immune-specialized region, SARS-CoV-2 infection may last longer there. The SARS-CoV-2 virus can also enter the central nervous system (CNS) by infecting blood cells that can cross the blood and brain barrier (BBB) after completing their initial replication into respiratory cells [48]. Since CSF-controlled RT-PCR resulted in a negative result, the current case does not indicate ongoing CNS disease.

Impaired Consciousness

Coronavirus is an infectious ailment caused by SARS-CoV-2 [49]. The significant worries about SARS-CoV-2 infections are pneumonic inconveniences, neurological indications, such as tipsiness, migraine, taste, and smell impairments, *etc.*, [50]. Additionally, SARS-CoV-2 RNA was found in the cerebrospinal fluid of an encephalitis patient [7]. The first signs of COVID-19 can frequently be neurological symptoms. Several theories have been put forth to explain the virus's capacity for neuroinvasion, including its affinity for ACE2 receptors and prior reports of neuroinvasion by other coronaviruses [29]. Damage to the nervous system can also be caused by indirect mechanisms [7]. A 73-year-old Caucasian man with a history of steroid ataxia, confusion, high blood pressure, and type 2 diabetes presented with these symptoms. The patient was mentally healthy, engaged in his profession, and had no prior neurological history. Meningeal symptoms were not detected during neurological examination, but background alpha activity in the posterior areas of the EEG was responsive, unstable, and symmetrical. The EEG also showed that intermittent spikes occur in the frontotemporal lobe without obvious epilepsy, mainly on the left side, and random, low voltage, central polymorph delta components in the anterior frontal left cortex. Hyperventilation or short photic stimulation did not affect activity [51].

Movement Disorders

There is evidence that SARS-CoV-2, the trigger of the COVID-19 pandemic, is increasing the spread of psychiatric disorders. Even among previously healthy individuals, there have been reports of new cases of mental health conditions such as reactive psychosis, anxiety, insomnia, panic, and obsessive-compulsive disorder. In the following case study, the patient experienced unusual movements while sitting, walking, and resting, as well as lower limb tremors with irregular frequency and amplitude [52]. The patient was later identified as having functional movement disorder. After seven days, the patient showed mild symptoms of COVID-19, including fever, loss of smell, muscle pain and gastrointestinal discomfort, as well as when two of the patient's family members also tested positive for SARS-CoV-2, these symptoms began to appear. Several serum tests were performed on the patient, who was then referred to a neurologist. However, none of the results indicated the presence of any underlying disease or infection [53].

CNS Vasculitis

Patients with severe COVID-19 reported symptoms of unifocal and multifocal lesions as well as CNS vasculitis, but histological studies are required to confirm the precise nature of the pathology. Some studies claim that the simultaneous occurrence of diffuse skin lesions and severe ischemic injuries in the brain on MRI may indicate cerebral vasculitis that targets the endothelium, whereas other studies support thromboembolism on vasculitis [54]. Six of the 20 COVID-19 victims had their brain tissue examined by a neuropathologist; the majority of the lesions were characterized as "small and patchy peripheral and deep perineal ischemic infarcts" and lacked any histological signs of vasculitis [55]. Finally, a potential mechanism for CNS disease in serious respiratory diseases, particularly COVID-19, is suggested by the variable viral RNA presence in the brains of patients with acute immune-thrombosis of the pulmonary artery area and neurological disease related to COVID-19 [56].

Cranial Nerves Disorder

Increasing research suggests that COVID-19 can affect the nervous system, with encephalopathy, severe cerebral artery diseases, severe polyradiculopathy, and neuropathies being the most common manifestations of this effect [57]. The CNS and PNS neurotropism of SARS-CoV-2 can directly cause these symptoms, or immune-mediated para-infectious or post-infectious mechanisms can cause them systematically. The effects on the CNS and PNS are believed to occur when the virus enters cells through ACE-2 receptors. It is thought that the virus can reach the CNS through retrograde neuronal transmission or hematological spread [58]. Although it is unclear whether this is the result of an immune response or direct invasion, reports suggest that COVID-19 may also cause the involvement of cranial nerves in addition to the neurological symptoms mentioned above. The role of the cranial nerves in COVID-19 is becoming more widely understood, and reports of various cranial nerve deficits linked to the condition have been made [58, 59]. These include dysphagia brought on by injuries to the vestibulocochlear, facial, oculomotor, abducens, trochlear, optic, and olfactory nerves [60 - 65], as well as dysphagia brought on by damage to the glossopharyngeal, vagus, and hypoglossal nerves [57]. It is not yet known, though, whether the involvement of the cranial nerves is an indirect result of viral invasion or an immune-mediated reaction brought on by the infection. To fully comprehend the type and degree of cranial nerve involvement in COVID-19, more investigation is required [66]. The current literature describes cranial nerve involvement in COVID-19 patients, including dysphagia brought on by damage to the glossopharyngeal, vagus, and hyoglossus [60], as well as injury to the vestibulocochlear [61], facial [62], oculomotor [63], abducens [64], trochlearis [50], optics [65], and olfactories [61].

The prevalence of cranial nerve expression in COVID-19 patients has not been specifically studied, but there are case reports and small case series describing these phenomena. For example, in a case report published in the Journal of Medical Virology, a COVID-19 patient suffered from severe bilateral optic neuritis and cranial nerve VI paralysis [7, 68]. A patient with COVID-19 who developed multiple cranial neuropathies, including facial, oculomotor, and abducens nerve palsies, was the subject of another case report that was published in JAMA Neurology [68]. In addition, three COVID-19 patients who presented with peripheral facial nerve palsy were described in a case series that was published in the Journal of Neurology [69]. To fully understand some aspects, however, more research is still needed; for example, on the precise mechanism underlying the more frequent cranial nerve involvement, which is unknown when the disease is in its early stages. At the beginning of infection, COVID-19 patients frequently report losing their sense of taste and smell, whereas ophthalmo-paresis, dysphagia, and problems with vision and hearing are uncommon. According to a multi-center study conducted in Europe, 85.6% and 88.0% of COVID-19 patients had a loss of taste and smell, respectively. The virus is thought to primarily harm cranial nerves through local immune responses and direct nerve invasion in the respiratory tract based on this information. We would expect loss of smell and taste to occur as frequently as the involvement of other cranial nerves if it is caused by CNS damage or a systemic immune response. However, although N. facialus and N. ophthalmicus, the cranial nerves that protrude in this area and are closest to the respiratory tract, are often predictable, N. hypoglossus, N. glosopharyngius, N. vagus, and N. trigeminus are involved less frequently, raising additional questions that need to be addressed. It is now known that the way these nerves can penetrate the respiratory tract will naturally increase their exposure, which is an important point when trying to understand the current situation. Additionally, it has been discovered that COVID-19 patients who have difficulty swallowing due to the absorption of their vagal and glossopharyngeal nerves experience a more severe disease course and require longer hospital stays [50].

Acute Disseminated Encephalomyelitis

ADEM is a rare disease that is often post-viral and affects children more than adults. Clinically, it varies widely, typically leading to encephalopathy and multifocal deficits. Flare hypertensives are often seen on MRI in the dark white matter and where the white and grey matter combine. While this happens occasionally, post-contrast improvement is usually puncture or edge upgrading. Spread restrictions can be observed, especially early during the disease [65]. The etiology of intraventricular hemorrhage in this case is unclear, but ADEM lesions may be hemorrhagic [67]. Blood pressure is kept under control overall, and anticoagulation is not used. With a severe demyelinating event, the location and progression of lesions on MRI, the development of fewer contraindications, clinical examinations, and CSF are reliable indicators. Weeks after a severe viral infection, the clinical situation in this case is encouraging for the development of ADEM. ADEM was identified in a child who recovered from a coronavirus infection. Early diagnosis and treatment may prevent further neurological damage, so it is important to be aware of the possibility of this complication. Patients should be monitored for the development of neurological symptoms and, if needed, referred for further evaluation and treatment.

Seizures

Animals and humans both contract enteric and respiratory diseases from coronaviruses enveloped in non-segmented positive-sense RNA infections [7]. Since the viral structure and disease pathway of the majority of coronaviruses are similar, recently discovered mechanisms of infection for other coronaviruses may also apply to SARS-CoV-2. Neurotropism is one of the fundamental components of coronaviruses, according to growing evidence [7]. One study specifically looked at the neurological symptoms of COVID-19 and found that 25 percent of patients had headaches (13 percent), fatigue (17 percent), impaired cognition (8 percent), severe cerebral artery problems (3 percent), ataxia (0.5 percent) and seizures (0.5 percent) as manifestations of the CNS. Additionally, a report of meningitis/meningitis caused by SARS-CoV-2 was prepared with seizures. SARS-CoV-2 RNA was found in CSF. Another report described a COVID-19 patient as having focal status epilepsy.

Neuromuscular Abnormalities

Myalgia

The prevalence of myalgia was 35.8% (range 11 to 50%) according to a meta-analysis of clinical characteristics (10 examinations, 1995 patients, 10 examinations published between December 2019 and February 2020). Among the symptoms that recurred were fever (88.5%), hack (68.6%), expectoration (28.2%), and dyspnea (21.9%). Tipsiness, loose bowels, sickness, and heaving were more unusual symptoms. However, in COVID-19 patients, the casualty rate was 5%, and the discharge rate was 52% [7]. According to another meta-analysis, myalgia was found in 21.9% of COVID-19 patients (55 investigations, 8,697 patients, spread between January 1, 2020 and March 16, 2020). Fever (78.4%), fatigue (34%), pregnancy (23.7%), loss of appetite (22.9%), chest tightness (22.9%) and dyspnea (20.6%) were other common symptoms. For the patients who were analyzed, fever was more common before January 31. According to this theory, unusual phenomena became more common as the pandemic progressed [49].

More than 50% of COVID-19 patients who participated in Lichen *et al.*'s study had myelgia. Muscle pain was one of the independent indicators of non-improvement in COVID-19 patients in a review by Zhang *et al.* Men, extreme COVID-19 status, expectation, and low albumin at admission were other independent indicators [24]. The recurrence of known side effects of COVID-19 infection in pregnant patients is similar to common symptoms. According to the study, there was no evidence of vertical COVID-19 disease transmission [69]. Fever was equally common in a study comparing the clinical characteristics of COVID-19 disease and SARS-CoV-1 infection, but myalgia and loose stools were more frequent in COVID-19 than in SARS-CoV-1. In a study on 1420 COVID-19 patients from Europe, older patients had higher rates of myalgia, fatigue, and fever than younger patients, who had higher rates of ear, nose, and throat symptoms. Patients who tested positive for COVID-19 and had respiratory illnesses experienced more severe side effects, such as fever (82% *vs* 44%), frailty (85% *vs* 50%), and myalgia (61% *vs* 27 days) than COVID-19-negative patients (average 7 *vs* 3 days). Myalgia persisted for an average of 23 days after the end of viral shedding. Heck, anosmia, anesthesia, and sore throat were among the various phenomena that persisted even after the viral shedding stopped [70].

Myositis/Rhabdomyolysis

There were nine patients (all male, ages 16 to 88) with myositis/rhabdomyolysis associated with COVID-19 [71]. Eight patients reported limb or generalized weakness. There were myalgias in four patients. One patient had myalgia fever and dyspnea but no muscle weakness [24]. One patient experienced regular muscle jerking, shivering, and leg numbness [72]. Only one patient had urine that was cola-coloured [73]. RBCs were found in the urine of three patients. CPK levels were elevated in all patients [72, 73]. The patient with the highest elevated CPK level (427,656 IU/L) provided urine that had cola in it. On chest imaging, six patients had abnormalities such as multifocal opacities, ground glass opacities, pneumonia, and lung effusion. Mechanical ventilation was necessary for some patients [73]. With traditional treatment, five patients got better.

Myasthenia Gravis

No new cases of Myasthenia gravis connected to COVID-19 have been reported. There were two reports of the severity of myasthenia gravis related to the COVID-19 epidemic in patients aged 42 to 90 years, four of whom were women [74]. Although only one patient had myasthenia gravis that tested positive for muscle-specific kinase (MuSK), five other patients had the disorder. The inconsistent grouping of patients first developed a cough, sore throat, fever, and shortness of breath, followed by an aggravation of all myasthenic symptoms in all patients. Steroids were started for four patients. Intravenous immunoglobulins were given to two patients. Two patients received mycophenolate mofetil, but it was temporarily stopped because of COVID-19 disease. MMF was continued after the two patients were discharged from the clinic. Five patients had improved at the time the report was published, while one patient was on a mechanical ventilator [38].

Neuropathy

Six COVID-19-related neuropathy patients were the subject of three reports. It was claimed that the neuropathy of their patients was not the same as GBS. A 68-year-old woman was initially reported to have upper breathing problems with motor neuron quadriparesis in her lower extremities. The patient lost consciousness due to respiratory entrapment, so electrophysiological tests were unable to be completed [75]. A 69-year-old man with gait ataxia and lower limb weakness had no COVID-19-related side effects. His nasopharyngeal swab was confirmed by RT-PCR for SARS-CoV-2. No electrophysiology test was performed. The patient suddenly recovered. These two cases of a particular type of neuropathy could not be treated without nerve conduction tests. Four patients (all male, aged 52 to 72) with quadriparesis and CNS manifestations were presented by Chaumont *et al.* [76] following or during the mechanical ventilator weaning stage.

Anosmia and Dysgeusia

Dysgesia and anosmia are common symptoms of COVID-19 and are extremely common in most patients. Anosmia was an early sensorineural reduction, and it gave simultaneous indications of anosmia and dysgesia in almost every patient (94%), especially during the most severe stages of the disease. Some observers have specifically considered how to examine the relationship between the temporary presentation of the mantle and the rapid deterioration and the severity of COVID-19 [77]. In a new meta-analysis of eight studies on 11,054 COVID-19 patients, we reported the expression of anosmia and dysgeusia in 74.89% and 81.3% of ambulatory and 81.3% of hospitalized patients, respectively. Overall, the data suggest that anosmia and dysgeusia may appear in isolation or simultaneously in varying degrees at all stages of the disease cycle [78].

However, there are other meta-analyses where rates of anosmia and dysgeusia were not as common. For example, an analysis of six studies published by Carrillo Larco *et al.* [79] showed that anosmia increased from 22% to 68% in COVID-19 patients, while taste disturbance, subclassified dyslexia, and distorted taste sensation were present in only 33%, 20% and 21% of patients, respectively. The third meta-analysis included five studies with dysgeusia. Due to the different results, which may be related to access to much less detailed studies in general since the pandemic in January 2020, concrete conclusions cannot be drawn from the past. To validate discoveries, long-term, upcoming studies with a larger cohort must be adopted [79].

Care and Management of Neurological Cases

The pandemic situation made it necessary to adopt procedures to admit patients to clinics for neurological care, such as stroke programs, emergency clinics, and pre-vast code stroke protocols, and to secure staff caring for these patients. Despite the existence of tele-stroke programs prior to the pandemic, it has also been important when making decisions about stroke patients who also have SARS-CoV-2 infection [80].

The application of previously exclusive tools occasionally used, like email and other electronic tools, has been prompted by the handling of crises [81].

Because of their advanced age or the characteristics of their illnesses, patients frequently choose not to use these developments. Neurologists may be able to evaluate clinical changes remotely with the help of photographs or videos that patients or their loved ones have taken. For instance, video may be used to evaluate balance changes, walking, and oculomotor function. These tactics have given neurologist divisions the ability to continue the patient follow-up and care plan despite the circumstances [82].

Operative Decisions

Patients frequently decide not to use these developments due to their advanced age or the characteristics of their illnesses. With the aid of pictures or videos that patients or their loved ones have taken, neurologists may be able to assess clinical changes remotely. Video could be used, for example, to assess changes in gait, balance, and oculomotor function. These strategies have enabled the neurologist divisions to carry out the patient follow-up and care plan despite the situation [82].

Operative Decisions Regarding Neurological Care Provision during the COVID-19 Pandemic

- Execution of a convenient overhauling plan or emergency course of action tending to the neurology department's assets and territories of responsibility.
- Organization of hospital confirmation and neurological emergencies
- Implementation of a telemedicine model for patients to conduct remote interviews and provide ongoing care, as well as to address any issues that may arise.
- Establishing a safe off-site care facility for patients experiencing sudden neurological crises, ailments requiring on-site treatment, or who need to receive critical medications during the visit.
- Developing protocols for the provision of essential in-hospital care.
- Clearly defining roles and responsibilities in the internal coordination of care nervous system science office
- Definition of explicit consideration pathways for crises

The relationship between neurological crises and hospital admissions becomes complex when many patients are infected with a disease. Initially, taking care of hospitalized patients through teams of doctors was not feasible due to the shortage of nervous system specialists who were busy helping patients in other fields of medicine. Moreover, with the inability to hold face-to-face departmental meetings, new forms of communication and coordination had to be implemented. Unfortunately, some healthcare providers also have to stay in quarantine. Nonetheless, a reasonable approach to caring for potentially infected patients is to maintain care continuity using telephone consultations and electronic resources [83-85].

This requirement results from the requirement for social isolation to stop the disease's spread, which has impacted clinical procedures. Healthcare facilities and transportation, however, are now potential sources of infection due to the rapid spread of the disease. Due to the importance of neurological decision-making, it has become necessary to concentrate on providing care through telephone consultations. These technical consultations should be instructive for both patients and doctors, who base clinical decisions on scant information. Due to preventative measures, speaking with patients right away is almost always possible, and follow-up interactions are more common than they were prior to the pandemic.

Patients express high levels of satisfaction with this individualized care, which benefits their wellbeing [85, 86].

Nervous system specialists should also be aware of any contamination among their patients, which may affect the diagnosis of underlying neurological conditions. Nervous system specialists must decide the best course of action for each case, weighing the risk/benefit ratio of the patient visiting the clinic, which should be avoided where possible if patients exhibit new symptoms or progression of a neurological infection. Remote follow-up involves making a case-by-case assessment of whether to delay routine complementary examinations that demand a hospital visit [86]. Nervous system specialists should also consider postponing clinic medications if necessary, weighing the effects of delaying or suspending treatment against the potential risks of infection transmission.

Neurological Complications of COVID-19-Related Treatments

Neurologists should be aware of the underlying sensory system symptoms of these treatments and constantly improve as COVID-19 treatment proceeds according to the latest evidence of viability and clinical preliminary studies. In addition to static medications, sedatives, and antivirals — last but not least in the relationship against thrombotic treatment — are medications that are frequently used for both children and adults. Antiviral therapies and drugs interact primarily with the nervous system and brain. Chloroquine and hydroxychloroquine have also been used in mild structures in COVID-19, although the use of both drugs has resulted in diametrically opposite results. Neurologists should be aware of the underlying sensory system symptoms of these treatments and stay up to date as COVID-19 treatment proceeds in response to the latest evidence of viability and clinical preliminary studies. Sedatives and antivirals, last but not least in the relationship against thrombotic treatment, are the drugs that are most commonly used in addition to static medications for both children and adults. Antiviral drugs and medications are fundamentally relevant for the nervous system and brain. Chloroquine and hydroxychloroquine have also been used in mild structures in COVID-19, even though the use of both drugs has yielded conflicting results. Furthermore, due to the involvement of CYP450, ritonavir can improve the absorption of phenytoin and other antiepileptic and antipsychotic tranquilizers. Furthermore, azithromycin in combination with hydroxychloroquine is feasible in COVID-19. Patients with Myasthenia gravis who are taking macrolides need to be monitored because it has been suggested that these medications may exacerbate symptoms or cause the onset of a new myasthenic disorder. Finally, monoclonal antibodies used in COVID-19 (mostly tocilizumab [87] and anakinra) have not demonstrated effects on the nervous system or association with sensory system infections [88].

Symptoms Related to the Peripheral Nervous System

Neurotropic viruses are those that can transduce and replicate in neurons, such as poliomyelitis, Japanese encephalitis, rabies, and coronaviruses [89, 90]. These viruses' neurovirulence mediates the disease pathogenesis in neurons [91]. Numerous neurotropic viruses have been found to infect the PNS as well as the CNS. Since all of these viruses fall under the same category, they all exhibit similar infectious behaviors on a larger scale. As a result, using SARS-CoV-2 as an example to list the neurological symptoms, especially PNS symptoms, is typical of this genre [92]. Neurological symptoms caused by SARS-CoV-2 are typically divided into CNS and PNS symptoms, as shown in Fig. (**1**).

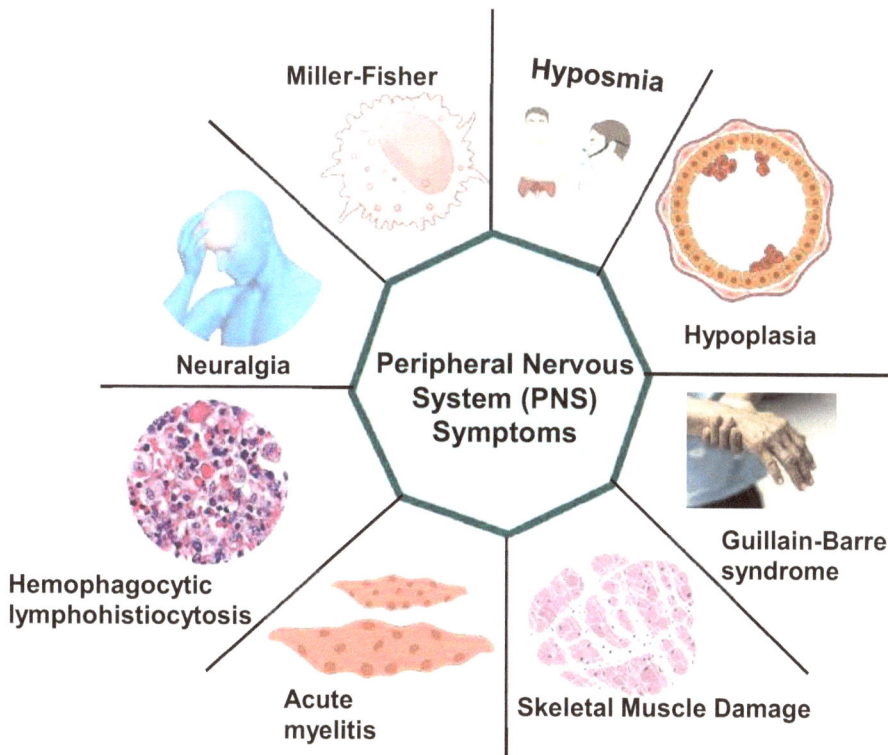

Fig. (1). PNS-related symptoms.

Anosmia struck a 48-year-old healthcare professional suddenly and without any warning signs. He had a COVID-19 infection but was unaware of any underlying comorbidities. He continued to exhibit no pulmonary or extrapulmonary manifestation symptoms, and a gradual recovery was anticipated. Ageusia and anosmia are frequently seen in asymptomatic individuals or are thought to be early disease symptoms that warrant concern. Since they might be carriers, these should be kept apart from others. Patients with SARS-CoV-2 infection typically regain their senses as they recover. The precise mechanisms underlying anosmia remain unknown. However, numerous explanations for the attack strategy have been proposed [93]. Research on animal models demonstrates coronavirus's capacity to transmurally spread into the brain *via* olfactory pathways and compromise the integrity of the olfactory neuroepithelium through the expression of ACE2 and TMPRSS2 in sustentacular cells. Anosmia is the result of the disruption of the olfactory neuroepithelium. Anosmia can also result from inflammation or pain in the olfactory nerves as opposed to structural damage to the receptors.

Some patients were reported as phantasmic and perismic. The use of nasal corticosteroids is not recommended due to their unexpected results. Dry cough was associated with cephalgia or myalgia due to bilateral inflammatory obstruction. PNS-related phenomena include a condition called GBS. This immune-mediated complication involves peripheral nerves and nerve roots. It is an autoimmune disorder that presents limb weakness and neurological paralysis [94]. The most common phenotype of GBS is "severe inflammatory demyelinating polyradiculoneuropathy". In this condition, autoantibodies attack the myelin membrane. In another condition known as "acute motor axonal neuropathy," autoantibodies attack the organ membranes of the peripheral nerve. Some patients have been described as paroxysms and phantomic. Due to the unexpected results of nasal corticosteroids, their use is not advised. Because of the bilateral inflammatory barrier of the mantle lungs, dry cough was associated with either cephalgia or myalgia. GBS is another condition whose manifestations are associated with PNS. In a condition known as GBS, the PNS is mistakenly attacked by the immune system. Peripheral nerves and nerve roots are involved in this immune-mediated complication. It is an autoimmune condition that causes paralysis of the nervous system and organ weakness. "Severe inflammatory demyelinating polyrediculoneuropathy" is the most common phenotype of GBS. In this condition, myelin membranes are attacked by autoantibodies. The nerve membranes of the peripheral nerve are attacked by autoantibodies called "acute motor axonal neuropathy". Its pathway mechanism shares a significant degree of similarity with the autoimmune disorder mechanism. This is the most common cause of severe paralysis. Early symptoms include tingling and weakness in the legs, but they quickly spread throughout the body and paralyze it. A lot of GBS cases infected with the coronavirus have been reported. Different symptoms were seen in these cases. On January 23, 2020, China received the GBS report on coronavirus for the first time. A 61-year-old woman was suffering from lower limb weakness. She suffered from respiratory disease and neurological symptoms after testing positive for SARS-CoV-2. Demyelination, a common symptom of

GBS, was also reported to cause peripheral neuropathy in some cases. The entire disorder is treated by giving IVIG as a treatment dose.

Different cases of GBS infected with SARS-CoV-2 showed different symptoms, for example, symmetrical ascending paralysis caused by bacteria or viruses after respiratory or gastrointestinal infection, respiratory inability, syphilis in both legs and legs, and the feeling of pinprick and light touch began to decrease remotely. Mild herniation of two intervertebral discs was also observed by MRI. The mechanism of SARS-CoV-2 in triggering GBS is not clear, but it has been suggested that SARS-CoV-2 may play a role in producing antibodies against specific gangliosides that participate in specific forms of GBS. Most patients contracted various infectious diseases within 4-6 weeks before the onset of GBS symptoms, such as Mycoplasma pneumonia, Herpes simplex virus, human immunodeficiency virus (HIV), chikungunya, dengue, hepatitis virus A, B and E, cytomegalovirus, zoster virus, Zika virus and Epstein-Barr virus. GBS was detected in 4 people living in a group of 23 people who had confirmed MERS-CoV.

Notably, complications related to the peripheral nervous system emerged 2-3 weeks after recovering from the respiratory infection. In comparison to the general population, including children, those who contracted the ZIKA virus had very poor prognoses. Additionally, reverse GBS because of possible SARS-Co--2 detection. A condition known as cytokine storm, which is brought on by PNS abnormalities, causes patients with SARS-CoV-2 to have acute transverse myelitis and acute necrotizing myelitis [95]. By releasing a large number of interleukins, macrophages, interferons, and chemokines during this cytokine storm, there is a severe inflammatory reaction [12]. An acute transverse myelitis case study involving a 60-year-old patient with SARS-CoV-2 infection was carried out. After discharge, respiratory illness and progressive neurological deficits, as well as deficits in both lower extremities and bladder dysfunction, appeared as symptoms. These symptoms progress to motor neuron lesion symptoms after a few days. Acute myelitis affected areas of the specific central part of the spinal cord that appear to be extremely intense on the T2 sequence, potentially demonstrating changes in bone swelling. This abnormality was treated with methylprednisolone. Another case involved neurological symptoms that appeared after fever and cough. Weakness, pain in the cervical region, balance problems, and apathy in the left hand were noted as symptoms. Upper motor neuron lesion (UMN) exposure was observed during a neurological examination [96]. There were gaps in research work for vitamins, autoimmune, and infectious etiologies. Spinal cord imaging revealed no changes in the brain, but expressions of patchy enhancer lesions spreading with T2 hyperintensity from the medulla to the C7 indicated severe transverse myelitis. Severe transverse myelitis in SARS-

CoV-2 patients also causes T1 central necrosis of the spinal cord. Bone muscle damage and myalgia have been observed in a variety of neurological complications associated with SARS-CoV-2 infection. Patients with SARS-Co--2 have a rapid increase in myalgia, which is linked to the severity of infection. Myalgia and fatigue were the most frequent and obvious symptoms seen in adults [97]. Patients also had increased levels of the enzyme creatinine kinase (CK) in both acute and mild SARS-CoV-2 infection. Patients receiving treatment experienced symptomatic relief from myalgia and a reduction in viral load [93]. Earlier studies from China reported that 40% of cases had dementia, consisting of both mild and severe cases.

A second prospective investigation examined cases of mild to moderate SARS-CoV-2. In this study, myalgia was present in 62.5% of patients [1]. According to one analysis, myalgia has no statistically significant relationship with SARS-CoV-2 patients and cannot be taken into account as a prognostic factor in patients with advanced illness. One observational series shows that severe cases of SARS-CoV-2 are more likely to cause muscle injury rather than mild, as evidenced by myalgia with serum creatin kinase levels (greater than 200 U/L). Patients with muscle damage are particularly prone to kidney and liver disorders, which can cause multi-organ failure. Rhabdomyolysis, a possible delayed complication, has only occasionally been documented [98]. Due to muscle inflammation caused by serious diseases such as myopathy and polyneuropathy, coronavirus-infected patients are more likely to develop certain diseases and muscle weakness, but still constructed analyses need to be planned. However, it is also likely that different types of bone muscle are possibly more vulnerable to SARS-CoV-2 because these muscles express more ACE2 receptors without the nervous system's involvement. A series of cytokines, including IL-6, released during muscle loss disrupt muscle metabolic homeostasis. SARS-CoV-2 infection represents such exclusion. Muscle injuries are a direct result of viral interactions with ACE2 receptors on muscle, or they may be the unexpected result of systemic cytokine-mediated disruption that causes homeostatic disruption without neuroinfection [99].

Care and Management of Neurological Cases

MERS, SARS-CoV-1, and COVID-19 are the most widespread members of this group of positive-sense, single-stranded RNA viruses. In the initial stages of an infection, these viruses have the potential to cause non-specific neurological symptoms [100]. Rarely has the infection been found to be asymptomatic or to have only minor symptoms like a lingering fever, a productive cough, and fatigue. They may be neuroinvasive, and side effects can result in encephalitis, acute disseminated encephalomyelitis, meningitis, and convulsive unconsciousness during seizures [101]. Retrospective studies suggest that neurological and neuromuscular symptoms may be brought on by the CNS and PNS tropism. Other than invading the pulmonary, renal, and hepatic systems, the Coronaviridae use the following mechanisms to attack the CNS:

1. Hematogenous virus transmission
2. PNS to CNS retrograde neural dissemination

Interleukin-6, C-reactive proteins, and coagulation tests (anti-thrombin iii, D-dimer) are examples of prognostic indicators that can be used under the mordancy of neurological signs. These viruses presumably invade the CNS's supportive cells, such as glial cells, astrocytes, and oligodendrocytes, in addition to the functional cells, such as neurons [102]. The MERS-CoV uses the following routes for coronavirus transmission:

1. Trans-synaptic neuroinvasion
2. Olfactory nerve transfer
3. Vascular endothelium invasion

Complex infections gradually become more confusing, signaling a change to a better strategy. Steps for supportive and therapeutic psychological treatment are part of proper management provided by neurorehabilitation units [100] to treat patients by administering particular therapeutic substances along with physical treatments.

1. Dysgeusia and anosmia caused by sensory symptoms
2. Include mild cases of olfactory dysfunction and
3. Chemo-sensory dysfunction.

SARS-COV-1

The virus briskly spreads trans-synoptically and may cause an axonal variant of GBS and ischemic strokes.

MERS-COV

Binds to the di-peptidyl peptidase 4 receptors on neural entry cells using cells, causing seizures, acute disseminated encephalomyelitis, Bickerstaff encephalitis, and diffused ischemic infarcts.

SARS-COV-2

The ACE2 receptor serves as the attachment site. Here, TMPRSS 2 primes the virus spikes before they are diffused in the CNS by sympathetic pathways in the brain stem, leading to delirium and impaired consciousness [103].

Immunoglobulins administered intravenously (IVIG) for GBS, corticosteroids administered as nasal saline irrigation for olfactory dysfunction, and steroid high-dose therapy (ribavirin, antivirals, and interferons) for critical polyneuropathies are all essential components of therapeutic management. The majority of improvements in critical case rehabilitation come from better management of advanced and complicated infections. This can be done in patients' homes or even in specialized neurorehabilitation facilities, offering them therapeutic, physiological, physical, and mental support. To provide a safe environment that ensures recovery, careful handling, the use of PPEs, and trial-based therapeutic chemical treatments must be well executed.

CONCLUSION AND FUTURE PERSPECTIVE

By being well developed, epidemic/epidemic virus control and prevention strategies can be upgraded or improved. Self-protection strategies such as hand washing, use of disinfectants, wearing masks, disinfecting surfaces with alcohol or bleach, and quarantining infected people are considered critical to a thorough plan that can be evaluated and encouraged that involves the entire community. SARS-CoV-2 is more contagious and spreads mainly through bronchial droplets. Hospitals have reported the highest transmission rate of SARS-CoV-2. A high level of infection in health was linked to inappropriate or inadequate infection-checking measures during the outbreak, such as the reuse of N95 masks and frequent use of personal protective equipment. In this way, the epidemic was effectively controlled in 2004. The WHO has published a framework that is divided into six phases of the epidemic, starting with preparation, planning and routine case surveillance, continuing with avoiding an upcoming international outbreak, and ending with disruption to global transmission. Since 2012, cases of MERS-CoV have been reported in 27 countries.

The World Health Organization (WHO), in partnership with the World Animal Health Organization (OIE) and the United Nations Food and Agriculture Organization (FAO), is collaborating with scientists from impacted nations to collect and exchange scientific evidence about former coronavirus outbreaks. This process of gathering information has improved the knowledge of the virus and the condition it causes and has helped in managing pandemic response priorities, clinical management strategies, and treatment methods. Learning from the SARS-

CoV/MERS-CoV and influenza pandemics has permitted researchers to evaluate the effectiveness of strategies in controlling the ongoing COVID-19 pandemic. However, preventing transmission of the COVID-19 virus has faced challenges, including low availability of medical facilities and equipment to diagnose the disease and the fact that patients can be completely asymptomatic. The International Health Regulations (IHR) has urged governments to provide comprehensive information about COVID-19 identification. A health collection platform was developed to assess the global response to the pandemic, to prevent its spread, and to limit morbidity and mortality. The principles of epidemic prevention include timely reporting of cases, patient care, provision of complete information, and real-time data analysis. The origin of the virus is believed to be from China, which has similarities to SARS-CoV and a history of contact with wild animals. MERS-CoV and SARS-CoV-2 have similarities in asymptomatic cases of the disease, while SARS-CoV-2 and influenza A have similar modes of transmission. Vaccine production is improving, and more people are getting vaccinated. Governments and health organizations worldwide are taking measures to combat this infectious disease and to help people recover and return to pre-pandemic normalcy.

REFERENCES

[1]   Sanyaolu A, Okorie C, Marinkovic A, *et al.* Comorbidity and its Impact on Patients with COVID-19. SN Compr Clin Med 2020; 2(8): 1069-76.
        [http://dx.doi.org/10.1007/s42399-020-00363-4] [PMID: 32838147]

[2]   Afzal Sajid H, Ali A, Razzaq Khan Y, *et al.* COVID-19: Third Wave Feared as Cases Soar and Precautionary Measures. Am J Liife Sci 2021; 9(2): 19-24.
        [http://dx.doi.org/10.11648/j.ajls.20210902.11]

[3]   Afzal Sajid H, Ali A, Afzal A. COVID-19: Recent Trends in the World and Precautionary Measures. Am J Liife Sci 2020; 8(3): 41-4.
        [http://dx.doi.org/10.11648/j.ajls.20200803.12]

[4]   Alhazzani W, Møller MH, Arabi YM, *et al.* Surviving Sepsis Campaign: guidelines on the management of critically ill adults with Coronavirus Disease 2019 (COVID-19). Intensive Care Med 2020; 46(5): 854-87.
        [http://dx.doi.org/10.1007/s00134-020-06022-5] [PMID: 32222812]

[5]   Tian S, Hu N, Lou J, *et al.* Characteristics of COVID-19 infection in Beijing. J Infect 2020; 80(4): 401-6.
        [http://dx.doi.org/10.1016/j.jinf.2020.02.018] [PMID: 32112886]

[6]   Zegarra-Valdivia J, Vilca BNC, Tairo T, Munive V, Lastarria C. Neurological component in coronaviruses induced disease: systematic review of sars-cov, mers-cov, and SARS-CoV-2 2020.
        [http://dx.doi.org/10.31219/osf.io/2fqtz]

[7]   Li L, Huang T, Wang Y, *et al.* COVID-19 patients' clinical characteristics, discharge rate, and fatality rate of meta-analysis. J Med Virol 2020; 92(6): 577-83.
        [http://dx.doi.org/10.1002/jmv.25757] [PMID: 32162702]

[8]   Baig AM, Khaleeq A, Ali U, Syeda H. Evidence of the COVID-19 virus targeting the CNS: tissue distribution, host–virus interaction, and proposed neurotropic mechanisms. ACS Chem Neurosci 2020; 11(7): 995-8.

[http://dx.doi.org/10.1021/acschemneuro.0c00122] [PMID: 32167747]

[9] Guo YR, Cao QD, Hong ZS, *et al.* The origin, transmission and clinical therapies on coronavirus disease 2019 (COVID-19) outbreak – an update on the status. Mil Med Res 2020; 7(1): 11.
[http://dx.doi.org/10.1186/s40779-020-00240-0]

[10] Paniz-Mondolfi A, Bryce C, Grimes Z, *et al.* Central nervous system involvement by severe acute respiratory syndrome coronavirus-2 (SARS-CoV-2). J Med Virol 2020; 92(7): 699-702.
[http://dx.doi.org/10.1002/jmv.25915] [PMID: 32314810]

[11] Brann DH, Tsukahara T, Weinreb C, *et al.* Non-neuronal expression of SARS-CoV-2 entry genes in the olfactory system suggests mechanisms underlying COVID-19-associated anosmia. Sci Adv 2020; 6(31): eabc5801.
[http://dx.doi.org/10.1126/sciadv.abc5801] [PMID: 32937591]

[12] Wang L, Shen Y, Li M, *et al.* Clinical manifestations and evidence of neurological involvement in 2019 novel coronavirus SARS-CoV-2: a systematic review and meta-analysis. J Neurol 2020; 267(10): 2777-89.
[http://dx.doi.org/10.1007/s00415-020-09974-2] [PMID: 32529575]

[13] Valderas JM, Starfield B, Sibbald B, Salisbury C, Roland M. Defining comorbidity: implications for understanding health and health services. Ann Fam Med 2009; 7(4): 357-63.
[http://dx.doi.org/10.1370/afm.983] [PMID: 19597174]

[14] Jakovljević M, Ostojić L. Comorbidity and multimorbidity in medicine today: challenges and opportunities for bringing separated branches of medicine closer to each other. Psychiatr Danub 2013; 25 (Suppl. 1): 18-28.
[PMID: 23806971]

[15] Aleebrahim-Dehkordi E, Soveyzi F, Deravi N, Rabbani Z, Saghazadeh A, Rezaei N. Human coronaviruses SARS-CoV, MERS-CoV, and SARS-CoV-2 in children. J Pediatr Nurs 2021; 56: 70-9.
[http://dx.doi.org/10.1016/j.pedn.2020.10.020] [PMID: 33186866]

[16] Lau JTF, Fung KS, Wong TW, *et al.* SARS transmission among hospital workers in Hong Kong. Emerg Infect Dis 2004; 10(2): 280-6.
[http://dx.doi.org/10.3201/eid1002.030534] [PMID: 15030698]

[17] Balasubramanian S, Rao NM, Goenka A, Roderick M, Ramanan AV. Coronavirus disease 2019 (COVID-19) in children-what we know so far and what we do not. Indian Pediatr 2020; 57(5): 435-42.
[http://dx.doi.org/10.1007/s13312-020-1819-5] [PMID: 32273490]

[18] Das KM, Lee EY, Enani MA, *et al.* CT correlation with outcomes in 15 patients with acute Middle East respiratory syndrome coronavirus. AJR Am J Roentgenol 2015; 204(4): 736-42.
[http://dx.doi.org/10.2214/AJR.14.13671] [PMID: 25615627]

[19] Heymann DL, Shindo N. COVID-19: what is next for public health? Lancet 2020; 395(10224): 542-5.
[http://dx.doi.org/10.1016/S0140-6736(20)30374-3] [PMID: 32061313]

[20] Zu ZY, Jiang MD, Xu PP, *et al.* Coronavirus disease 2019 (COVID-19): a perspective from China. Radiology 2020; 296(2): E15-25.
[http://dx.doi.org/10.1148/radiol.2020200490] [PMID: 32083985]

[21] Nigeria COVIDN. Nigeria Centre for Disease Control. 2020 n.

[22] Mohamed S, Abo El-Hassan O, Rizk M, Ismail JH, Baioumy A. Death due to cardiac arrest in a young female with highly suspected COVID-19: A case report. Cureus 2020; 12(8): e10127.
[http://dx.doi.org/10.7759/cureus.10127] [PMID: 33005541]

[23] Berry M, Gamieldien J, Fielding B. Identification of new respiratory viruses in the new millennium. Viruses 2015; 7(3): 996-1019.
[http://dx.doi.org/10.3390/v7030996] [PMID: 25757061]

[24] Zhang J, Wang X, Jia X, *et al.* Risk factors for disease severity, unimprovement, and mortality in

COVID-19 patients in Wuhan, China. Clin Microbiol Infect 2020; 26(6): 767-72.
[http://dx.doi.org/10.1016/j.cmi.2020.04.012] [PMID: 32304745]

[25] Corman VM, Muth D, Niemeyer D, Drosten C. Hosts and sources of endemic huma coronaviruses. Adv Virus Res 2018; 100: 163-88.
[http://dx.doi.org/10.1016/bs.aivir.2018.01.001] [PMID: 29551135]

[26] Helms J, Kremer S, Merdji H, *et al.* Neurologic features in severe SARS-CoV-2 infection. N Engl J Med 2020; 382(23): 2268-70.
[http://dx.doi.org/10.1056/NEJMc2008597] [PMID: 32294339]

[27] Mao L, Wang M, Chen S, He Q, Chang J, Hong C, *et al.* Neurological manifestations of hospitalized patients with COVID-19 in Wuhan, China: a retrospective case series study. MedRxiv 2020.
[http://dx.doi.org/10.1101/2020.02.22.20026500]

[28] Pletcher MJ, Tice JA, Pignone M. Use of coronary calcification scores to predict coronary heart disease. JAMA 2004; 291(15): 1831-2.
[PMID: 15100194]

[29] Zhao H, Shen D, Zhou H, Liu J, Chen S. Guillain-Barré syndrome associated with SARS-CoV-2 infection: causality or coincidence? Lancet Neurol 2020; 19(5): 383-4.
[http://dx.doi.org/10.1016/S1474-4422(20)30109-5] [PMID: 32246917]

[30] Helmich RC, Bloem BR. The impact of the COVID-19 pandemic on Parkinson's disease: hidden sorrows and emerging opportunities. J Parkinsons Dis 2020; 10(2): 351-4.
[http://dx.doi.org/10.3233/JPD-202038] [PMID: 32250324]

[31] Rothstein A, Oldridge O, Schwennesen H, Do D, Cucchiara BL. Acute cerebrovascular events in hospitalized COVID-19 patients. Stroke 2020; 51(9): e219-22.
[http://dx.doi.org/10.1161/STROKEAHA.120.030995] [PMID: 32684145]

[32] Poissy J, Goutay J, Caplan M, *et al.* Pulmonary embolism in patients with COVID-19: awareness of an increased prevalence. Circulation 2020; 142(2): 184-6.
[http://dx.doi.org/10.1161/CIRCULATIONAHA.120.047430] [PMID: 32330083]

[33] Yaghi S, Ishida K, Torres J, Mac Grory B, Raz E, Humbert K, *et al.* SARS-CoV-2 y accidente cerebrovascular en un sistema de salud de Nueva York. Stroke 2020; 51(7): 2002-11.
[http://dx.doi.org/10.1161/STROKEAHA.120.030335]

[34] Dhamoon MS, Thaler A, Gururangan K, *et al.* Acute cerebrovascular events with COVID-19 infection. Stroke 2021; 52(1): 48-56.
[http://dx.doi.org/10.1161/STROKEAHA.120.031668] [PMID: 33280551]

[35] Aggarwal G, Lippi G, Michael Henry B. Cerebrovascular disease is associated with an increased disease severity in patients with Coronavirus Disease 2019 (COVID-19): A pooled analysis of published literature. Int J Stroke 2020; 15(4): 385-9.
[http://dx.doi.org/10.1177/1747493020921664] [PMID: 32310015]

[36] Lodigiani C, Iapichino G, Carenzo L, *et al.* Venous and arterial thromboembolic complications in COVID-19 patients admitted to an academic hospital in Milan, Italy. Thromb Res 2020; 191: 9-14.
[http://dx.doi.org/10.1016/j.thromres.2020.04.024] [PMID: 32353746]

[37] Beyrouti R, Adams ME, Benjamin L, Cohen H, Farmer SF, Goh YY, *et al.* Characteristics of ischaemic stroke associated with COVID-19. J Neurol Neurosurg Psychiatry 2020; 91(8): 889-91.
[http://dx.doi.org/10.1136/jnnp-2020-323586]

[38] Alberti P, Beretta S, Piatti M, *et al.* Guillain-Barré syndrome related to COVID-19 infection. Neurol Neuroimmunol Neuroinflamm 2020; 7(4): e741.
[http://dx.doi.org/10.1212/NXI.0000000000000741] [PMID: 32350026]

[39] Toscano G, Palmerini F, Ravaglia S, *et al.* Guillain–Barré syndrome associated with SARS-CoV-2. N Engl J Med 2020; 382(26): 2574-6.
[http://dx.doi.org/10.1056/NEJMc2009191] [PMID: 32302082]

[40]   Poyiadji N, Shahin G, Noujaim D, Stone M, Patel S, Griffith B. COVID-19–associated acute hemorrhagic necrotizing encephalopathy: imaging features. Radiology 2020; 296(2): E119-20.
[http://dx.doi.org/10.1148/radiol.2020201187] [PMID: 32228363]

[41]   Bernard-Valnet R, Pizzarotti B, Anichini A, *et al.* Two patients with acute meningoencephalitis concomitant with SARS-CoV-2 infection. Eur J Neurol 2020; 27(9): e43-4.
[http://dx.doi.org/10.1111/ene.14298] [PMID: 32383343]

[42]   Moriguchi T, Harii N, Goto J, *et al.* A first case of meningitis/encephalitis associated with SARS-Coronavirus-2. Int J Infect Dis 2020; 94: 55-8.
[http://dx.doi.org/10.1016/j.ijid.2020.03.062] [PMID: 32251791]

[43]   Baggett TP, Keyes H, Sporn N, Gaeta JM. COVID-19 outbreak at a large homeless shelter in Boston: implications for universal testing. MedRxiv 2020.
[http://dx.doi.org/10.1101/2020.04.12.20059618]

[44]   Yeh EA, Collins A, Cohen ME, Duffner PK, Faden H. Detection of coronavirus in the central nervous system of a child with acute disseminated encephalomyelitis. Pediatrics 2004; 113(1 Pt 1): e73-6.
[PMID: 14702500]

[45]   Dong Y, Mo X, Hu Y, *et al.* Epidemiology of COVID-19 among children in China. Pediatrics 2020; 145(6): e20200702.
[http://dx.doi.org/10.1542/peds.2020-0702] [PMID: 32179660]

[46]   Domingues RB, Mendes-Correa MC, de Moura Leite FBV, *et al.* First case of SARS-COV-2 sequencing in cerebrospinal fluid of a patient with suspected demyelinating disease. J Neurol 2020; 267(11): 3154-6.
[http://dx.doi.org/10.1007/s00415-020-09996-w] [PMID: 32564153]

[47]   Netland J, Meyerholz DK, Moore S, Cassell M, Perlman S. Severe acute respiratory syndrome coronavirus infection causes neuronal death in the absence of encephalitis in mice transgenic for human ACE2. J Virol 2008; 82(15): 7264-75.
[http://dx.doi.org/10.1128/JVI.00737-08] [PMID: 18495771]

[48]   Morrow SA, Fraser JA, Day C, *et al.* Effect of treating acute optic neuritis with bioequivalent oral *vs* intravenous corticosteroids: a randomized clinical trial. JAMA Neurol 2018; 75(6): 690-6.
[http://dx.doi.org/10.1001/jamaneurol.2018.0024] [PMID: 29507942]

[49]   Zhu J, Zhong Z, Ji P, *et al.* Clinicopathological characteristics of 8697 patients with COVID-19 in China: a meta-analysis. Fam Med Community Health 2020; 8(2): e000406.
[http://dx.doi.org/10.1136/fmch-2020-000406] [PMID: 32371463]

[50]   Lechien JR, Chiesa-Estomba CM, De Siati DR, *et al.* Olfactory and gustatory dysfunctions as a clinical presentation of mild-to-moderate forms of the coronavirus disease (COVID-19): a multicenter European study. Eur Arch Otorhinolaryngol 2020; 277(8): 2251-61.
[http://dx.doi.org/10.1007/s00405-020-05965-1] [PMID: 32253535]

[51]   Balestrino R, Rizzone M, Zibetti M, *et al.* Onset of COVID-19 with impaired consciousness and ataxia: a case report. J Neurol 2020; 267(10): 2797-8.
[http://dx.doi.org/10.1007/s00415-020-09879-0] [PMID: 32462348]

[52]   Shigemura J, Ursano RJ, Morganstein JC, Kurosawa M, Benedek DM. Public responses to the novel 2019 coronavirus (2019-nCoV) in Japan: Mental health consequences and target populations. Psychiatry Clin Neurosci 2020; 74(4): 281-2.
[http://dx.doi.org/10.1111/pcn.12988] [PMID: 32034840]

[53]   Baizabal-Carvallo JF, Alonso-Juarez M, Jankovic J. Functional gait disorders, clinical phenomenology, and classification. Neurol Sci 2020; 41(4): 911-5.
[http://dx.doi.org/10.1007/s10072-019-04185-8] [PMID: 31832998]

[54]   McGonagle D, Bridgewood C, Ramanan AV, Meaney JFM, Watad A. COVID-19 vasculitis and novel vasculitis mimics. Lancet Rheumatol 2021; 3(3): e224-33.

[http://dx.doi.org/10.1016/S2665-9913(20)30420-3] [PMID: 33521655]

[55] Hanafi R, Roger PA, Perin B, *et al.* COVID-19 neurologic complication with CNS vasculitis-like pattern. AJNR Am J Neuroradiol 2020; 41(8): 1384-7.
[http://dx.doi.org/10.3174/ajnr.A6651] [PMID: 32554425]

[56] Neumann B, Schmidbauer ML, Dimitriadis K, *et al.* Cerebrospinal fluid findings in COVID-19 patients with neurological symptoms. J Neurol Sci 2020; 418: 117090.
[http://dx.doi.org/10.1016/j.jns.2020.117090] [PMID: 32805440]

[57] Ellul MA, Benjamin L, Singh B, *et al.* Neurological associations of COVID-19. Lancet Neurol 2020; 19(9): 767-83.
[http://dx.doi.org/10.1016/S1474-4422(20)30221-0] [PMID: 32622375]

[58] Lima MA, Silva MTT, Soares CN, *et al.* Peripheral facial nerve palsy associated with COVID-19. J Neurovirol 2020; 26(6): 941-4.
[http://dx.doi.org/10.1007/s13365-020-00912-6] [PMID: 33006717]

[59] Yachou Y, El Idrissi A, Belapasov V, Ait Benali S. Neuroinvasion, neurotropic, and neuroinflammatory events of SARS-CoV-2: understanding the neurological manifestations in COVID-19 patients. Neurol Sci 2020; 41(10): 2657-69.
[http://dx.doi.org/10.1007/s10072-020-04575-3] [PMID: 32725449]

[60] Homma Y, Watanabe M, Inoue K, Moritaka T. Coronavirus disease-19 pneumonia with facial nerve palsy and olfactory disturbance. Intern Med 2020; 59(14): 1773-5.
[http://dx.doi.org/10.2169/internalmedicine.5014-20] [PMID: 32669517]

[61] Xydakis MS, Dehgani-Mobaraki P, Holbrook EH, *et al.* Smell and taste dysfunction in patients with COVID-19. Lancet Infect Dis 2020; 20(9): 1015-6.
[http://dx.doi.org/10.1016/S1473-3099(20)30293-0] [PMID: 32304629]

[62] Belghmaidi S, Nassih H, Boutgayout S, *et al.* Third cranial nerve palsy presenting with unilateral diplopia and strabismus in a 24-year-old woman with COVID-19. Am J Case Rep 2020; 21: e925897-1.
[http://dx.doi.org/10.12659/AJCR.925897] [PMID: 33056942]

[63] Falcone MM, Rong AJ, Salazar H, Redick DW, Falcone S, Cavuoto KM. Acute abducens nerve palsy in a patient with the novel coronavirus disease (COVID-19). J AAPOS 2020; 24(4): 216-7.
[http://dx.doi.org/10.1016/j.jaapos.2020.06.001] [PMID: 32592761]

[64] Bagheri SH, Asghari A, Farhadi M, *et al.* Coincidence of COVID-19 epidemic and olfactory dysfunction outbreak in Iran. Med J Islam Repub Iran 2020; 34: 62.
[http://dx.doi.org/10.47176/mjiri.34.62] [PMID: 32974228]

[65] Marin SE, Callen DJA. The magnetic resonance imaging appearance of monophasic acute disseminated encephalomyelitis: an update post application of the 2007 consensus criteria. Neuroimaging Clin N Am 2013; 23(2): 245-66.
[http://dx.doi.org/10.1016/j.nic.2012.12.005] [PMID: 23608688]

[66] Selvaraj V, Sacchetti D, Finn A, Dapaah-Afriyie K. Acute vision loss in a patient with COVID-19. MedRxiv 2020.
[http://dx.doi.org/10.1101/2020.06.03.20112540]

[67] Tenembaum S, Chamoles N, Fejerman N. Acute disseminated encephalomyelitis. Neurology 2002; 59(8): 1224-31.
[http://dx.doi.org/10.1212/WNL.59.8.1224] [PMID: 12391351]

[68] Vollono C, Rollo E, Romozzi M, *et al.* Focal status epilepticus as unique clinical feature of COVID-19: A case report. Seizure 2020; 78: 109-12.
[http://dx.doi.org/10.1016/j.seizure.2020.04.009] [PMID: 32344366]

[69] Peyronnet V, Sibiude J, Deruelle P, *et al.* [SARS-CoV-2 infection during pregnancy. Information and proposal of management care. CNGOF]. Gynécol Obstét Fertil Sénol 2020; 48(5): 436-43.

[http://dx.doi.org/10.1016/j.gofs.2020.03.014] [PMID: 32199996]

[70] Corsini Campioli C, Cano Cevallos E, Assi M, Patel R, Binnicker MJ, O'Horo JC. Clinical predictors and timing of cessation of viral RNA shedding in patients with COVID-19. J Clin Virol 2020; 130: 104577.
[http://dx.doi.org/10.1016/j.jcv.2020.104577] [PMID: 32777762]

[71] Betul BU, Hande I, Serap Y, Mehmet SI, Mahir C. Case Report: A COVID-19 Patient Presenting With Mild Rhabdomyolysis. Am J Trop Med Hyg 2020; 103(2): 847-50.
[http://dx.doi.org/10.4269/ajtmh.20-0583]

[72] Chan KH, Farouji I, Abu Hanoud A, Slim J. Weakness and elevated creatinine kinase as the initial presentation of coronavirus disease 2019 (COVID-19). Am J Emerg Med 2020; 38(7): 1548.e1-3.
[http://dx.doi.org/10.1016/j.ajem.2020.05.015] [PMID: 32414522]

[73] Gefen AM, Palumbo N, Nathan SK, Singer PS, Castellanos-Reyes LJ, Sethna CB. Pediatric COVID-19-associated rhabdomyolysis: a case report. Pediatr Nephrol 2020; 35(8): 1517-20.
[http://dx.doi.org/10.1007/s00467-020-04617-0] [PMID: 32447505]

[74] Ramaswamy SB, Govindarajan R. COVID-19 in refractory myasthenia gravis-a case report of successful outcome. J Neuromuscul Dis 2020; 7(3): 361-4.
[http://dx.doi.org/10.3233/JND-200520] [PMID: 32508329]

[75] Ghiasvand F, Ghadimi M, Ghadimi F, Safarpour S, Hosseinzadeh R, SeyedAlinaghi S. Symmetrical polyneuropathy in coronavirus disease 2019 (COVID-19). IDCases 2020; 21: e00815.
[http://dx.doi.org/10.1016/j.idcr.2020.e00815] [PMID: 32514394]

[76] Chaumont H, San-Galli A, Martino F, *et al.* Mixed central and peripheral nervous system disorders in severe SARS-CoV-2 infection. J Neurol 2020; 267(11): 3121-7.
[http://dx.doi.org/10.1007/s00415-020-09986-y] [PMID: 32533322]

[77] Giacomelli A, Pezzati L, Conti F, *et al.* Self-reported olfactory and taste disorders in patients with severe acute respiratory coronavirus 2 infection: a cross-sectional study. Clin Infect Dis 2020; 71(15): 889-90.
[http://dx.doi.org/10.1093/cid/ciaa330] [PMID: 32215618]

[78] Samaranayake LP, Fakhruddin KS, Mohammad OE, Panduwawala C, Bandara N, Ngo HC. Attributes of dysgeusia and anosmia of coronavirus disease 2019 (COVID-19) in hospitalized patients. Oral Dis 2022; 28 Suppl 1: 891-8.
[http://dx.doi.org/10.1111/odi.13713] [PMID: 33176049]

[79] Carrillo-Larco RM, Altez-Fernandez C. Anosmia and dysgeusia in COVID-19: A systematic review. Wellcome Open Research 2020.
[http://dx.doi.org/10.12688/wellcomeopenres.15917.1]

[80] Khosravani H, Rajendram P, Notario L, Chapman MG, Menon BK. Protected code stroke: hyperacute stroke management during the coronavirus disease 2019 (COVID-19) pandemic. Stroke 2020; 51(6): 1891-5.
[http://dx.doi.org/10.1161/STROKEAHA.120.029838] [PMID: 32233980]

[81] Dorsey ER, Glidden AM, Holloway MR, Birbeck GL, Schwamm LH. Teleneurology and mobile technologies: the future of neurological care. Nat Rev Neurol 2018; 14(5): 285-97.
[http://dx.doi.org/10.1038/nrneurol.2018.31] [PMID: 29623949]

[82] Matías-Guiu J, Porta-Etessam J, Lopez-Valdes E, Garcia-Morales I, Guerrero-Solá A, Matias-Guiu JA. Management of neurological care during the COVID-19 pandemic. Neurología (English Edition) 2020; 35(4): 233-7.
[http://dx.doi.org/10.1016/j.nrleng.2020.04.001] [PMID: 32336528]

[83] Greenhalgh T, Wherton J, Shaw S, Morrison C. Video consultations for covid-19 BMJ 2020; 368: m998.
[http://dx.doi.org/10.1136/bmj.m998]

[84]   Carlotti AP de CP. Carvalho WB de, Johnston C, Rodriguez IS, Delgado AF. COVID-19 diagnostic and management protocol for pediatric patients. Clinics (Sao Paulo) 2020; 75: e1894.
[http://dx.doi.org/10.6061/clinics/2020/e1894]

[85]   Cortegiani A, Ingoglia G, Ippolito M, Giarratano A, Einav S. A systematic review on the efficacy and safety of chloroquine for the treatment of COVID-19. J Crit Care 2020; 57: 279-83.
[http://dx.doi.org/10.1016/j.jcrc.2020.03.005] [PMID: 32173110]

[86]   del Farmaco AI. AIFA sospende l'autorizzazione all'utilizzo di idrossiclorochina per il trattamento del COVID-19 al di fuori degli studi clinici https://www. aifa. gov

[87]   Jean SS, Lee PI, Hsueh PR. Treatment options for COVID-19: The reality and challenges. J Microbiol Immunol Infect 2020; 53(3): 436-43.
[http://dx.doi.org/10.1016/j.jmii.2020.03.034] [PMID: 32307245]

[88]   Cao B, Wang Y, Wen D, *et al.* A trial of lopinavir–ritonavir in adults hospitalized with severe Covid-19. N Engl J Med 2020; 382(19): 1787-99.
[http://dx.doi.org/10.1056/NEJMoa2001282] [PMID: 32187464]

[89]   Gautret P, Lagier JC, Parola P, *et al.* Hydroxychloroquine and azithromycin as a treatment of COVID-19: results of an open-label non-randomized clinical trial. Int J Antimicrob Agents 2020; 56(1): 105949.
[http://dx.doi.org/10.1016/j.ijantimicag.2020.105949] [PMID: 32205204]

[90]   Orsini A, Corsi M, Santangelo A, *et al.* Challenges and management of neurological and psychiatric manifestations in SARS-CoV-2 (COVID-19) patients. Neurol Sci 2020; 41(9): 2353-66.
[http://dx.doi.org/10.1007/s10072-020-04544-w] [PMID: 32767055]

[91]   Giraudon P, Bernard A. Inflammation in neuroviral diseases. J Neural Transm (Vienna) 2010; 117(8): 899-906.
[http://dx.doi.org/10.1007/s00702-010-0402-y] [PMID: 20390431]

[92]   Azhideh A. COVID-19 neurological manifestations. Int Clin Neurosci J 2020; 7: 54-4.
[http://dx.doi.org/10.34172/icnj.2020.20]

[93]   Padda I, Khehra N, Jaferi U, Parmar MS. The neurological complexities and prognosis of COVID-19. SN Compr Clin Med 2020; 2(11): 2025-36.
[http://dx.doi.org/10.1007/s42399-020-00527-2] [PMID: 33015552]

[94]   Eliezer M, Hamel AL, Houdart E, *et al.* Loss of smell in patients with COVID-19. Neurology 2020; 95(23): e3145-52.
[http://dx.doi.org/10.1212/WNL.0000000000010806] [PMID: 32917809]

[95]   Ahmad I, Rathore FA. Neurological manifestations and complications of COVID-19: A literature review. J Clin Neurosci 2020; 77: 8-12.
[http://dx.doi.org/10.1016/j.jocn.2020.05.017] [PMID: 32409215]

[96]   Tang W, Cao Z, Han M, *et al.* Hydroxychloroquine in patients with mainly mild to moderate coronavirus disease 2019: open label, randomised controlled trial. BMJ 2020; 369: m1849.
[http://dx.doi.org/10.1136/bmj.m1849] [PMID: 32409561]

[97]   Lippi G, Wong J, Henry BM. Myalgia may not be associated with severity of coronavirus disease 2019 (COVID-19). World J Emerg Med 2020; 11(3): 193-4.
[http://dx.doi.org/10.5847/wjem.j.1920-8642.2020.03.013] [PMID: 32351656]

[98]   Jin M, Tong Q. Rhabdomyolysis as potential late complication associated with COVID-19. Emerg Infect Dis 2020; 26(7): 1618-20.
[http://dx.doi.org/10.3201/eid2607.200445] [PMID: 32197060]

[99]   Ferrandi PJ, Alway SE, Mohamed JS. The interaction between SARS-CoV-2 and ACE2 may have consequences for skeletal muscle viral susceptibility and myopathies. J Appl Physiol 2020; 129(4): 864-7.

[http://dx.doi.org/10.1152/japplphysiol.00321.2020] [PMID: 32673162]

[100] Orsucci D, Caldarazzo Ienco E, Nocita G, Napolitano A, Vista M. Neurological features of COVID-19 and their treatment: a review. Drugs Context 2020; 9: 1-12.
[http://dx.doi.org/10.7573/dic.2020-5-1] [PMID: 32587625]

[101] Berlit P, Bösel J, Gahn G, *et al.* "Neurological manifestations of COVID-19" - guideline of the German society of neurology. Neurol Res Pract 2020; 2(1): 51.
[http://dx.doi.org/10.1186/s42466-020-00097-7] [PMID: 33283160]

[102] Al-Ramadan A, Rabab'h O, Shah J, Gharaibeh A. Acute and post-acute neurological complications of COVID-19. Neurol Int 2021; 13(1): 102-19.
[http://dx.doi.org/10.3390/neurolint13010010] [PMID: 33803475]

[103] Castro VM, Sacks CA, Perlis RH, McCoy TH. Development and external validation of a delirium prediction model for hospitalized patients with coronavirus disease 2019. J Acad Consult Liaison Psychiatry 2021; 62(3): 298-308.
[http://dx.doi.org/10.1016/j.jaclp.2020.12.005] [PMID: 33688635]

CHAPTER 10

Artificial Intelligence and Coronaviruses

Shafeeq Ur Rehman[1,#], Furqan Shafqat[1,#], Momin Khan[2], Alam Zeb[2], Ijaz Ahmad[3] and Kamal Niaz[4,*]

[1] *Department of Microbiology, Cholistan University of Veterinary and Animal Sciences (CUVAS), Bahawalpur 63100, Pakistan*

[2] *Directorate of Livestock and Dairy Development Department, Khyber Pakhtunkhwa, Peshawar, Pakistan*

[3] *Department of Human, Legal and Economic Sciences, Telematic University "Leonardo da Vinci", Chieti, Italy*

[4] *Department of Pharmacology and Toxicology, Faculty of Bio-Sciences, Cholistan University of Veterinary and Animal Sciences (CUVAS), Bahawalpur 63100, Pakistan*

Abstract: For the third time in the last few decades, novel coronavirus-19 (2019-nCoV or COVID-19) has been described as the most fatal coronavirus ever, capable of infecting not just animals but even humans all over the world. Healthcare policy makes use of advanced technologies such as artificial intelligence (AI), big data, the internet of things (IoT), and deep machine learning to tackle and forecast emerging diseases. AI is increasingly being used to help in disease identification, prevention, reaction, rehabilitation, and clinical analysis. Since these developments are currently in their initial phases of development, slow improvement in their application for significant deliberation at local and foreign strategy levels is being made. Nevertheless, a current case shows that AI-driven technologies are improving in reliability. Companies like BlueDot and Metabiota used AI technology to predict the coronavirus disease-19 (COVID-19) in China before it surprised the world in late 2019 by spying on its effects and propagation. One approach is to use computational techniques to discover new target drugs and vaccines in silico. Machine learning-based algorithms trained on particular biomolecules have provided affordable and quick-to-implement tools for the development of successful viral treatments during the last decade. Drug repurposing is a technique for finding new uses for accepted or experimental drugs. For novel diseases like COVID-19, a drug repurposing approach is a viable approach. Future directions of AI are drug discovery and vaccination, biological research, remote video diagnosis, tracking patient contacts, COVID-19 recognition and therapy *via* smart robots, and identification of non-contact infection. This chapter aims to explore AI-based techno-

[*] **Corresponding author Kamal Niaz:** Department of Pharmacology and Toxicology, Faculty of Bio-Sciences, Cholistan University of Veterinary and Animal Sciences (CUVAS), Bahawalpur 63100, Pakistan; Tel: +923129360054; E-mails: kamalniaz@cuvas.edu.pk, kamalniaz1989@gmail.com
[#] Shafeeq Ur Rehman and Furqan Shafqat have equal contribution

logy for diagnosis, management, drug repurposing medications, novel drug discovery, and vaccines for coronaviruses (SARS-CoV and MERS), including during the COVID-19 pandemic.

Keywords: Artificial intelligence, Drug, MERS, SARS-CoV, SARS-CoV-2.

INTRODUCTION

Coronaviruses are a group of viruses that can cause a variety of infections, from mild flu to severe acute syndrome. Coronaviruses are members of the Coronaviridae group. Its order is divided into two subfamilies: (1) *Coronavirinae*, which includes the genera *Alphacoronavirus*, *Betacoronavirus*, *Gammacoronavirus*, and *Deltacoronavirus*, and (2) *Torovirinae*, which includes the genera *Torovirus* and *Bafinivirus*, as well as an unidentified genus. The Middle East respiratory syndrome coronavirus (MERS-CoV) virus has been found in camels [1]. MERS-CoV is thought to be transferred to humans from camels *via* pulmonary particle spit or the consumption of raw camel flesh or dairy. The virus's pathogenic status was verified utilizing viral bioinformatics tools [2]. One way to learn more about the virus and develop detection and management methods is through artificial intelligence (AI).

The introduction of modern computer simulation techniques and their widespread acceptance in many industries worldwide have resulted in better risk analysis for local and global markets. The healthcare sector, in particular, has been developed with a rise in health knowledge assisted by the existence of different techniques such as machine learning, the IoT, Big Data, AI, and many others. Prognostic computing tools' accessibility and corresponding use in the medical industry globally have resulted in noteworthy changes in surgical procedures, personalized healthcare, and epidemiology. These are supposed to improve accuracy in this domain, particularly regarding diagnostic precision [3]. Forecasting technologies are still used in the healthcare workforce's recruiting and evaluation, and they are being bolstered to incorporate questions about inclusivity and meritocracy [4]. AI is one of the tools for understanding the virus and developing prevention and management strategies. From symptomatic monitoring to early diagnostic tests and quicker drug production, AI can assist at any level of the healthcare process. In China, AI-based technologies are being used to detect coronavirus outbreaks [5]. Computer vision, speech detection, natural linguistic processing, and digital anatomy knowledge processing are only a few AI technologies. Similarly, AI has transformed drug development by uncovering secret trends and facts in biomedical data. AI has been used by pharmaceutical firms and start-ups for drug research and production [6].

For instance, IBM's Watson health platform scans large quantities of text information, such as lab results, clinical reports, and scientific papers, to locate drugs [7]. AI approaches for a particular field in drug development and drug repurposing provide quick and efficient therapeutic design strategies. These benefits are particularly evident in the COVID-19's worldwide outbreak induced by the severe acute respiratory syndrome-coronavirus-2 (SARS-CoV-2), where novel drug development is almost impossible. For drug repurposing, the outbreak is a great time to introduce improved AI algorithms and network treatment. The AI-based approach is simple and accurate, as it has previously examined molecules and provided recommendations for the most effective molecules to combat the virus. The AI-based program looks up data about COVID-19 on the internet to determine where the infection is spreading. As a result, the device encourages identifying epidemic sites and expanded knowledge and understanding of possible remedies [8]. AI radiologists employ deep learning to create a template that learns from familiarity with a sample to make decisions relying on clinical and medical imaging [9]. Artificial neural networks (ANNs) are the most commonly employed deep learning template, with an artificial neuron as the fundamental building block that converts the weighed aggregate of input function parameters non-linearly. AI may be used to divide patients into classes based on the severity of their illnesses, genetic makeup, and medical history, allowing for more effective treatment options. Through remotely monitoring cases and gathering patient data in subclinical cases or those with mild symptoms, AI in telemedicine may be used to reduce the need for frequent and unnecessary doctor's visits. Remdesivir has therapeutic effects against COVID-19, urging FDA permission for emergency usage, but only for serious diseases. Mefuparib (CVL218) is a suppressor of poly ADP-ribose polymerase 1 and inhibits SARS-CoV-2 reproduction in the laboratory with no clear toxicity consequences, according to machine learning trials and statistical testing techniques. Mefuparib has much more effective antiviral activity at virus entry and equivalent antiviral activity at subsequent viral entry compared to remdesivir, indicating that it may be a choice for an anti-SARS-CoV-2 drug [10].

The operational approach to COVID-19 on the front lines is similar to SARS, with one big variation: 17 years after SARS, a new effective technology (AI) has arisen that may theoretically be influential in holding this virus inside acceptable lines of AI. AI can aid in the battle against this virus by providing community monitoring, clinical assistance warning, and disease prevention guidelines [11, 12]. Despite having many advantages, AI has several limitations, including inadequate information, there are not enough multimodal AI assessments, benefits are not realized straight away, internal and external validation is also lacking, inability to be seen by non-technical people, and ethical Issues. From the next available pathways, AI will continue the battle against COVID-19. Future directions are biological research, drug discovery vaccination, remote video diagnosis, consultations, assessment and measurement of the consequences, tracking patient contacts, COVID-19 recognition, therapy *via* smart robots, and identification of non-contact infection [13].

AI and Coronaviruses

AI is a subdivision of computer science that can analyze and interpret complex medical data. In several clinical scenarios, its ability to extract concrete relationships from a data set can be used in diagnosis, treatment, and outcome prediction. The word AI is also known as machine intelligence. The imitation of human intelligence in an appliance to act like a human is known as AI [8, 14]. AI is used by any computer that interacts with humans. It may be included in problem-solving or determining the source of the problem. AI plays a variety of roles in our everyday lives, with numerous promising stories. AI has also helped to deal with different types of coronaviruses around the globe. The developed countries always have directed this technology for a different kind of purpose [15]. However, emerging and reemerging diseases like SARS-CoV-2 or COVID-19, MERS-CoV, and SARS-CoV make it difficult to control. However, with the help of AI, the healthcare systems are creating new prognostic and preventive systems to overcome various diseases, in particular, COVID-19, the latest emerging disease. AI is aiding people to live stronger by tackling these diseases through many processes [16].

Coronaviruses are a group of viruses that can cause a variety of infections, from mild flu to severe acute syndrome. AI is one of the ways to learn more about the virus and improve prevention and control strategies. The use of mathematical models to better understand the spread of viruses, structural biology to detect and refine vaccines, computational science for a greater explanation of viral developments, and studies of docking to identify drugs and blockers are included in this report [5, 17]. Coronaviruses belong to the family *Coronaviridae.* There are two subfamilies of its order: (1) Coronavirinae, which includes Alphacoronavirus, Betacoronavirus, Deltacoronavirus and Gammacoronavirus (2) Torovirinae, which comprises *Torovirus* and *Bafinivirus* genera. Five swine coronaviruses are recognized: transmissible gastroenteritis virus (TGEV) is the 1st type of swine coronavirus first described in Europe in 1946; porcine hemagglutinating encephalomyelitis virus (pHEV) was discovered in 1962; porcine epidemic diarrhea virus (PEDV) isolated in 1977; porcine respiratory coronavirus (PRCV) identified in 1984, and porcine delta coronavirus (PDCoV) detected in 2012 [18].

SARS is a sickness caused by SARS-CoV-1 [19]. It is an enveloped RNA virus that affects the epithelial cells of the lungs [20]. This virus can affect humans, bats, and palm civets [21]. There was an outbreak of SARS in Asia and other countries on 16 April 2003 [19]. The United States and Canada recognized the SARS-CoV-1 in April 2003 [22, 23]. SARS-CoV-1 satisfied Koch's postulates, and it was confirmed as a causative agent. An experiment on macaque showed symptoms similar to human symptoms infected with SARS-CoV-1 [24].

MERS-CoV

Respiratory infections in humans are also caused by viruses other than SARS-CoV-1 and SARS-CoV-2. MERS-CoV also affects the respiratory system in humans [25]. This virus is a zoonotic virus that is transmitted from animal to human and vice versa. The first case was reported in June 2012 in Saudia Arabia [26]. It is also known as camel flu [27]. The route of transmission is not understood, but it is believed that those closely related to camels found symptoms of this disease. Symptoms vary from none to life-threatening [28]. The diseases are more severe in immunocompromised persons. This virus does not pass easily from human to human unless there is close contact with no preventive measures.

Machine learning algorithms were used to identify the essential factors linked to viral diseases. The tests were conducted. The R programming language was used to incorporate them. The device supports vector machines, naive Bayes, and other learning methods J48. This research used logistic regression and conditional inference trees to find the most powerful determinants [29 - 31]. The differential significance linked to recovery from MERS-CoV infection indicates the relevance of the factors. Machine learning techniques are used to discover patterns, conduct sentiment research, give insight into the origins of fake information, and help eliminate rumors and propaganda [32]. To find the statistically relevant variables, researchers used univariate and multivariate analysis with logistic regression [33]. To analyze MERS-CoV data from Saudi Arabia, Al-Turaiki *et al*. used statistical models such as naive Bayes and J48 [31].

SARS-CoV-2

In December 2019, in Wuhan, China, a similar causative agent to SARS was found that affects the respiratory system in humans. This virus was named SARS-CoV-2, which triggered the COVID-19 pandemic [34]. The symptoms of SARS-CoV-2 vary from person to person, ranging from none to fatal conditions. This virus is transmitted from one person to another through the air when they are near each other and *via* mouth, nose, and eyes. COVID-19 is primarily spread from person to person *via* direct contact with airborne routes during coughing or sneezing, as well as *via* indirect contact with fomites and frequently touched surfaces [35]. SARS-CoV-2 can survive on different external materials for a few hours to days [36]. In a medical or laboratory setting, airborne transmission is possible. In a hospital environment, some processes produce aerosols. Sometimes, this virus remains hidden in one person and may spread to another without showing symptoms [37].

Big data and AI are assisting at an astounding level to combat the COVID-19 pandemic. In the battle against COVID-19, AI can be extremely useful. AI is used to effectively identify disease occurrences, track cases, forecast potential diseases, assess higher mortality, diagnose COVID-19, handle infection by allocating resources, facilitate training, maintain records, and analyze trends. In COVID-19, AI can supplement mobile health applications in which electronic devices such as watches, tablets, cameras, and a variety of portable devices are used for efficient monitoring and touch tracing [38]. Telemedicine applications such as AI4 COVID-19, which insists on voice recorder specimens of cough, can be used [39]. By prioritizing the need for ventilators and respiratory services in the emergency ward, AI can provide critical knowledge for resource utilization and evaluation [40]. AI can also be used to forecast the likelihood of recovery or death in COVID-19, as well as to support regular alerts, collection and pattern analysis, and care tracking.

Role of BlueDot

The software company Bluedot is based in Canada. Insights, the company's flagship product, is a software-as-a-service tool for tracking the spread of infectious diseases. BlueDot depends heavily on AI and machine learning technology to detect outbreaks of infectious diseases. The organization can collect data from various sources, like media sources and international aircraft ticketing data, utilizing these and many natural language processing strategies [41]. When it comes to battling a pandemic, the pace is almost everything. A small group of doctors and technologists claim to have discovered the critical speed needed to combat the COVID-19 AI's computing ability. Their new weapon is named "outbreak research", and it can potentially transform the way we battle future epidemics. In the year 2013, BlueDot was created. According to the company's founder, the consequences of the SARS outbreak in 2002–2004 influenced BlueDot's initial business model [42]. During the COVID-19 pandemic, BlueDot and its software got much attention. COVID-19 outbreaks are being tracked using BlueDot software [42, 43]. BlueDot's technology detected rare pneumonia cases in Wuhan, China, and warned its clients on December 31st, nine days before the WHO issued its first alerts about a new coronavirus. As a result, BlueDot correctly predicted that twelve of the twenty cities would be affected after Wuhan was struck. BlueDot is currently collaborating with the Canadian government to monitor the virus's progress [44 - 46]. BlueDot has previously predicted the worldwide propagation of the Zika virus from Brazil [45]. Throughout any epidemic, the pace of data collection and dissemination is vital to the threat's containment [46]. BlueDot's paper shows how a huge range and data validity can be collated to create precise epidemiologic estimates using AI.

The international data set is another means of information that Bluedot uses. This beginning claims to analyze big data every day from over 10,000 official and media outlets in 60 languages. Landmass data from regional enumeration, The World Factbook, and national statistical records, among other outlets, are used in its data collection. The international communicable diseases warning, actual weather patterns, pathogenic organisms, and infection reserves in animals are some of the data sources that Bluedot uses. The organization then utilizes screening techniques to narrow down regions of concern and efficient grouping methods to enable the fast invention of fields that may be considered hot spots, cold spots, and geographical outliers using information from these data sources [47]. The organization then uses the information to improve the network using machine learning and natural language processing (NLP) technology, and it is now possible to send frequent warnings to its customers, especially in cases of rare infections and the dangers they pose, as well as the potential destinations most likely to develop epidemics. The system is trained by utilizing a hazard analysis method that includes vast data sources derived from different disciplines to detect, banner, and show rhythms illustrating possible infection hazards, as well as estimate the propagation of diseases. BlueDot accurately estimated the Zika pandemic in Florida six months ago, in 2016 [48]. In 2020, nine days before the actual declaration of the COVID-19 epidemic, BlueDot, using air transportation information from Wuhan, was capable of predicting the outbreak and, as a consequence, effectively identifying the urban areas that were at increased risk of getting the flu pandemic [49].

Role of Metabiota

Metabiota is a threat monitoring firm that works in animal and human health. In 2008, Nathan Wolfe formed the company in San Francisco, California. Metabiota makes assumptions about contagious disease infection distributions, strategies, and incident magnitude using AI, Machine Learning, Big Data, and NLP approaches [41]. This San Francisco-based organization collects vast volumes of information from both formal and informal outlets, as well as those from genetic, social, democratic, and ecological frontiers. It uses sophisticated analysis and simulation of epidemic rates, magnitude, and length to make precise judgments [50].

Except for BlueDot, which seldom uses social networks for information, Metabioita has been found to gather and use social networking information to make forecasts, such as in the past situation of the COVID-19 outbreak. Metabiota also utilizes these predictive analytics on where and how diseases affect human nature and the extent of anxiety they create based on AI and machine learning. Such forecasts are critical for this firm, which notes that its primary investors are finance firms that are especially concerned with these data, particularly in terms of reducing investment threats and insurance providers. Metabiota's work supports federal organizations anti-associations, consultants, and charities, including others that depend upon these data to enable smart judgments in the case of infections. Metabiota's tale began in 2009, but it was brought to light in 2014 during the West African Ebola epidemic. Prior to the virus's emergence, the organization analyzed data in Africa to determine the relationship between human and animal welfare. It was included in the Ebola epidemic, particularly through the United States government, and was on the front lines of the war, but once the virus was handled, the funding forwarded to the organization was brought to an end.

As a result, the organization widened its reach to include insurers, and it now has a robust infection database. It now hires new predictive technology such as AI, big data, and Machine Learning to make forecasts. Regarding that, when COVID-19 was identified, it was at the forefront in estimating the following affected regions beyond Wuhan, which was the first place where the virus was discovered. This forecast was made a few days before the earliest incidents were recorded in those locations, thanks to these technologies [51]. This was achieved by the application of NLP, through which the organization was capable to monitor the propagation of the virus using communication platforms' information from diverse sources, resulting in even more accurate forecasts [52].

AI-Based Algorithms and Bioinformatics for Coronaviruses

In a pandemic, early diagnosis is critical for preventing disease severity and human mortality. The SARS outbreak, induced by the SARS-CoV, took the lives of 774 people from 17 countries. All over the world, some of these fatalities might have been prevented if Chinese authorities had not delayed exchanging details. Consequently, it took about four months to discover the SARS epidemic, initially recorded in November 2002 in wildlife purchased as meals in a Guangdong marketplace in China (February 2003) [52]. For the time being in China, due to disorganized bureaucracies, the first response by government authorities was to refuse that an epidemic had occurred, resulting in silence and the virus spreading rapidly. Chinese researchers traced the virus's origins to horseshoe bats in Yunnan Territory through Asian Palm Civets (Paradoxurus Hermaphroditus). The Institute of Medicine (US) states that the lack of details and delayed administrative reaction due to the data being regarded as "state secret," and anybody who wanted to share or write on the epidemic in any manner, even doctors and journalists, risked being punished. The virus was spread to 29 countries when the information was shared [53].

China seems to have acquired from the experience of 2002–2003, and the local government's response to the SARS-CoV-2 has been much more prompt and clearer [52]. Another example of slow diagnosis was the epidemic of MERS-CoV. In 2012, it was known as camel flu, which killed 858 people [52]. MERS-related mortalities were reported between 2012 and 2016, mostly in the Arabian Peninsula but also in South Korea, Kenya, the Philippines, and the United Kingdom, including 1841 cases confirmed by laboratory analysis [52, 54].

In contrast to these events, the latest COVID-19 outbreak has been perceived in just a week, which is expected to aid in disseminating knowledge about the outbreak. The availability of Big Data analytics, which is having a substantial effect on the health sector, is being attributed in part to the early identification of such cases in recent years. The collection of information in this field is aided by the accessibility of a variety of health-wearable technologies that can collect information on vital signs. Gaille believes that such devices are crucial in deciding the future development of this field. Big data is being hailed as the next "gold rush" of the 21st century, with benefits influencing geopolitical position in both commercial and traditional governing domains of the country. There is a huge conflict among powerful nations to ensure that they also have access to big data [55]. Smart Cities innovations 'push and pull', especially Huawei's 5G implementation, demonstrate it [52, 56]. It has been stated that data management and handling by a few companies should not be geared primarily for personal benefit or to support the realms in which they are registered [57]. Thus, geopolitical and technological competition between big data-rich companies will positively impact the economic environment and the health sector. There will be a big improvement in health information because of the large number of these devices, which, when evaluated, have the power to alter the healthcare system [52 - 58]. However, this study likely faced several difficulties, especially when using AI and machine learning. Both approaches are in their early stages of development, and medical information is heavily protected due to security, political, and public sensitivities [59]. Furthermore, managing such forms of information raises concerns about data breaches and moral concerns related to data collection and misuse, particularly when it comes to entire genome data [60]. Allam and Jones explained how it could potentially be accomplished through networks on a local, regional, and global scale [61]. Given the above, there are several ways set by national legislation that can be used to anonymize health records securely. This requires measures to guarantee that a patient's privacy is not at risk. These approaches include scenarios in which the data in question is being used for rational reasons, such as analysis that does not reveal the patient's identity or promote stigmatization. Due to the existence of large databases, approaches such as k-anonymity (having a database without any combinations of user attributes) [62] and the technique of anonymization may contribute to improved AI processing [63]. Datasets and protocols must be standardized to enable a diverse range of devices to connect through networks and ensure that the data is truly anonymized. Though this argument could be prolonged, considering challenges such as exclusive possession by certain gadget makers and the loss of revenues by companies that can get profit from the management of these kinds of information, the possibility for data analysis from an open dataset is infinite [61]. Accordingly, this will be highly beneficial to the health sector in raising challenges such as diagnosis, individualized treatment, and finding treatments for diseases that plague the worldwide population [52 - 64].

SARS-CoV-2's adverse impact on their economies is well-known in Hong Kong and China. Consequently, it seems that China's nationwide initialization to COVID-19 by ceasing human activity within China, air travel, ships, buses, trains, and other means pose not only a danger to the economy in general but also a risk faced externally by an epidemic during Chinese New Year cultural celebrations. Internal and international travel and means of transportation had already been adversely affected by the end of January 2020 [52, 65]. Many experts believe that using AI to process data would significantly facilitate diverse approaches that would assist in rapidly diagnosing an outbreak and be important for maintaining local economies when such outbreaks occur. Furthermore, such perspectives can help guide initiatives that will potentially affect the development of public health strategies, ensuring outbreaks are dealt with more effectively and systematically, with knowledge exchanged more efficiently and faster [52].

Application of AI for Coronavirus Diagnosis

AI is one of the ways to learn more about the virus and improve control measures. This involves, but is not restricted to, numerical techniques to examine virus propagation, structural biology to better understand virus processes and enhance vaccines, analytical genetics to better explain infection development, and docking research to understand medications and antagonists. From symptomatic monitoring to rapid diagnostic and faster drug production, AI can aid in all stages of healthcare. In China, AI-based technologies are still being used to determine coronavirus disease. A device built by YITU technologies for the Shanghai Public Health Clinical Center (SPHCC) called the "Coronavirus Chest CT Smart Assessment System" can now detect suspicious infections in milliseconds [5].

SARS CoV-1

Although AI in healthcare has been frequently reported as a useful tool for detecting infection and designing treatment strategies, this current pandemic highlights the requirement for and potential for AI to forecast epidemics. However, professional epidemiologists and healthcare professionals cannot be substituted. AI can help public medical officials make difficult decisions by compiling rapidly changing data. During an epidemic, the pace at which data is collected and disseminated is vital to the threat's management [8]. The writers of a scientific journal by BlueDot show how a wide number and validity of information can be collated to enable reliable epidemiologic forecasts using AI. AI in medicare was already mainly known as a valuable tool for detecting infection and making clinical predictions. This current period highlights the use and potential of using AI to anticipate diseases, although professional physiologists and healthcare professionals cannot be substituted, AI can help public health officials make complex decisions by compiling quickly shifting data. The accumulation of social networks, news organizations, constantly changing health records, and other fragmented data is a difficult challenge that AI is designed to solve. There was no real-time data usable throughout initial encounters, such as the SARS epidemic in China in 2003. The continually transforming nature of pathogens like SARS-CoV, SARS-CoV-2, and MERS-CoV makes keeping ahead of the game hard. However, with the assistance of AI, the healthcare industry or technology continues to develop new forecasting, therapeutic, and protective technologies to manage these latest innovative infections, particularly COVID-19, to improve citizens' safety and longer stay [8, 66].

The AI-based platform will look up knowledge on SARS CoV mostly on the internet and determine where the illness is spreading. As a result, the device aids in the identification of epidemic hotspots while also promoting enhanced enlightenment and understanding of possible remedies [8]. Data-driven predictive technology is altering the way people think about data. New features are used to handle outbreaks, and further improvements often accompany these upgrades. Investigators and experts use AI to forecast zones where new diseases might arise [67, 68]. AI is about speed and size to prevent a SARS-CoV disease outbreak. It immediately senses adjustments in the situation, making AI a more effective tool in the battle against the SARS-CoV epidemic [8].

MERS-CoV

MERS-CoV is a significant contagious agent that has afflicted communities in the Middle East, particularly the Kingdom of Saudi Arabia (KSA). Coronaviruses are a type of virus that can cause a range of illnesses, from minor infections to serious illnesses. SARS Co-V, HCoV-NL63, HCoV-HKU1, and other new coronaviruses have been identified since the beginning of the twenty-first century [69].

The key factors correlated with viral strains were discovered using machine learning techniques. R program code was used to carry out the trials. Machine learning approaches such as naive Bayes, support vector machines, J48, conditional inference trees, and logistic regression were used to find the significant predictor variables [33]. The naive Bayes is built on the presumption that the variables in the database under consideration are unrelated. It is built on Bayes' principle, which calculates the category result's conditional possibility depending on independent variables [70, 71]. J48 creates C4.5 trees that can be trimmed or unpruned. C4.5 is a judgment chain approach based on Iterative Dichotomiser 3. (ID3). C4.5 can handle both static and dynamic attributes. A conditional inference tree is a tree-based sorting methodology that is commonly implemented. The technique used to pick parameters when extracting the tree varies from RPart. The VereCoV detection system kit, a portable Lab-on-Chip platform capable of detecting MERS-CoV, SARS-CoV, and COVID-19, has been launched by Veredus Research labs, a Singapore-based manufacturer of innovative biological testing equipment. VereChip™ computing, a Labon-Chip platform that combines two essential molecular genomic networks, polymerase chain reaction (PCR) and a microarray, will be ready to identify and differentiate MERS-CoV, SARS-CoV, and COVID-19 with extreme accuracy and accessibility in two hours [72]. Early infection status, pre-existing infections, age, and whether or not the person is a health professional are the four most common factors associated with MERS Co-V persistence, as seen in different plots. Scientific studies such as multivariate regression and univariate analysis were used to identify the significant aspects correlated with MERS remediation.

COVID-19

AI is often used to assist in disease analysis identification, reaction, rehabilitation, and diagnostic testing (Power of AI to diagnose and prevent further COVID-19 outbreak: a short communication). AI will assist us in combating this virus by providing community monitoring, medical assistance, warning, and infectious management advice [11, 12, 73]. In contrast to 15 minutes by human physicians, the AI-based device can classify COVID-19 from computerized tomography (CT) scan photos in around 15 seconds with 90% precision. BlueDot, an AI innovation organization, created an intelligence network that transcribes data regarding people to assess the likelihood of human infection [8]. Healthcare delivery includes new techniques such as AI, the IoT, big data, and machine learning to tackle and predict emerging diseases. We want to look at how AI can analyze, plan for, and combat COVID-19 and other outbreaks. AI easily detects suspicious signs and other "red flags", alerting clinicians and healthcare officials. It assists in premium judgment. It contributes to creating a new evaluation and intervention system for COVID-19 conditions by providing valuable parameters. AI may assist in diagnosing diseases using medical imaging techniques such as magnetic resonance imaging (MRI) and CT scans of animal parts. This technology will monitor and predict the virus's existence, as well as the infection's risks and likely distribution, using historical data, social networks, and internet sites. It may also estimate the number of effective outcomes and mortalities in a specific field. AI would aid in determining the more susceptible territories, people, and regions so that immediate steps can be taken [74]. AI is utilized in drug testing by evaluating the existing current information on COVID-19. It can be used in the production and layout of drug delivery systems.

This technique is utilized to accelerate drug screening in real-time, whereas routine screening takes a long time and thus helps to accelerate significantly this method, which would be impossible for a person to do [75, 76]. The collection of social media platforms, news organizations, rapidly evolving health information, and other distributed information is a challenging task AI intends to address. There was no real-time data to work with during early experiences, such as the SARS outbreak in China in 2003. Health professionals became overworked due to a rapid and unprecedented rise in the rate of clinicians during the COVID-19 outbreak. AI is being used to help medical practitioners decrease their responsibilities [77, 78]. It assists in earlier detection and care by utilizing modern techniques and management sciences. It also offers the best instruction to students and physicians on this lethal infection [79, 80]. The BlueDot community explained that the knowledge provided by its networks anticipated the COVID-19 pandemic long before the Chinese and WHO made public statements [8]. The machine expected an outbreak of COVID-19, which was right. The machine detected the COVID-19 disease in December 2019, which later proved correct as the pandemic began to spreadin February, 2020 [8, 49]. The organization is creating a collection of ingredients that research scientists have used in their experiments, intending to use the resource to stop the COVID-19 from spreading more [8]. The AI-based system looked up COVID-19 details on the internet and find out where the disease was spreading. As a result, the framework made it easier to find disease hotspots and raised the perception of possible solutions.

While AI has been widely documented in healthcare as a useful tool for predicting infection and developing treatment plans, the current pandemic highlights the need for AI's ability to predict epidemics. Investigators and scientists use AI to forecast zones where new diseases may arise [67, 68]. It immediately senses shifts in a situation, making AI a more effective weapon in the battle against the

COVID-19 pandemic [8]. While AI cannot replace trained epidemiologists and healthcare practitioners, it can assist public health officials in making tough decisions by compiling rapidly changing data. On a median, an AI network screens 60 people every day; thus, with 1000 systems, 60,000 individuals can be screened every day. As a result, there are currently no human materials sufficient to sustain this amount of evaluation in an effective and timely manner [15, 81].

AI, COVID-19, and Healthcare Workers

The current COVID-19 is a viral infection caused by SARS-CoV-2. According to the World Health Organization (WHO), most people will experience mild to severe respiratory disease and will heal despite the need for further care [82]. David Heymann supervised the global reaction to SARS as Executive Director of the Contagious Diseases Cluster, WHO. He describes that whether AI is used or not, multiple main aspects are needed for an effective community health response to a new disease epidemic [83]. Recognizing transmissibility and threat communities, determining the evolutionary background of the disease, comprising incubation duration and death rates, defining and categorizing the pathogenic species, and, in some cases, observational analysis to indicate effective preventive and management strategies are all among these aspects [83]. This data can be gathered from all those operating in epidemic areas connected to WHO. He emphasizes that this technique operated for SARS and will again be a significant basis of knowledge for COVID-19. This information can be combined to develop and optimize the AI program. It is a devoted mission. There is no way to substitute the human mind, nor the infectious disease specialist or virologist, with something that can diagnose and act quickly when an epidemic occurs [83].

Linear forecasting models [84, 85] AI methods [86, 87], and hybrid forecasting models [88, 89] have all been shown to be valuable resources for predicting COVID-19 instances. The benefits of AI techniques for time sequence prediction include the versatility of operating with various types of reaction parameters and the ability of these techniques to understand information dynamical action, sophistication, and manage non-linearity, such as that found in epidemiological data [90]. AI will assist us in fighting this virus by providing public monitoring, medical assistance, warning and infection prevention recommendations [11, 12, 73]. AI-based systems can assist medical personnel and nursing professionals in minimizing their workload by automating systems such as providing instruction to physicians, deciding the mode of treatment and care by analyzing clinical information utilizing pattern detection methods, digitizing patient records, and providing interventions that minimize their interaction with the patient Neurol Res Pract [91-93].

AI would be able to distinguish individuals into minimal, medium, and severe categories depending on the intensity of their signs, biological makeup, and clinical outcomes, allowing for the most appropriate treatment possible. In machine-learning patients or individuals with slight symptoms, AI in telemedicine may also reduce the requirement for repetitive and unwanted hospital visits by remotely tracking conditions and documenting patient information. AI-based healthcare mobile applications may often be utilized for appointments, minimizing hospital overcrowding and disease transmission and thus stopping intensive care systems from running smoothly [94, 95].

Sufferers in remote locations can get much help from chatbots like Clara from the Centers for Epidemic Management and Zini [96]. Utilizing machine learning techniques and derived characteristics obtained from the information of other patients as a learning database, a diagnostic suggested scheme estimated the death threat of patients [97]. A related tool was found to determine whether or not someone will experience acute respiratory distress syndrome [98]. In hospital environments, service machines and anthropocentric robots with AI cores can also be used for regular washing, sanitizing, and screening [99, 100].

Application of AI in COVID-19 Disease Management

Big data and AI are driving action to overcome the COVID-19 disease. Many AI offshoots have previously been used in infectious diseases. In the battle against COVID-19, AI can be useful. AI is being used effectively in detecting illness clusters, case tracking, epidemic forecasting, COVID-19 detection, and outbreak control by resource distribution. It is essential to keep track of records and identify patterns to research the disease phenomenon. The following are a few AI implementations generating a lot of passion and raising aspiration in the battle against COVID-19 [101].

AI-assisted Assessment and Surveillance

By collecting data from public networks, calls, and media sources, AI can be used to predict infection transmission, improve countermeasures, and provide valuable data about affected communities and the prognosis of disease burden and death. Utilizing machine learning, Bluedot detected a group of pneumonia cases and estimated the COVID-19 epidemic and geographical area based on the facts. HealthMap compiles publicly accessible COVID-19 information and makes it readily available to aid in accurately monitoring the virus propagation [38, 102].

AI in Contact Tracing

In COVID-19, AI may reinforce mobile health applications in which computing devices such as watches, smartphones, cameras, and a variety of portable devices are used for detection, contact tracing, and efficient management. Telemedicine software such as AI4COVID-19, which depends on a voice recording specimen of a 2-second cough, can be used [39].

AI in COVID-19 Cases Tracking

In the medical context, AI approaches are used to track patients and estimate health outcomes. AI can provide important data for the distribution of resources and choices in the intensive care unit by highlighting the need for artificial ventilation therapies by analyzing the data retrieved from vital statistics and clinical parameters. AI can also be used to forecast the rehabilitation or fatality of COVID-19, as well as to provide regular alerts, storage, trend monitoring, and medication tracking [40].

AI in Early Diagnosis

COVID-19 cases were quantitated using AI from chest X-rays and CT scan images. Experts created COVID-19 detection neural network (COVNet) to distinguish between COVID-19 and pneumonia using visual 2D and 3D characteristics derived from a chest CT scan [103]. Singh *et al.* used multi-objective differential evolution (MODE) and CNN to build a new deep-learning system for COVID-19 detection using a chest CT scan. COVID-ResNet, which used an automated and discriminative learning rate as well as gradual image resizing to identify COVID-19, surpassed COVID-Net [104]. COVID MTNet is a tool for identifying and standardizing relevant features in x-ray images and chest CT scans that employ improved genesis of recurrent, residual neural network (RCNN) and NABLA-3 network models [105].

AI in Reducing the Workload of Healthcare Professionals

AI-based triage systems can assist medical personnel and health professionals in minimizing their workload by automating certain activities like providing training to physicians, deciding the method of cure and support by reviewing epidemiological records using pattern recognition strategies, digitizing patient records, and providing ways to reduce their interaction with patients [91]. AI can be used to classify patients based on the severity of their conditions, genetic makeup, and medical records, such that alternative steps can be taken to treat them effectively [92]. In subclinical cases or those with moderate symptoms, AI in telemedicine may also be used to minimize the need for regular and unwanted doctor visits by remotely tracking the cases and collecting patient data [97].

AI in the Prediction of Protein Structure

AI can assist in the prognosis of the essential protein structure necessary for virus entrance and reproduction, as well as provide valuable information that can open the way for quick drug discovery. Google Deep Mind's AlphaFold algorithm used deep residual networks (DRN) named ResNets to bring massive momentum for drug development to estimate the protein structures of membrane protein, protein 3a, nsp2, nsp4, nsp6, and papain-like C-terminal domain of SARS-CoV-2 [106]. DeepTracer, a software based on a customized CNN, was designed to extract the protein structure of SARS-CoV-2 from high-resolution cryo-electron microscopy density data and amino acid sequences [107].

AI in Therapeutical Growth

By accelerating lead detection and simulated sampling, AI strategies can aid traditional methods by drastically reducing the time needed to bring a drug from the bench to bedside. AI will also help with drug repurposing and repositioning by scanning characteristics of accepted and tested drugs using molecular descriptors, something a professional would not be ready to do. BenevolentAI used machine learning techniques to accelerate its drug development project, and Baricitinib was recognized as a promising drug for COVID-19 [108]. Using AI, *in silico* medicine discovered many small molecules that are effective against COVID-19 [109]. Another research used virtual sampling and supervised learning to find new COVID-19 drugs [110]. Other AI-based projects, such as inclProject IDentif.AI (identifying infectious disease hybrid therapy with AI) and PolypharmDB, have efficiently found candidates for COVID-19 [111].

AI in Vaccine Production

There has never been a race like this in human history to discover a vaccine for such a virus. The rate of development can be significantly accelerated by using AI's capabilities. Using the Vaxign reverse vaccinology-machine learning technique, Ong *et al.* [112] projected potential COVID-19 vaccine targets through supervised classification models.

AI to Stop Rumors from Spreading

As a result of the influx of information, this outbreak has morphed into an infodemic. Acknowledging COVID-19 data, perceptions, and behaviors, as well as evidence from social media sites and other sources, will help implement a strategy to collect and propagate reliable and timely data to minimize COVID-19's impact [113]. Machine learning techniques may be used to identify trends, pursue attitudes, give data about the source of false news, and help dispel myths and propaganda [32].

AI in Genomics

Randhawa *et al.* [108] used machine learning algorithms on known genomic signatures to develop a tool for rapidly and correctly categorizing accessible SARS-CoV-2 genomes. Wang *et al.* used an ontology-based side effect prediction framework (OSPF) and ANN to test the adverse effects of traditional Chinese medicines to cure SARS-CoV-2 [114].

AI in COVID-19 Drug Repurposing

The technique in which former drugs are reconfigured to tackle novel diseases such as COVID-19 is called drug repurposing. Drug repurposing has been a preferred technology because of the faster production and low expenditures. AI and network medicine are highly advanced applications in particular science that define pathology, therapeutics, and target diagnosis with the minimum amount of error in the age of information [10].

Deep Learning Architecture

Deep learning is a branch of machine learning that applies layers of linear and non-linear transformations to explore data. ANN is the most commonly used deep learning model [115]. The highly interconnected feedforward neural network (FNN) is a model that uses artificial neurons to map data input to output objectives. Each link has a weight enhanced by using backpropagation on test data to reduce the forecast loss of the desired outcomes. For datasets described as vectors, FNNs are often used. Aliper and colleagues, for example, used FNN to categorize medications according to their transcriptomic vectors into the pharmaceutical therapeutic groups. When images are used as the input, and each pixel is a function vector, FNNs become impractical as the weights increase [116].

On the other hand, the convolutional neural network (CNN; panel) is specifically fit for image processing. Rather than completely linking neurons in corresponding layers, CNN employs filters that implement a convolution operation on an image, considerably limiting the number of weights. Chemical images are processed using CNN to give a perspective on pharmaceutical therapeutic functions [117]. For example, based on structural detail obtained by CNN, AtomNet estimates that tiny molecules are linked to proteins. Biological sequences are yet another form of information for drug repurposing that has gained a lot of interest [118]. Both FNN and CNN cannot be used to process such types of information.

Recurrent neural networks (RNNs) are built primarily for sequences, with a recurrent cell existing at a particular time or sequence position to maintain previous data while studying new data in the sequence. RNN models are used to build oriented molecule libraries for drug discovery, and the molecules are identified as sequences using basic molecular input line entry system codes [119]. Beck and colleagues established the molecule transformer-drug target interaction model, a combination of the CNN and RNN model that determines if any currently produced antiviral drugs could serve in SARS-CoV-2 [119].

Learning Graphic Representation

The development of medical information graphs involving association between various areas of clinical entities (*e.g* ., disorders, therapeutics, and proteins) and the estimation of the possible relationship between authorized drugs and diseases (*e.g* ., COVID-19) is a typical way to repurpose drugs. Methods based on graph embedding have gained popularity for projection in graphs where nodes and edges are expressed as low-dimensional feature vectors [120]. We can simply estimate the resemblance between drugs and diseases using feature vectors and thus differentiate productive drugs for a particular disease [121]. Scalability is a problem for the graph embedding process. The scale of actual knowledge graphs is typically huge. In a medical information graph, the number of individuals can be millions. PyTorch and TensorFlow are deep learning systems built for information with normal frameworks, not for large graphs. As a result, various models have been built that are specially developed for studying large-scale graph interpretations. Zhu and collaborators, for instance, designed GraphVite, a highly efficient apparatus capable of processing millions of nodes, which might be useful for upcoming drug repurposing [122].

Antiviral Drugs

Remdesivir was found as a monophosphate medicine to cure Ebola virus disease using an active C-adenosine nucleoside triphosphate precursor [123]. The FDA accepted the fact based on initial findings, which indicated that the drug could aid faster recovery of under-medication COVID-19 patients. Remdesivir has therapeutic potential against COVID-19, encouraging FDA approval for emergency use, but the recommendation is only for serious illnesses. The mechanism of remdesivir has been proved to stop the viral RNA-dependent RNA polymerase [124]. A double-blind experiment of injecting remdesivir intravenously in patients infected with SARS-COV-2 noticed that the treatment time was reduced to 11 days for patients treated with remdesivir in contrast to patients with no dose of the same drug [125]. These tentative results justify the application of remdesivir in COVID-19 cases who need adequate oxygen therapy in the hospital. Nevertheless, there was no substantial variation between a five-day treatment plan and a ten-day treatment plan in another open-label study covering patients with no artificial ventilation [126]. To identify the shortest successful therapy time, it is essential to carry out a deeper study on the therapeutic benefits for COVID-19 patients in various sub-groups of patients with or without oxygen therapy. Furthermore, it is not sure if remdesivir will reduce the rehabilitation process of early COVID-19 individuals.

Mefuparib (CVL218), a suppressor of poly ADP-ribose polymerase 1, inhibits SARS-CoV-2 reproduction in the laboratory with no clear toxicity consequences, according to machine learning trial and statistical testing techniques [127]. Compared to Remdesivir, Mefuparib has much more effective antiviral activity at the entry of the virus and equivalent antiviral activity at subsequent viral entry, showing that the drug may be a possible anti-SARS-CoV-2 drug candidate (Fig. **1**). In 1997, toremifene, a non-steroidal first-generation specific for estrogenic receptor modulation, was recommended to cure breast cancer [128]. Toremifene was listed as a strong candidate for the cure of COVID-19 in the research on network medicine [109]. Multiple viral infections, such as MERS-CoV, SARS-CoV, and SARS-CoV-2, were restricted *in vitro* at very minute concentrations by toremifene. Another research showed that toremifene could block nonstructural protein 14 of SARS-CoV-2 and suppress the interaction between the SARS-Co-2 spike protein and ACE2, promoting the drug's antiviral activity [129].

Host-targeting Therapy

SARS-CoV-2 induces inflammation in the body, which may lead to a cytokine storm in some cases, highlighting the significant potential for treatment efficacy with drugs that target the immune system and inflammation (such as Baricitinib, dexamethasone, and melatonin) [130], as shown in Fig. (**1**). Scientists discovered that melatonin consumption was correlated with a 50–60% lower risk of positive laboratory examination reports for SARS-CoV-2 after integrating data from network therapy and extensive individual information review from the COVID-19 patient database at the Cleveland Clinic, Cleveland, OH, USA [131]. The US FDA has certified dexamethasone as a glucocorticoid receptor agonist for several inflammatory and autoimmune disorders [132]. CoV-KGE listed dexamethasone as a potential repurposed drug. According to a randomized study on COVID-19 treatment, dexamethasone minimized mortality by a third in those requiring oxygen therapy and a fifth in those who do not require artificial ventilation [133].

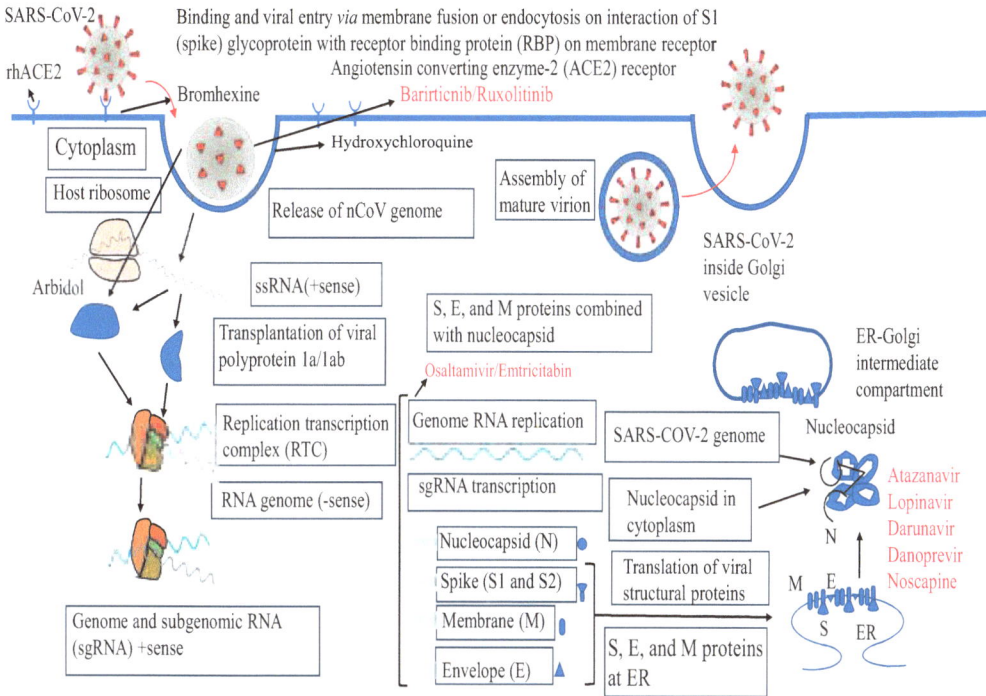

Fig. (1). Repurposing drug for SARS-CoV-2.

COVID-19 Drug Combinations

Patients with COVID-19 have demonstrated slight therapeutic success from monotherapies such as hydroxychloroquine and remdesivir [125, 134]. Since the immune system plays a crucial role in COVID-19 patients' deteriorating health and death, integrating inflammatory or immune boosters with antiviral drugs can be a potent therapy for COVID-19 patients [135]. Drug formulations with enhanced therapeutic efficiency and lower toxicity, such as remdesivir plus Baricitinib [NCT04401579], play a significant role in curing diseases involving COVID-19 [136]. Nevertheless, significant growth in the number of available drug combinations limits our capability to recognize and verified successful combinations. Scientists discovered three possible COVID-19 drug formulations by applying a network-based methodology, sirolimus plus dactinomycin, mercaptopurine plus melatonin, and toremifene plus emodin [109]. The same researchers also found that adding melatonin and toremifene could help treat COVID-19 [137]. The Cleveland Clinic is undertaking a selective estrogen regulation and melatonin in early COVID-19 (SENTINEL; NCT04531748) study to determine the therapeutic effectiveness of integrating melatonin and toremifene for cure in patients with early COVID-19 [137]. Baricitinib was recognized as a possible therapy for COVID-19 through Benevolent AI's knowledge graph [138], as shown in Fig. (**1**).

Challenges in Drug Repurposing

As the drug repurposing can treat COVID-19, there are always roadblocks to clear. Likely, cellular or animal assays do not correctly represent the virus's host condition in humans. In their actual indications, repurposed medications could be modified for a certain purpose, dosage, or tissue. Intensive clinical trials of known antimalarial, antiviral and immunoregulatory drugs are against COVID-19. Due to their convenient nature, absence of therapeutic outcomes, limited patients, and other factors, several types of research did not optimize the medication's therapeutic outcomes and biological queries [139]. For instance, *in vitro* assays indicate that hydroxychloroquine has anti-SARS-CoV-2 activity [140]. In preclinical and clinical trials, hydroxychloroquine exhibits small or no efficacy [134]. COVID-19 studies may also fail to produce therapeutic effects due to a lack of reproducible experimental animal models and clinical result interventions. The prevalence of heterogeneous groups of varying genetic profiles can also affect clinical outcomes. Attacking the incorrect biological or physiological pathways in COVID-19, utilizing medications that will not interfere with the target site, and interacting at the incorrect stage of the infection, such as quickly, medium, and late, are all issues related to these clinical research outcomes that must be considered in future experiments [10].

Detection of Novel Drugs Discovery and Vaccine Using AI For SARS-CoV-2

Protein-Based COVID-19 Drug Discovery

The virtual study on all repurposed new drugs and novel chemical agents is one of the most recent implementations of AI for COVID-19. During one of the first efforts, Gordon *et al.* experimentally discovered human proteins bound to SARS-CoV-2 proteins, opening the way for drug repurposing [141]. In contrast to wet-lab techniques, the network-based modeling approach seems to be the primary analytical method for studying the virus-host interactome. By studying the genomic sequence of three major coronavirus family members and comparing them to human infection-based mechanisms, Li *et al.* found 30 drugs for repurposing [142]. BenevolentAI used its AI-derived information graph to aggregate health data from structured and non-structured domains [143]. Baricitinib, an authorized drug for treating rheumatoid arthritis, was found to block the host protein AAK1 [110]. Beck *et al.* used their deep learning-based drug–target interaction model to identify currently accessible antiviral medications that could affect the SARS-COV-2-associated protease and helicase in related research [119]. Atomwise recently worked on attacking many SARS-CoV-2 protein binding positions that are highly conserved across many coronavirus groups to make new broad-spectrum antivirals. Atomwise is testing lots of virtual substances against different targets using its AtomNet CNN algorithm, as well as 15 different collaborations with academic scientists who would check the proposed compounds through *in vitro* studies [118]. Multi-task learning (MTL) models are also being used to classify known medicines that could target central viral proteins, such as protease (3CLpro) and spike protein [144]. Off-target activities of thirty conventional medications were discovered, for example, against the 3CLpro and ACE2 target proteins, due to Cyclica's development and exploration of PolypharmDB, a database of proven drugs and their possible attachment to host target proteins [111]. The dissemination of recently proposed chemical structures is one of the implementations of deep learning-based virtual screening for the SARS-CoV-2 primary protease reported. Amongst the most widely used methods for virtual screening is machine learning-aided molecular docking. Using docking, several molecules have been found that match the target affinity of different SARS-CoV-2 proteins necessary for viral multiplication and disease. Ton *et al.*, for example, developed and used the Deep Docking (DD) network technology to find a minimum of one thousand protease inhibitors [145]. Viral protease inhibitors as a cure for many other viruses have also been properly studied. Deep learning-aided methods have also become the center of attention since their automated feature extraction speeds up research [146].

RNA-Based COVID-19 Drug Discovery

In the life spans of coronaviruses, conserved structural elements have been exhibited to play important functional parts [147]. Structural elements add a variety of values to the regulatory data in viral RNA by interfering exclusively with target proteins that bind to RNA and helicases. Direct interruption of such structural elements' regulatory mechanisms offers a relatively undiscovered approach for minimizing viral loads with limited effects on typical cell biology [148]. Although this concept seemed unlikely, only five years earlier, developments in AI-based computational techniques and high-throughput observational RNA structure studies have more or less eliminated the major obstacles [149]. Various viral groups have greatly conserved RNA structural elements, most of which are being practically tested. A few stem-loops found in the 5′UTR of SARS-CoV-2's structural elements have been shown to affect viral growth in beta coronaviruses [147]. Several active RNA structural elements can be found in the coding region and the 3′UTR [150]. Scientists discovered 106 structurally similar sequences that could be used as bio targets for antiviral drugs that have yet to be discovered [150]. The discovery of novel and advanced targets is possible by learning RNA data changes. A new strategy demonstrates whether remdesivir, a currently FDA-approved drug, might attach to the novel coronavirus's RNA-binding network [151]. They found more potential drugs by focusing on the proteins involved in RNA synthesis and processes. The genetic material of the virus, RdRP, and processed mRNA seem to be important drug repurposing strategies.

Generative Approaches

Due to the introduction of AI, molecule synthesis has become one of the most popular domains of therapeutics in the last decade. In collaboration with IBM Research, Chenthamarakshan *et al.* showed a VAE that collects elements in a latent space. VAE stands for Variational Auto-Encoders, and it is a generative system that improves the variety of derived results. Molecules are encoded into vectors by autoencoders, which collect characteristics like molecule, bond order, and functional group [152]. After the molecule vectors have been collected, changes are made depending on the required characteristics. After that, they can also be decoded into new molecules [153]. Quantitative engineering design (QED), LogP regressors, and synthetic accessibility were used to optimize the latent space differences to improve the models.

Tang *et al.* [154] proposed a new strategy, designing a new advanced deep Q-learning network with fragment-based drug design (ADQN-FBDD) to resolve most problems with conventional generative models. They showed a reliable approach for developing unique, high-binding molecules based on the SARS-CoV-2 3CLPro structure. Researchers were able to discover space more deeply by integrating SARS-CoV-2 molecules one fraction at that same time instead of depending on latent space variations. A pharmacophore and filter descriptor is used to optimize the collection after generating interactions and rewarding molecules to the most drug-like associations. For novel drug development, the primary protease seems to focus on researchers using target-based virtual screening [154].

COVID-19 Vaccine Discovery

It is important to find the best potential targets for vaccine production to overcome a virus's rapid infection rate. The host's immune system of the host attacks the cells infected by the virus either through humoral or cell-mediated responses [155]. Major histocompatibility complex (MCH-I and MCH-II) proteins are regulated by the human leukocyte antigen (HLA) gene that introduces epitopes as antigenic determinants [156]. These molecules aid B-cell and T-cell antibodies attach to pathogens and destroy them. Machine learning techniques such as support vector machine (SVM), random forest (RF), and recursive feature selection (RFE) are used to distinguish foreign substances from protein sequences [157]. Because of their poor responsiveness in forecasting locally clustered associations in certain circumstances, deep convolutional neural networks (DCNN) have become a valid option for the attachment detection of MHC and proteins [158].

Since the first coronavirus outbreak, various AI-based techniques have been used to forecast possible epitopes and develop vaccines. To find possible SARS-CoV-2 T-cell epitopes and the SARS-CoV-2 spike receptor-binding domain, Fast and Chen used two supervised DNN-driven approaches, NetMHCPan4 (RBD) and MARIA [159, 160]. The LSTM (Long Short-Term Memory) has too yielded good results. This form of RNN was used by Abbasi *et al.* [161] to estimate epitopes for the spike. A similar strategy is using RNN and virtual Spike sequences to find potential vaccine targets [162]. RNN presented sequences for a specific protein that matched the basic local alignment search tool (BLAST) result with a high degree of sequence identity. Feng *et al.* developed a vaccine that included both B-cell and T-cell epitopes using the iNeo method. SARS-CoV-2 could be combated in a new way with this polypeptide vaccine. They also found 17 vaccine peptides that included B-cell and T-cell [163]. Vaxign-RV was employed by Ong *et al.* [164] to consider non-structural peptides as SARS-CoV-2 vaccine targets. Nsp3, the coronavirus family's most significant non-structural protein, was identified as one of the most important potential vaccine targets after Spike [112]. Malone *et al.* [165] developed an epitope chart for distinct HLA alleles, as well as the whole SARS-CoV-2 proteome other than spike, using the NEC immune profiler, immune epitope database (IEDB), and BepiPred techniques to give a detailed vaccine blueprint for SARS-CoV-2. In COVID-19 vaccine development, NLP models, especially language modeling approaches, have an influence. Sah *et al.* looked at how the seq-2-seq model based on LSTM could be used to forecast the secondary structure of SARS-COV-2 proteins [166]. Beck *et al.* [119] have used transformers to repurpose currently accessible drugs by anticipating how they will interact with SARS-COV-2 viral proteins. When all of this research is taken into account, it is obvious that spike protein has become the most successful target for simulated vaccine development. These approaches could develop virtual sequences that can be used as a roadmap for developing the new SARS-CoV-2 vaccine and other future diseases [167].

Limitations, Challenges, and Future Perspective of AI

Despite having many advantages, AI has many limitations to its application. AI requires a massive quantity of training data to produce effective predictive algorithms. On the other hand, this amount of knowledge might not be accessible in the initial stages of the infection when the projection is the most essential [102]. As a result, early in such an infection outbreak, depending on AI could be unrealistic. However, even though a significant quantity of data is accessible, AI is not flawed, as GoogleFlu illustrated, a big data processing platform for influenza epidemiological trending. Besides a large amount of data, collecting good-quality inputs can be extremely hard [168]. Many types of research focused on specific kinds of data to implement AI-driven functions, such as using only radiological images to detect COVID-19 [169]. Patients' evaluations focused on a particular data type can be biased, reinforcing the demand for a single AI system designed to measure various data types. Since there is a massive crossover in how the pulmonary organ responds to different pathological insults, and since radiological appearance is always the result of a complicated interaction of causes, non-image-based clinical information can help CT-based AI algorithms reach their maximum potential [170]. As AI can help assist in the discovery of COVID-19 drugs and vaccines, these remedies are difficult to become readily available soon, exactly where they are the most essential. Comprehensive medical testing is necessary before medications or vaccinations are approved that cause significant delays, and developing a vaccine can take 12 to 18 months [171]. Most of the trials had weak internal validity, making it difficult to identify AI's therapeutic or progressive benefit over traditional approaches. The success of AI augmentation of CT-scan and simple radiographs in research did not equate AI to radiologists' assessments, nor did they characterize the datasets used for validation [172]. External validation might be better as well. Most of the trials were limited to cases seen in a particular center or populations within the same territory. This suggests that algorithms that have been shown to become effective for the population tested perform poorly in other scenarios [173].

Although the application of the AI approach in the clinical environment looks to be simple, the basic principle and mechanism of how such algorithms work is often ambiguous to the unskilled layperson, especially healthcare personnel who are new to AI. for instance, one of the underlying limitations of deep learning, is its deficiency of interpretability [174]. To develop trends, make prognoses, and analyze data, AI may need an approach to personal data. Furthermore, personal medical data has been made available on various websites. Privacy and personal privileges can be violated if such material is shared. While collecting personal information for outbreak control could be appropriate, issues occur where the information is used for malicious purposes [175]. Automatic image categorization in X-ray and CT imaging will probably stop the spread of infection from patients to radiologists during the COVID-19 pandemic. AI-based machine learning and deep learning systems can determine patient pose, X-ray and CT image identification, and camera capabilities. Various forms of simulations can measure the influence of different social control modes on the distribution of infection using AI-based machine learning and deep learning systems. They could also be used to analyze appropriate and research-based approaches to control an infectious disease. By developing social networks and information charts, an AI-based machine learning and deep learning system will control and track the attributes of individuals living around COVID-19 patients, precisely projecting and observing the disease's possible propagation [13, 74].

Intelligent robots are intended to be utilized in public hygienic services, product distribution, and patient care that do not require human resources. To include COVID-19 patient examination, AI, with the cooperation of NLP approaches, can be used to create virtual video diagnostic and robot systems. This will prevent the propagation of the COVID-19 disease. Discovering the treatment for COVID-19 is much more important. We noted that most current AI-based machine learning and deep learning approaches are more focused on detecting the cure for COVID-19. However, in the future, more work will be focused on treating COVID-19 disease [13, 176]. In biological science, AI-based machine learning and deep learning systems may help classify protein content and viral factors using precise biomedical information analysis, including essential protein structures, genomic codes, and viral routes. AI-based machine learning and deep learning systems might be used to classify potential therapeutics and simulate drug-protein and vaccine-receptor associations, allowing for the assessment of likely drug and vaccine responses in patients with COVID-19 [13, 177, 178].

CONCLUSION

Coronaviruses are a class of viruses that can develop various diseases, from the common cold to SARS. The COVID-19 pandemic is wreaking havoc on people's lives and suffering. Due to the pandemic's fast transmission, much advanced scientific research and information exchange is in progress. Till now, AI's possible ability to quickly discover novel candidate drugs that can be put into drug testing is being utilized and, if acknowledged, AI will revolutionize healthcare, making it a focal point of emerging technology. As a result, AI holds promise for accelerating drug repurposing for human infections, particularly new evolving infections such as COVID-19. AI is an emerging and powerful tool for identifying initial coronavirus diseases and monitoring the health of those who have been infected [178]. AI is beneficial for the cure of COVID-19 and proper health monitoring. AI will aid in implementing effective treatment regimens, preventive measures, and drug and vaccine production. Among several advantages that AI can have, there are also significant drawbacks to its application, like data sharing and privacy, fake information, and unavailability of important information.

AUTHORS CONTRIBUTION

KN conceived the original idea and designed the outlines of the study. SR and F equally contributed and wrote the 1st draft of the manuscript. MK, AM and IA drew the figures and edited the manuscript. KN revised the whole manuscript and formatted it accordingly. All authors have read and approved the final manuscript.

ACKNOWLEDGEMENTS

The authors acknowledge the support of Cholistan University of Veterinary & Animal Sciences-Bahawalpur, Pakistan, during the write-up.

REFERENCES

[1]   Gossner C, Danielson N, Gervelmeyer A, *et al.* health, p., Human–dromedary camel interactions and the risk of acquiring zoonotic Middle East respiratory syndrome coronavirus infection. Zoonoses Public Health 2016; 63(1): 1-9.
       [http://dx.doi.org/10.1111/zph.12171] [PMID: 25545147]

[2]   Azhar EI, El-Kafrawy SA, Farraj SA, *et al.* Evidence for camel-to-human transmission of MERS coronavirus. N Engl J Med 2014; 370(26): 2499-505.
       [http://dx.doi.org/10.1056/NEJMoa1401505] [PMID: 24896817]

[3]   Allam Z, Tegally H, Thondoo MJSC. Redefining the use of big data in urban health for increased liveability in smart cities. Smart Cities 2019; 2(2): 259-68.
       [http://dx.doi.org/10.3390/smartcities2020017]

[4]   Watson KJDDLNY. NY, USA, Predictive Analytics in Health Care: Emerging Value and Risks. 2019.

[5]   Yassine HM, Shah Z. How could artificial intelligence aid in the fight against coronavirus? An interview with Dr Hadi M Yassine and Dr Zubair Shah by Felicity Poole, Commissioning Editor. Expert Review of Anti-Infective Therapy 2020; 18(6): 493-7.
       [http://dx.doi.org/10.1080/14787210.2020.1744275]

[6]   Fleming N. How artificial intelligence is changing drug discovery. Nature 2018; 557(7707): S55-7.
       [http://dx.doi.org/10.1038/d41586-018-05267-x] [PMID: 29849160]

[7]   Smalley E. AI-powered drug discovery captures pharma interest. Nature Biotechnology. 2017 Jul 1; 35(7): 604-6.

[8]   Jibril ML, Sharif USJa. Power of artificial intelligence to diagnose and prevent further COVID-19 outbreak: A short communication. 2020.
       [http://dx.doi.org/10.48550/arXiv.2004.12463]

[9]   Zhavoronkov A, Aladinskiy V, Zhebrak A, *et al.* Potential 2019-nCoV 3C-like protease inhibitors designed using generative deep learning approaches. Chem Rxiv 2020; 1182(9102): v1.
       [http://dx.doi.org/10.26434/chemrxiv.11829102.v1]

[10]   Zhou Y, Wang F, Tang J, Nussinov R, Cheng F. Artificial intelligence in COVID-19 drug repurposing. Lancet Digit Health 2020; 2(12): e667-76.
       [http://dx.doi.org/10.1016/S2589-7500(20)30192-8] [PMID: 32984792]

[11]   Haleem A, Javaid M, Vaishya R. Effects of COVID 19 pandemic in daily life. Current Medicine Research and Practice, 2020; 10(2): 78-79.
       [http://dx.doi.org/10.1016/j.cmrp.2020.03.011]

[12]   Bai HX, Hsieh B, Xiong Z, *et al.* Performance of radiologists in differentiating COVID-19 from non-COVID-19 viral pneumonia at chest CT. Radiology 2020; 296(2): E46-54.

[http://dx.doi.org/10.1148/radiol.2020200823] [PMID: 32155105]

[13]   Alafif T, Tehame AM, Bajaba S, Barnawi A, Zia S, Health P. Machine and Deep Learning towards COVID-19 Diagnosis and Treatment: Survey, Challenges, and Future Directions. Int J Environ Res Public Health 2021; 18(3): 1117.
[http://dx.doi.org/10.3390/ijerph18031117] [PMID: 33513984]

[14]   Hassani H, Silva ES, Unger S, TajMazinani M, Mac Feely S. Artificial intelligence (AI) or intelligence augmentation (IA): what is the future?. Ai. 2020 Apr 12; 1(2): 8.
[http://dx.doi.org/10.3390/ai1020008]

[15]   Long JB, Ehrenfeld JM. The role of augmented intelligence (AI) in detecting and preventing the spread of novel coronavirus. Journal of medical systems. 2020 Mar; 44: 1-2.
[http://dx.doi.org/10.1007/s10916-020-1536-6]

[16]   Jin C, Chen W, Cao Y, *et al.* Development and evaluation of an artificial intelligence system for COVID-19 diagnosis. Nat Commun 2020; 11(1): 5088.
[http://dx.doi.org/10.1038/s41467-020-18685-1]

[17]   Harrison C. Coronavirus puts drug repurposing on the fast track. Nat Biotechnol 2020; 38(4): 379-81.
[http://dx.doi.org/10.1038/d41587-020-00003-1] [PMID: 32205870]

[18]   Gozes O, Frid-Adar M, Greenspan H, *et al.* Rapid ai development cycle for the coronavirus (covid-19) pandemic: Initial results for automated detection & patient monitoring using deep learning ct image analysis. arXiv: 2003.05037.
[http://dx.doi.org/10.48550/arXiv.2003.05037]

[19]   Ksiazek TG, Erdman D, Goldsmith CS, Zaki SR, Peret T, Emery S, Tong S, Urbani C, Comer JA, Lim W, Rollin PE. A novel coronavirus associated with severe acute respiratory syndrome. New England journal of medicine. 2003 May 15; 348(20): 1953-66.

[20]   Fehr AR, Perlman S, Maier HJ, Bickerton E, Britton P.. An Overview of Their Replication and Pathogenesis; Section 2 Genomic Organization. Methods Mol Biol 2015; 1282: 1-23.
[http://dx.doi.org/10.1007/978-1-4939-2438-7_1]

[21]   Ge XY, Li JL, Yang XL, *et al.* Isolation and characterization of a bat SARS-like coronavirus that uses the ACE2 receptor. Nature 2013; 503(7477): 535-8.
[http://dx.doi.org/10.1038/nature12711] [PMID: 24172901]

[22]   Control CD. Remembering SARS: A Deadly Puzzle and the Efforts to Solve It. 2016; 25.

[23]   Remembering SJCDC. Prevention, A Deadly Puzzle and the Efforts to Solve It. 2013; 11.

[24]   Fouchier RAM, Kuiken T, Schutten M, *et al.* Koch's postulates fulfilled for SARS virus. Nature 2003; 423(6937): 240-0.
[http://dx.doi.org/10.1038/423240a] [PMID: 12748632]

[25]   Ahad MA. Coronavirus-A Global Emergency. Med Today 2020; 32(2): 138–142.
[PMID: 33552257]

[26]   Al-Tayib OA. An overview of the most significant zoonotic viral pathogens transmitted from animal to human in Saudi Arabia. Pathogens. 2019 Feb 22; 8(1): 25.

[27]   Parry RL. Travel alert after eighth camel flu death. The Times. 2015 Jun; 2(10).

[28]   Zumla A, Hui DS, Perlman S. Middle East respiratory syndrome. The Lancet. 2015 Sep 5; 386(9997): 995-1007.

[29]   Rivers CM, Majumder MS, Lofgren ET. Risks of death and severe disease in patients with Middle East respiratory syndrome coronavirus, 2012–2015. Am J Epidemiol 2016; 184(6): 460-4.
[http://dx.doi.org/10.1093/aje/kww013] [PMID: 27608662]

[30]   Ahmed AE. The predictors of 3- and 30-day mortality in 660 MERS-CoV patients. BMC Infect Dis 2017; 17(1): 615.

[http://dx.doi.org/10.1186/s12879-017-2712-2] [PMID: 28893197]

[31]   Al-Turaiki I, Alshahrani M, Almutairi T. Building predictive models for MERS-CoV infections using data mining techniques. J Infect Public Health 2016; 9(6): 744-8.
[http://dx.doi.org/10.1016/j.jiph.2016.09.007] [PMID: 27641481]

[32]   Khan R, Shrivastava P, Kapoor A, Tiwari A. Social media analysis with AI: sentiment analysis techniques for the analysis of twitter COVID-19 data. J Critic Review 2020; 7(9): 2761-74.

[33]   John M, Shaiba H. Main factors influencing recovery in MERS Co-V patients using machine learning. J Infect Public Health 2019; 12(5): 700-4.
[http://dx.doi.org/10.1016/j.jiph.2019.03.020] [PMID: 30979679]

[34]   Lau SK, Luk HK, Wong AC, *et al.* Possible bat origin of severe acute respiratory syndrome coronavirus 2. Emerg Infect Dis 2020; 26(7): 1542-7.
[http://dx.doi.org/10.3201/eid2607.200092]

[35]   Cai J, Sun W, Huang J, Gamber M, Wu J, He G. Indirect virus transmission in cluster of COVID-19 cases. Emerg Infect Dis 2020; 26(6): 1343-5.
[http://dx.doi.org/10.3201/eid2606.200412] [PMID: 32163030]

[36]   van Doremalen N, Bushmaker T, Morris DH, *et al.* Aerosol and surface stability of SARS-CoV-2 as compared with SARS-CoV-1. N Engl J Med 2020; 382(16): 1564-7.
[http://dx.doi.org/10.1056/NEJMc2004973] [PMID: 32182409]

[37]   Cheng VCC, Wong SC, Chuang VWM, *et al.* The role of community-wide wearing of face mask for control of coronavirus disease 2019 (COVID-19) epidemic due to SARS-CoV-2. J Infect 2020; 81(1): 107-14.
[http://dx.doi.org/10.1016/j.jinf.2020.04.024] [PMID: 32335167]

[38]   Maghded HS, Ghafoor KZ, Sadiq AS, Curran K, Rawat DB, Rabie K. A novel AI-enabled framework to diagnose coronavirus COVID-19 using smartphone embedded sensors: design study. In2020 IEEE 21st international conference on information reuse and integration for data science (IRI) 2020 Aug 11 pp. 180-187. IEEE.

[39]   Imran A, Posokhova I, Qureshi HN, *et al.* AI4COVID-19: AI enabled preliminary diagnosis for COVID-19 from cough samples *via* an app. Informatics in Medicine Unlocked 2020; 20: 100378.
[http://dx.doi.org/10.1016/j.imu.2020.100378] [PMID: 32839734]

[40]   Rahmatizadeh S, Valizadeh-Haghi S, Dabbagh A. The role of artificial intelligence in management of critical COVID-19 patients. J Cell Mol Anesth 2020; 5(1): 16-22.
[http://dx.doi.org/10.22037/jcma.v5i1.29752] [PMID: 33240422]

[41]   Heaven WD. AI could help with the next pandemic—but not with this one. MIT Technology Review. 2020 Mar 12.

[42]   Flynn S, Geiger C, Quintais JP, Margoni T, Sag M, Guibault L, Carroll MW. Implementing user rights for research in the field of artificial intelligence: A call for international action. Joint PIJIP/TLS Research Paper Series. 2020 (48).

[43]   Niiler E. An AI epidemiologist sent the first warnings of the Wuhan virus. wired. Available from: https://www. wired. com/story/ai-epidemiologist-wuhan-public-health-warnings/ Accessed. 2020 Dec;25.

[44]   Allam Z, Dey G, Jones DS. Artificial intelligence (AI) provided early detection of the coronavirus (COVID-19) in China and will influence future Urban health policy internationally. Ai. 2020 Apr 13; 1(2): 156-65.

[45]   Bogoch II, Brady OJ, Kraemer MUG, *et al.* Anticipating the international spread of Zika virus from Brazil. Lancet 2016; 387(10016): 335-6.
[http://dx.doi.org/10.1016/S0140-6736(16)00080-5] [PMID: 26777915]

[46]   Phelan AL, Katz R, Gostin LO. The novel coronavirus originating in Wuhan, China: challenges for

global health governance. JAMA 2020; 323(8): 709-10.
[http://dx.doi.org/10.1001/jama.2020.1097] [PMID: 31999307]

[47]   Allam Z. Underlining the Role of Data Science and Technology in Supporting Supply Chains, Political Stability and Health Networks During Pandemics. Surveying the COVID-19 Pandemic and its Implications 2020; 129-39.
[http://dx.doi.org/10.1016/B978-0-12-824313-8.00010-3]

[48]   Benny D, Virdi K. Application of Big Data in Analysis and Management of Coronavirus (COVID-19). Impact of AI and Data Science in Response to Coronavirus Pandemic. 2021: 149-68.

[49]   Bowles J. How Canadian AI start-up BlueDot spotted Coronavirus before anyone else had a clue. 2020.

[50]   Allam Z. The Rise of Machine Intelligence in the COVID-19 Pandemic and Its Impact on Health Policy. Surveying the COVID-19 Pandemic and its Implications 2020; 8996-96.
[http://dx.doi.org/10.1016/B978-0-12-824313-8.00006-1]

[51]   Tong SJMo. Big Data Predicted the Coronavirus Outbrea and Where It Would Spread. 2020.

[52]   Allam Z, Dey G, Jones DS. Artificial intelligence (AI) provided early detection of the coronavirus (COVID-19) in China and will influence future Urban health policy internationally. AI 2020; 1(2): 156-65.
[http://dx.doi.org/10.3390/ai1020009] [PMID: 33552274]

[53]   Oberholtzer K, Sivitz L, Mack A, Lemon S, Mahmoud A, Knobler S. Learning from SARS: preparing for the next disease outbreak: workshop summary. National Academies Press 2004.

[54]   Organization WH. WHO MERS global summary and assessment of risk, July 2019. World Health Organization 2019.

[55]   Alsunaidi SJ, Almuhaideb AM, Ibrahim NM, Shaikh FS, Alqudaihi KS, Alhaidari FA, Khan IU, Aslam N, Alshahrani MS. Applications of big data analytics to control COVID-19 pandemic. Sensors. 2021 Mar 24; 21(7): 2282.

[56]   Kharpal A. China 'has the Edge'in the War for 5g and the Us and Europe Could Fall Behind. 2018.

[57]   Allam Z, Dhunny ZA. On big data, artificial intelligence and smart Cities. Cities 2019; 89: 80-91.
[http://dx.doi.org/10.1016/j.cities.2019.01.032]

[58]   Allam Z. In Cities and the digital revolution. Springer 2020; pp. 85-106.
[http://dx.doi.org/10.1007/978-3-030-29800-5_4]

[59]   Vayena E, Blasimme A. Health research with big data: Time for systemic oversight. J Law Med Ethics 2018; 46(1): 119-29.
[http://dx.doi.org/10.1177/1073110518766026] [PMID: 30655746]

[60]   Allam Z. In Cities and the Digital Revolution. Springer 2020; pp. 1-29.
[http://dx.doi.org/10.1007/978-3-030-29800-5]

[61]   Allam Z, Jones DS. On the coronavirus (COVID-19) outbreak and the smart city network: universal data sharing standards coupled with artificial intelligence (AI) to benefit urban health monitoring and management. InHealthcare, 2020 Feb 27; 8(1), 46.
[http://dx.doi.org/10.3390/healthcare8010046]

[62]   Sweeney L. K-anonymity: a model for protecting privacy. Int J Uncertainty Fuzziness and Knowledge-Based Systems 2002; 10(05): 557-70.
[http://dx.doi.org/10.1142/S0218488502001648]

[63]   de Montjoye Y-A, Farzanehfar A, Hendrickx J, Rocher L. Solving artificial intelligence's privacy problem. 2017; 17: 80.

[64]   Ellahham S, Ellahham N, Simsekler MCE. Application of artificial intelligence in the health care safety context: opportunities and challenges. Am J Med Qual 2020; 35(4): 341-8.

[http://dx.doi.org/10.1177/1062860619878515] [PMID: 31581790]

[65] Liu P, Beeler P, Chakrabarty RKJm. COVID-19 progression timeline and effectiveness of response-t--spread interventions across the United States. 2020.

[66] Muhammad L, Haruna AA, Mohammed IA, Abubakar M, Badamasi BG, Amshi JM. 2019.

[67] Chen J, Wu L, Zhang J, *et al.* Deep learning-based model for detecting 2019 novel coronavirus pneumonia on high-resolution computed tomography. Sci Rep 2020; 10(1): 19196.
[http://dx.doi.org/10.1038/s41598-020-76282-0] [PMID: 33240407]

[68] Shi H, Han X, Jiang N, *et al.* Radiological findings from 81 patients with COVID-19 pneumonia in Wuhan, China: a descriptive study. Lancet Infect Dis 2020; 20(4): 425-34.
[http://dx.doi.org/10.1016/S1473-3099(20)30086-4] [PMID: 32105637]

[69] Zaki AM. van BS, Bestebroer TM, Osterhaus AD, Fouchier RA. Isolation of a novel coronavirus from a man with pneumonia in Saudi Arabia. N Engl J Med 2012; 367(19): 1814-20.
[http://dx.doi.org/10.1056/NEJMoa1211721]

[70] Wiemken TL, Furmanek SP, Mattingly WA, *et al.* Predicting 30-day mortality in hospitalized patients with community-acquired pneumonia using statistical and machine learning approaches. J Respiratory 2017; 1(3): 10.
[http://dx.doi.org/10.18297/JRI/VOL1/ISS3/10/]

[71] Morens DM, Folkers GK, Fauci AS. The challenge of emerging and re-emerging infectious diseases. Nature 2004; 430(6996): 242-9.
[http://dx.doi.org/10.1038/nature02759] [PMID: 15241422]

[72] Kim KH, Tandi TE, Choi JW, Moon JM, Kim MS. Middle East respiratory syndrome coronavirus (MERS-CoV) outbreak in South Korea, 2015: epidemiology, characteristics and public health implications. J Hosp Infect 2017; 95(2): 207-13.
[http://dx.doi.org/10.1016/j.jhin.2016.10.008] [PMID: 28153558]

[73] Hu Z, Ge Q, Li S, Jin L, Xiong MJ. Artificial intelligence forecasting of COVID-19 in china. 2020.

[74] Vaishya R, Javaid M, Khan IH, Haleem A, Research MSC. Artificial Intelligence (AI) applications for COVID-19 pandemic. Diabetes Metab Syndr 2020; 14(4): 337-9.
[http://dx.doi.org/10.1016/j.dsx.2020.04.012] [PMID: 32305024]

[75] Haleem A, Vaishya R, Javaid M, Khan IH. Artificial Intelligence (AI) applications in orthopaedics: An innovative technology to embrace. J Clin Orthop Trauma 2020; 11 (Suppl. 1): S80-1.
[http://dx.doi.org/10.1016/j.jcot.2019.06.012] [PMID: 31992923]

[76] Biswas K, Sen PJ. Space-time dependence of corona virus (COVID-19) outbreak. 2020.

[77] Smeulders AW, van Ginneken AM. An analysis of pathology knowledge and decision making for the development of artificial intelligence-based consulting systems. Anal Quant Cytol Histol 1989; 11(3): 154-65.
[PMID: 2663007]

[78] Gozes O, Frid-Adar M, Greenspan H, *et al.* Rapid ai development cycle for the coronavirus (covid-19) pandemic: Initial results for automated detection & patient monitoring using deep learning ct image analysis. arXiv 2020.
[http://dx.doi.org/10.48550/arXiv.2003.05037]

[79] Gupta R, Misra A. Contentious issues and evolving concepts in the clinical presentation and management of patients with COVID-19 infectionwith reference to use of therapeutic and other drugs used in Co-morbid diseases (Hypertension, diabetes *etc*). Diabetes Metab Syndr 2020; 14(3): 251-4.
[http://dx.doi.org/10.1016/j.dsx.2020.03.012] [PMID: 32247213]

[80] Gupta R, Ghosh A, Singh AK, Misra A. Clinical considerations for patients with diabetes in times of COVID-19 epidemic. Diabetes Metab Syndr 2020; 14(3): 211-2.
[http://dx.doi.org/10.1016/j.dsx.2020.03.002] [PMID: 32172175]

[81]   Heymann DL. Data sharing and outbreaks: best practice exemplified. Lancet 2020; 395(10223): 469-70.
[http://dx.doi.org/10.1016/S0140-6736(20)30184-7] [PMID: 31986258]

[82]   Sharma A, Tiwari S, Deb MK, Marty JL. Severe acute respiratory syndrome coronavirus-2 (SARS-CoV-2): a global pandemic and treatment strategies. International journal of antimicrobial agents. 2020 Aug 1; 56(2): 106054.

[83]   McCall B. COVID-19 and artificial intelligence: protecting health-care workers and curbing the spread. Lancet Digit Health 2020; 2(4): e166-7.
[http://dx.doi.org/10.1016/S2589-7500(20)30054-6] [PMID: 32289116]

[84]   Zhang X, Ma R, Wang L. Predicting turning point, duration and attack rate of COVID-19 outbreaks in major Western countries. Chaos Solitons Fractals 2020; 135: 109829.
[http://dx.doi.org/10.1016/j.chaos.2020.109829] [PMID: 32313405]

[85]   Ceylan Z. Estimation of COVID-19 prevalence in Italy, Spain, and France. Sci Total Environ 2020; 729: 138817.
[http://dx.doi.org/10.1016/j.scitotenv.2020.138817] [PMID: 32360907]

[86]   Ribeiro MHDM, da Silva RG, Mariani VC, Coelho LS. Short-term forecasting COVID-19 cumulative confirmed cases: Perspectives for Brazil. Chaos Solitons Fractals 2020; 135: 109853.
[http://dx.doi.org/10.1016/j.chaos.2020.109853] [PMID: 32501370]

[87]   Chimmula VKR, Zhang L. Time series forecasting of COVID-19 transmission in Canada using LSTM networks. Chaos Solitons Fractals 2020; 135: 109864.
[http://dx.doi.org/10.1016/j.chaos.2020.109864] [PMID: 32390691]

[88]   Chakraborty T, Ghosh I. Real-time forecasts and risk assessment of novel coronavirus (COVID-19) cases: A data-driven analysis. Chaos Solitons Fractals 2020; 135: 109850.
[http://dx.doi.org/10.1016/j.chaos.2020.109850] [PMID: 32355424]

[89]   Singh S, Parmar KS, Kumar J, Makkhan SJS. Development of new hybrid model of discrete wavelet decomposition and autoregressive integrated moving average (ARIMA) models in application to one month forecast the casualties cases of COVID-19. Chaos Solitons Fractals 2020; 135: 109866.
[http://dx.doi.org/10.1016/j.chaos.2020.109866] [PMID: 32395038]

[90]   Ribeiro MH, da Silva RG, Fraccanabbia N, Mariani VC, Coelho LS. Forecasting epidemiological time series based on decomposition and optimization approaches. In14th Brazilian computational intelligence meeting (CBIC), Belém, Brazil, PA 2019; 1-8.

[91]   Rasheed J, Jamil A, Hameed AA, *et al.* A survey on artificial intelligence approaches in supporting frontline workers and decision makers for COVID-19 pandemic. Chaos Solitons Fractals 2020; 141: 110337.
[http://dx.doi.org/10.1016/j.chaos.2020.110337]

[92]   Wu J, Zhang P, Zhang L, *et al.* Rapid and accurate identification of COVID-19 infection through machine learning based on clinical available blood test results. medRxiv 2020.
[http://dx.doi.org/10.1101/2020.04.02.20051136]

[93]   Iwendi C, Bashir AK, Peshkar A, *et al.* COVID-19 patient health prediction using boosted random forest algorithm. Front Public Health 2020; 8: 357.
[http://dx.doi.org/10.3389/fpubh.2020.00357] [PMID: 32719767]

[94]   Miner AS, Laranjo L, Kocaballi AB. Chatbots in the fight against the COVID-19 pandemic. NPJ Digit Med 2020; 3: 65.
[http://dx.doi.org/10.1038/s41746-020-0280-0] [PMID: 33240407]

[95]   Battineni G, Chintalapudi N, Amenta F. AI chatbot design during an epidemic like the novel coronavirus. In Healthcare 2020 Jun 3 8(2), 154.

[96]   Sarbadhikari S, Sarbadhikari S. The global experience of digital health interventions in COVID-19

management. Indian J Public Health 2020; 64(6) (Suppl.): 117.
[http://dx.doi.org/10.4103/ijph.IJPH_457_20] [PMID: 32496240]

[97]   Yan L, Zhang H, Goncalves J, *et al.* A machine learning-based model for survival prediction in patients with severe COVID-19 infection. medRxiv 2020.
[http://dx.doi.org/10.1101/2020.02.27.20028027]

[98]   Jiang X, Coffee M, Bari A, *et al.* Towards an artificial intelligence framework for data-driven prediction of coronavirus clinical severity. Computers, Materials & Continua 2020; 63(1): 537-51.
[http://dx.doi.org/10.32604/cmc.2020.010691]

[99]   Yang GZ, Nelson BJ, Murphy RR, Choset H, Christensen H, Collins SH, Dario P, Goldberg K, Ikuta K, Jacobstein N, Kragic D. Combating COVID-19-The role of robotics in managing public health and infectious diseases. Science Robotics, 5 (40) [Internet]. 2020.

[100] Zeng Z, Chen P-J, Lew A. From high-touch to high-tech: COVID-19 drives robotics adoption. Tourism Geographies 2020; 22(3): 724-34.
[http://dx.doi.org/10.1080/14616688.2020.1762118]

[101] Arora N, Banerjee AK, Narasu ML. The role of artificial intelligence in tackling COVID-19. Future Virology. 2020 Nov 1; 15(11): 717-24.

[102] Santosh KC. AI-driven tools for coronavirus outbreak: need of active learning and cross-population train/test models on multitudinal/multimodal data. J Med Syst 2020; 44(5): 93.
[http://dx.doi.org/10.1007/s10916-020-01562-1] [PMID: 32189081]

[103] Li L, Qin L, Xu Z, *et al.* Artificial intelligence distinguishes COVID-19 from community acquired pneumonia on chest CT. Radiology 2020; 200905.
[http://dx.doi.org/10.1148/radiol.2020200905]

[104] Farooq M, Hafeez A. Covid-resnet: A deep learning framework for screening of covid19 from radiographs. arXiv 2020.
[http://dx.doi.org/10.48550/arXiv.2003.14395]

[105] Alom MZ, Rahman M, Nasrin MS, Taha TM, Asari VK. Covid_mtnet: COVID-19 detection with multi-task deep learning approaches. arXiv 2020.
[http://dx.doi.org/10.48550/arXiv.2004.03747]

[106] Senior AW, Evans R, Jumper J, *et al.* Improved protein structure prediction using potentials from deep learning. Nature 2020; 577(7792): 706-10.
[http://dx.doi.org/10.1038/s41586-019-1923-7] [PMID: 31942072]

[107] Pfab J, Phan NM, Si DJb. DeepTracer: Automated Protein Complex Structure Prediction from CoV-related Cryo-EM Density Maps. bioRxiv 2020.
[http://dx.doi.org/10.1101/2020.07.21.214064]

[108] Randhawa GS, Soltysiak MPM, El Roz H, de Souza CPE, Hill KA, Kari L. Machine learning using intrinsic genomic signatures for rapid classification of novel pathogens: COVID-19 case study. PLoS One 2020; 15(4): e0232391.
[http://dx.doi.org/10.1371/journal.pone.0232391] [PMID: 32330208]

[109] Zhou Y, Hou Y, Shen J, Huang Y, Martin W, Cheng F. Network-based drug repurposing for novel coronavirus 2019-nCoV/SARS-CoV-2. Cell Discov 2020; 6(1): 1-18.
[http://dx.doi.org/10.1038/s41421-020-0153-3] [PMID: 33240407]

[110] Stebbing J, Phelan A, Griffin I, *et al.* COVID-19: combining antiviral and anti-inflammatory treatments. Lancet Infect Dis 2020; 20(4): 400-2.
[http://dx.doi.org/10.1016/S1473-3099(20)30132-8] [PMID: 32113509]

[111] Chauhan N. Possible drug candidates for COVID-19. 2020.
[http://dx.doi.org/10.26434/chemrxiv.11985231.v1]

[112] Ong E, Wong MU, Huffman A, He Y. COVID-19 coronavirus vaccine design using reverse

vaccinology and machine learning. Front Immunol 2020; 11: 1581.
[http://dx.doi.org/10.3389/fimmu.2020.01581] [PMID: 32719684]

[113] Rashid MT, Wang D. CovidSens: a vision on reliable social sensing for COVID-19. Artif Intell Rev 2021; 54(1): 1-25.
[http://dx.doi.org/10.1007/s10462-020-09852-3] [PMID: 32836651]

[114] Wang Z, Li L, Song M, Yan J, Shi J, Yao Y. Evaluating the traditional chinese medicine (TCM) officially recommended in China for COVID-19 using ontology-based side-effect prediction framework (OSPF) and deep learning. J Ethnopharmacol 2021; 272: 113957.
[http://dx.doi.org/10.1016/j.jep.2021.113957] [PMID: 33631276]

[115] LeCun Y, Bengio Y, Hinton G. Deep learning. Nature 2015; 521(7553): 436-44.
[http://dx.doi.org/10.1038/nature14539] [PMID: 26017442]

[116] Aliper A, Plis S, Artemov A, Ulloa A, Mamoshina P, Zhavoronkov A. Deep learning applications for predicting pharmacological properties of drugs and drug repurposing using transcriptomic data. Mol Pharm 2016; 13(7): 2524-30.
[http://dx.doi.org/10.1021/acs.molpharmaceut.6b00248] [PMID: 27200455]

[117] Meyer JG, Liu S, Miller IJ, Coon JJ, Gitter A. modeling, Learning drug functions from chemical structures with convolutional neural networks and random forests. J Chem Inf Model 2019; 59(10): 4438-49.
[http://dx.doi.org/10.1021/acs.jcim.9b00236] [PMID: 31518132]

[118] Wallach I, Dzamba M, Heifets A. AtomNet: a deep convolutional neural network for bioactivity prediction in structure-based drug discovery. arXiv 2015.
[http://dx.doi.org/10.48550/arXiv.1510.02855]

[119] Beck BR, Shin B, Choi Y, Park S, Kang K. Predicting commercially available antiviral drugs that may act on the novel coronavirus (SARS-CoV-2) through a drug-target interaction deep learning model. Comput Struct Biotechnol J 2020; 18: 784-90.
[http://dx.doi.org/10.1016/j.csbj.2020.03.025] [PMID: 32280433]

[120] Cai H, Zheng VW, Chang KC. A comprehensive survey of graph embedding: Problems, techniques, and applications. IEEE transactions on knowledge and data engineering. 2018 Feb 19; 30(9): 1616-37.

[121] Tang J, Qu M, Wang M, Zhang M, Yan J, Mei Q. Proceedings of the 24th international conference on world wide web 2015; 1067-77.
[http://dx.doi.org/10.48550/arXiv.1503.03578]

[122] Gunturu LN, Dornadula G, Nimbagal RN. Reconsideration of drug repurposing through artificial intelligence program for the treatment of the novel coronavirus. Artificial Intelligence in Healthcare and COVID-19. 2023 Jan 1: 45-68.

[123] Sanders JM, Monogue ML, Jodlowski TZ, Cutrell JB. Pharmacologic treatments for coronavirus disease 2019 (COVID-19): a review. JAMA 2020; 323(18): 1824-36.
[http://dx.doi.org/10.1001/jama.2020.6019] [PMID: 32282022]

[124] Yin W, Mao C, Luan X, *et al.* Structural basis for inhibition of the RNA-dependent RNA polymerase from SARS-CoV-2 by remdesivir. Science 2020; 368(6498): 1499-504.
[http://dx.doi.org/10.1126/science.abc1560] [PMID: 32358203]

[125] Beigel JH, Tomashek KM, Dodd LE, *et al.* Remdesivir for the treatment of Covid-19—preliminary report. 2020.

[126] Godman B. Combating COVID-19: Lessons learnt particularly among developing countries and the implications. Bangladesh J Med Sci 2020; 103-S: 108.
[http://dx.doi.org/10.3329/bjms.v19i0.48413]

[127] Ge Y, Tian T, Huang S, *et al.* A data-driven drug repositioning framework discovered a potential therapeutic agent targeting COVID-19. Sig Transduct Target Ther 2021; 6: 165.
[http://dx.doi.org/10.1101/2020.03.11.986836]

[128] Wiseman LR, Goa KL. Toremifene. Drugs 1997; 54(1): 141-60.
[http://dx.doi.org/10.2165/00003495-199754010-00014] [PMID: 9211086]

[129] Martin WR, Cheng F. Repurposing of FDA-approved toremifene to treat COVID-19 by blocking the Spike glycoprotein and NSP14 of SARS-CoV-2. J Proteome Res 2020; 19(11): 4670-7.
[http://dx.doi.org/10.1021/acs.jproteome.0c00397] [PMID: 32907334]

[130] Gupta A, Madhavan MV, Sehgal K, *et al.* Extrapulmonary manifestations of COVID-19. Nat Med 2020; 26(7): 1017-32.
[http://dx.doi.org/10.1038/s41591-020-0968-3] [PMID: 32651579]

[131] Moreno A, Romero AR, Neochoritis C, Groves M, Velázquez M, Dömling A. Gliptin repurposing for COVID-19. ChemRxiv 2020.
[http://dx.doi.org/10.26434/chemrxiv.12110760.v1]

[132] Ramamoorthy S, Cidlowski JA. Corticosteroids: mechanisms of action in health and disease. Rheum Dis Clin North Am 2016; 42(1): 15-31, vii.
[PMID: 26611548]

[133] Chenot C, Robiette R, Collin S. chemistry, f., First evidence of the cysteine and glutathione conjugates of 3-sulfanylpentan-1-ol in hop (Humulus lupulus L.). J Agric Food Chem 2019; 67(14): 4002-10.
[http://dx.doi.org/10.1021/acs.jafc.9b00225] [PMID: 30874436]

[134] Rosenberg ES, Dufort EM, Udo T, *et al.* Association of treatment with hydroxychloroquine or azithromycin with in-hospital mortality in patients with COVID-19 in New York State. JAMA 2020; 323(24): 2493-502.
[http://dx.doi.org/10.1001/jama.2020.8630] [PMID: 32392282]

[135] Tay MZ, Poh CM, Rénia L, MacAry PA, Ng LF. The trinity of COVID-19: immunity, inflammation and intervention. Nat Rev Immunol 2020; 20(6): 363-74.
[http://dx.doi.org/10.1038/s41577-020-0311-8]

[136] Cheng F, Kovács IA, Barabási AL. Network-based prediction of drug combinations. Nat Commun 2019; 10(1): 1197.
[http://dx.doi.org/10.1038/s41467-019-09186-x]

[137] Cheng F, Rao S, Mehra R. COVID-19 treatment: Combining anti-inflammatory and antiviral therapeutics using a network-based approach. Cleve Clin J Med 2020.
[http://dx.doi.org/10.3949/ccjm.87a.ccc037] [PMID: 32606050]

[138] Richardson P, Griffin I, Tucker C, *et al.* Baricitinib as potential treatment for 2019-nCoV acute respiratory disease. Lancet 2020; 395(10223): e30-1.
[http://dx.doi.org/10.1016/S0140-6736(20)30304-4] [PMID: 32032529]

[139] Mehta HB, Ehrhardt S, Moore TJ, Segal JB, Alexander GC. Characteristics of registered clinical trials assessing treatments for COVID-19: a cross-sectional analysis. BMJ Open 2020; 10(6): e039978.
[http://dx.doi.org/10.1136/bmjopen-2020-039978] [PMID: 32518212]

[140] Liu J, Cao R, Xu M, *et al.* Hydroxychloroquine, a less toxic derivative of chloroquine, is effective in inhibiting SARS-CoV-2 infection *in vitro*. Cell Discov 2020 :6:16 doi: 101038/s41421-020-0156-0 2020; 6: 16.
[http://dx.doi.org/10.1038/s41421-020-0156-0] [PMID: 33240407]

[141] Gordon D, Jang G, Bouhaddou M, *et al.* A SARS-CoV-2-Human Protein-Protein Interaction Map Reveals Drug Targets and Potential Drug-Repurposing. bioRxiv Prepr.
[http://dx.doi.org/10.1101/2020.03.22.002386]

[142] Liu X. Deep recurrent neural network for protein function prediction from sequence. arXiv 2017.
[http://dx.doi.org/10.48550/arXiv.1701.08318]

[143] Richardson P, Griffin I, Tucker C, *et al.*, Baricitinib as potential treatment for 2019-nCoV acute respiratory disease. Lancet (London, England). 2020 Feb 15; 395(10223): e30.

[144]   Hu F, Jiang J, Yin P. Prediction of potential commercially inhibitors against SARS-CoV-2 by multi-task deep model. arXiv 2020.
[http://dx.doi.org/10.48550/arXiv.2003.00728]

[145]   Ton AT, Gentile F, Hsing M, Ban F, Cherkasov A. Rapid identification of potential inhibitors of SARS-CoV-2 main protease by deep docking of 1.3 billion compounds. Mol Inform 2020; 39(8): 2000028.
[http://dx.doi.org/10.1002/minf.202000028] [PMID: 32162456]

[146]   Ewing TJA, Makino S, Skillman AG, Kuntz ID. DOCK 4.0: search strategies for automated molecular docking of flexible molecule databases. J Comput Aided Mol Des 2001; 15(5): 411-28.
[http://dx.doi.org/10.1023/A:1011115820450] [PMID: 11394736]

[147]   Yang D, Leibowitz JL. The structure and functions of coronavirus genomic 3′ and 5′ ends. Virus Res 2015; 206: 120-33.
[http://dx.doi.org/10.1016/j.virusres.2015.02.025] [PMID: 25736566]

[148]   Park SJ, Kim YG, Park HJ. Identification of RNA pseudoknot-binding ligand that inhibits the -1 ribosomal frameshifting of SARS-coronavirus by structure-based virtual screening. J Am Chem Soc 2011; 133(26): 10094-100.
[http://dx.doi.org/10.1021/ja1098325] [PMID: 21591761]

[149]   Alipanahi B, Delong A, Weirauch MT,Frey BJ.. Predicting the sequence specificities of DNA-and RNA-binding proteins by deep learning. Nat Biotechnol 2015; 33: 831-8.
[http://dx.doi.org/10.1038/nbt.3300]

[150]   Plant EP, Dinman JD. The role of programmed-1 ribosomal frameshifting in coronavirus propagation. Front Biosci 2008; 13(13): 4873-81.
[http://dx.doi.org/10.2741/3046] [PMID: 18508552]

[151]   Paraskevis D, Kostaki EG, Magiorkinis G, Panayiotakopoulos G, Sourvinos G, Tsiodras S. Full-genome evolutionary analysis of the novel corona virus (2019-nCoV) rejects the hypothesis of emergence as a result of a recent recombination event. Infect Genet Evol 2020; 79: 104212.
[http://dx.doi.org/10.1016/j.meegid.2020.104212] [PMID: 32004758]

[152]   Bjerrum EJ, Sattarov B. Improving chemical autoencoder latent space and molecular *de novo* generation diversity with heteroencoders. Biomolecules 2018; 8(4): 131.
[http://dx.doi.org/10.3390/biom8040131] [PMID: 30380783]

[153]   Chenthamarakshan V, Das P, Padhi I, *et al.* CogMol: Target-Specific and Selective Drug Design for COVID-19 Using Deep Generative Models. arXiv 2020.
[http://dx.doi.org/10.48550/arXiv.2004.01215]

[154]   Tang B, He F, Liu D, Fang M, Wu Z, Xu D. AI-aided design of novel targeted covalent inhibitors against SARS-CoV-2. bioRxiv 2020.
[http://dx.doi.org/10.1101/2020.03.03.972133] [PMID: 32511346]

[155]   Pillaiyar T, Meenakshisundaram S, Manickam M. Recent discovery and development of inhibitors targeting coronaviruses. Drug Discov Today 2020; 25(4): 668-88.
[http://dx.doi.org/10.1016/j.drudis.2020.01.015] [PMID: 32006468]

[156]   Dangi M. Kumari, R.; Singh, B.; Chhillar, A.K. Bioinformatics: Sequences, Structures, Phylogeny. Springer 2018; pp. 329-57.
[http://dx.doi.org/10.1007/978-981-13-1562-6_15]

[157]   Fernandez-Lozano C, Fernández-Blanco E, Dave K, *et al.*, Improving enzyme regulatory protein classification by means of SVM-RFE feature selection. Molecular Biosystems. 2014; 10(5): 1063-71.

[158]   Han Y, Kim D. Deep convolutional neural networks for pan-specific peptide-MHC class I binding prediction. BMC Bioinformatics 2017; 18(1): 585.
[http://dx.doi.org/10.1186/s12859-017-1997-x] [PMID: 29281985]

[159] Chen B, Khodadoust MS, Olsson N, *et al.* Predicting HLA class II antigen presentation through integrated deep learning. Nat Biotechnol 2019; 37(11): 1332-43.
[http://dx.doi.org/10.1038/s41587-019-0280-2] [PMID: 31611695]

[160] Jurtz V, Paul S, Andreatta M, Marcatili P, Peters B, Nielsen M. NetMHCpan-4.0: improved peptide–MHC class I interaction predictions integrating eluted ligand and peptide binding affinity data. J Immunol 2017; 199(9): 3360-8.
[http://dx.doi.org/10.4049/jimmunol.1700893] [PMID: 28978689]

[161] Abbasi BA, Saraf D, Sharma T, *et al.*, Identification of vaccine targets & design of vaccine against SARS-CoV-2 coronavirus using computational and deep learning-based approaches. PeerJ. 2022 May 19;10: e13380.

[162] Crossman LCJb. Leverging Deep Learning to Simulate Coronavirus Spike proteins has the potential to predict future Zoonotic sequences. bioRxiv 2020.
[http://dx.doi.org/10.1101/2020.04.20.046920]

[163] Feng Y, Qiu M, Zou S, *et al.* Multi-epitope vaccine design using an immunoinformatics approach for 2019 novel coronavirus in China (SARS-CoV-2). bioRxiv 2020.
[http://dx.doi.org/10.1101/2020.03.03.962332]

[164] Dona MSI, Prendergast LA, Mathivanan S, Keerthikumar S, Salim A. Powerful differential expression analysis incorporating network topology for next-generation sequencing data. Bioinformatics 2017; 33(10): 1505-13.
[http://dx.doi.org/10.1093/bioinformatics/btw833] [PMID: 28172447]

[165] Bala PC, Eisenreich BR, Yoo SBM, Hayden BY, Park HS, Zimmermann JJ. Automated markerless pose estimation in freely moving macaques with OpenMonkeyStudio. Nat Commun 2020; 11(1): 4560.
[http://dx.doi.org/10.1038/s41467-020-18441-5] [PMID: 32917899]

[166] Sah S, Surendiran B, Dhanalakshmi R, Mohanty SN. Mutation prediction and phylogenetic analysis of SARS-CoV2 protein sequences using LSTM based encoder-decoder model. Arab Journal of Basic and Applied Sciences. 2023 Mar 13; 30(1): 103-21.

[167] Lyu L, Huang L, Huang T, Xiang W, Yuan JD, Zhang C. Cell-penetrating peptide conjugates of gambogic acid enhance the antitumor effect on human bladder cancer EJ cells through ROS-mediated apoptosis. Drug Des Devel Ther 2018; 12: 743-56.
[http://dx.doi.org/10.2147/DDDT.S161821] [PMID: 29670331]

[168] Lazer D, Kennedy R, King G, Vespignani A. Big data. The parable of Google Flu: traps in big data analysis. Science 2014; 343(6176): 1203-5.
[http://dx.doi.org/10.1126/science.1248506] [PMID: 24626916]

[169] Bouchareb Y, Khaniabadi PM, Al Kindi F, Al Dhuhli H, Shiri I, Zaidi H, Rahmim A. Artificial intelligence-driven assessment of radiological images for COVID-19. Computers in biology and medicine. 2021 Sep 1;136: 104665.

[170] Li Y, Xia L. Coronavirus disease 2019 (COVID-19): role of chest CT in diagnosis and management. AJR Am J Roentgenol 2020; 214(6): 1280-6.
[http://dx.doi.org/10.2214/AJR.20.22954] [PMID: 32130038]

[171] Khamsi R. If a coronavirus vaccine arrives, can the world make enough? Nature 2020; 580(7805): 578-80.
[http://dx.doi.org/10.1038/d41586-020-01063-8] [PMID: 32273621]

[172] Hurt B, Kligerman S, Hsiao A. Deep learning localization of pneumonia: 2019 coronavirus (COVID-19) outbreak. J Thorac Imaging 2020; 35(3): W87-9.
[http://dx.doi.org/10.1097/RTI.0000000000000512] [PMID: 32205822]

[173] Yang Z, Zeng Z, Wang K, *et al.* Modified SEIR and AI prediction of the epidemics trend of COVID-19 in China under public health interventions. J Thorac Dis 2020; 12(3): 165-74.

[http://dx.doi.org/10.21037/jtd.2020.02.64] [PMID: 32274081]

[174] Kallianos K, Mongan J, Antani S, *et al.* How far have we come? Artificial intelligence for chest radiograph interpretation. Clin Radiol 2019; 74(5): 338-45.
[http://dx.doi.org/10.1016/j.crad.2018.12.015] [PMID: 30704666]

[175] Naudé W. Artificial intelligence *vs* COVID-19: limitations, constraints and pitfalls. AI Soc 2020; 35(3): 761-5.
[http://dx.doi.org/10.1007/s00146-020-00978-0] [PMID: 32346223]

[176] Nguyen TT. Artificial intelligence in the battle against coronavirus (COVID-19): a survey and future research directions. arXiv 2020.
[http://dx.doi.org/10.48550/arXiv.2008.07343]

[177] Bragazzi NL, Dai H, Damiani G, Behzadifar M, Martini M, Wu J. How big data and artificial intelligence can help better manage the COVID-19 pandemic. Int J Environ Res Public Health 2020; 17(9): 3176.
[http://dx.doi.org/10.3390/ijerph17093176] [PMID: 32370204]

[178] Rehman SU, Shafqat F, Niaz K. Recent artificial intelligence methods and coronaviruses. In: Application of Natural Products in SARS-CoV-2. 2023; pp. 353-80.
[http://dx.doi.org/10.1016/B978-0-323-95047-3.00009-5]

SUBJECT INDEX

www.ingramcontent.com/pod-product-compliance
Lightning Source LLC
Chambersburg PA
CBHW050817220326
41598CB00006B/237